Global Maternal and Child Health

Medical, Anthropological, and Public Health Perspectives

Series Editor:

David A. Schwartz
Department of Pathology
Medical College of Georgia
Augusta University
Augusta, GA, USA

Global Maternal and Child Health: Medical, Anthropological, and Public Health Perspectives is a series of books that will provide the most comprehensive and current sources of information on a wide range of topics related to global maternal and child health, written by a collection of international experts. The health of pregnant women and their children are among the most significant public health, medical, and humanitarian problems in the world today. Because in developing countries many people are poor, and young women are the poorest of the poor, persistent poverty exacerbates maternal and child morbidity and mortality and gender-based challenges to such basic human rights as education and access to health care and reproductive choices. Women and their children remain the most vulnerable members of our society and, as a result, are the most impacted individuals by many of the threats that are prevalent, and, in some cases, increasing throughout the world. These include emerging and re-emerging infectious diseases, natural and man-made disasters, armed conflict, religious and political turmoil, relocation as refugees, malnutrition, and, in some cases, starvation. The status of indigenous women and children is especially precarious in many regions because of ethnic, cultural, and language differences, resulting in stigmatization, poor obstetrical and neonatal outcomes, limitations of women's reproductive rights, and lack of access to family planning and education that restrict choices regarding their own futures. Because of the inaccessibility of women to contraception and elective pregnancy termination, unsafe abortion continues to result in maternal deaths, morbidity, and reproductive complications. Unfortunately, maternal deaths remain at unacceptably high levels in the majority of developing countries, as well as in some developed ones. Stillbirths and premature deliveries result in millions of deaths annually. Gender inequality persists globally as evidenced by the occurrence of female genital mutilation, obstetrical violence, human trafficking, and other forms of sexual discrimination directed at women. Many children are routinely exposed to physical, sexual, and psychological violence. Childhood and teen marriages remain at undesirably high levels in many developing countries.

Global Maternal and Child Health: Medical, Anthropological, and Public Health Perspectives is unique in combining the opinions and expertise of public health specialists, physicians, anthropologists and social scientists, epidemiologists, nurses, midwives, and representatives of governmental and non governmental agencies to comprehensively explore the increasing challenges and potential solutions to global maternal and child health issues.

More information about this series at http://www.springer.com/series/15852

Series Editorial Advisory Board

Kim Gutschow • Robbie Davis-Floyd
Betty-Anne Daviss

Editors

Sustainable Birth
in Disruptive Times

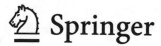 Springer

Editors
Kim Gutschow (iD)
Department of Anthropology and Religion
Williams College
Williamstown, MA, USA

Robbie Davis-Floyd (iD)
Department of Anthropology
The University of Texas at Austin
Austin, TX, USA

Betty-Anne Daviss
Women's and Gender Studies
The Pauline Jewett Institute
Carleton University
Ottawa, ON, Canada

ISSN 2522-8382   ISSN 2522-8390   (electronic)
Global Maternal and Child Health
ISBN 978-3-030-54777-6   ISBN 978-3-030-54775-2   (eBook)
https://doi.org/10.1007/978-3-030-54775-2

This Springer imprint is published by the registered company Springer Nature Switzerland AG
The registered company address is: Gewerbestrasse 11, 6330 Cham, Switzerland

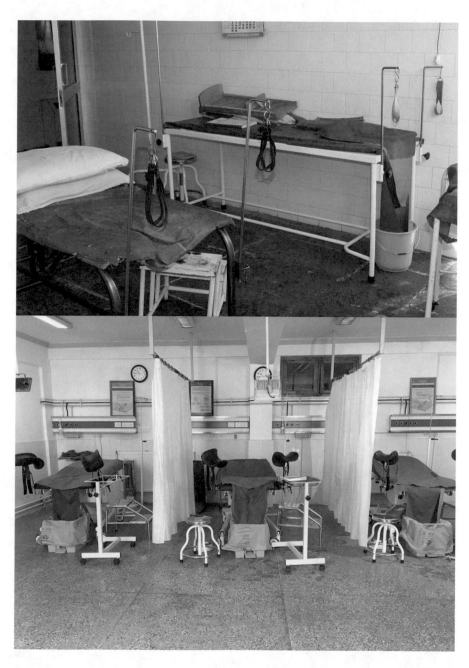

The Labor & Delivery room at Sonam Norbu Memorial Hospital in Leh, Ladakh, India in 2006 (top) and 2019 (bottom). The upper image shows two tables for delivery, the stirrups that women were required to use for most deliveries, buckets for absorbing blood, and other bodily fluids during the delivery, as well as wooden tray used to measure newborns on the right-hand table. The lower image shows the brand new Labor & Delivery room that was part of an entirely new hospital construction that followed partial destruction of the hospital during the catastrophic Leh flash floods in 2010. Published with permission from © Kim Gutschow. All Rights Reserved.

From Kim Gutschow:
This book is dedicated to the childbearers,
providers, and babies, born and unborn,
past, present, future,
for their care and compassion.

From Robbie Davis-Floyd:
This book is dedicated to my culture heroes
Robin Lim and Vicki Penwell, who have
developed and practiced sustainable models
of birth, saved countless lives, and brought
love, light, and joy to the thousands of people
who experienced their care, even in the most
disruptive of times.

From Betty-Anne Daviss:
This book is dedicated to all of our
grandchildren in the hope that they will
understand that social activism is as
important as education, regulation, and
association.

Acknowledgments

Kim Gutschow is profoundly grateful to the women and providers—midwives, obstetricians, nurses, neonatologists in the USA, India, Germany, Nepal, and elsewhere—who have participated in countless conversations on maternity care and MNCH (maternal, neonatal, and child health) over the past 16 years. She deeply thanks the doctors—Dr. Michelle Lauria, Dr. Torren Rhodes, and Dr. George Little (coauthor of Chapter 19)—who helped steward her vaginal delivery of 26-week-old breech twins who spent 77 days in the NICU at Dartmouth-Hitchcock Hospital in 2004. Subsequent conversations with these and other providers helped shape her research into the anthropology of maternal and newborn health and reproduction. She is so very grateful to Robbie and Betty-Anne for their inspirational work and wonderful friendship, cemented in 2015 on a train journey from Bad Wildbad, Germany, that helped conceive this book. Last but not least, she thanks her family—her children Tashi, Krishan, and Yeshe as well as her partner Robin Sears—for their support and many questions about how the book was coming to fruition in past years.

Robbie Davis-Floyd is deeply grateful to lead editor Kim Gutschow for her long-term dedication to seeing this book through to completion, for her international understanding of the issues surrounding sustainable birth—which enabled her to invite just the right authors for the chapters in this collection–for her outstanding editing skills, and for her ongoing friendship. She is also grateful for that train trip from Bad Wildbad—it is amazing what people can come up with when their brains are moving as fast as that fast-moving train!

Betty-Anne Daviss would like to thank her coeditors for their patience with her as they did the main work on this book while she was finishing another book, *Birthing Models on the Human Rights Frontier: Speaking Truth to Power* (BMHRF). She sees BMHRF as highly complementary to this volume, yet different in that it often takes a more iconoclastic approach and proactively calls people to action. Both styles are needed. She finds that a book focusing on sustainability is critical, given that some of the optimal birth models in BMHRF have already been threatened by the neoliberal economic values that plague healthcare funding. Betty-Anne would also like to thank a casualty of those problems, traditional midwives the world over, whose work often goes unnoticed and disrespected at best; at worst, many are being persecuted and arrested. Finally, she would like to thank her husband, Ken Johnson, a steadfast support, who reminds her, when she engages with Kim and Robbie in trying to fix everything in the world, that Marshall Klaus said: "Opinion divides, data unites."

Contents

1   **Introduction: Sustainable Birth in Disruptive Times**   1
    Kim Gutschow and Robbie Davis-Floyd

Part I   Sustainable Maternity Solutions in High-Income Countries

2   **Sustainable Midwifery**   29
    Elizabeth Davis

3   **Bringing Back Breech by Reframing the Language of Risk**   43
    Betty-Anne Daviss, Anita Hedditch, Vijaya Krishnan,
    and Helen Dresner Barnes

4   **From Home to Hospital: Sustainable Transfers
    of Care in the United States**   61
    Bria Dunham and Sara Hall

5   **Structures for Sustainable Collaboration Between Midwives
    and Obstetricians in the Netherlands: The Obstetric
    and Midwifery Manual and Perinatal Care Partnerships**   73
    Rachael Kulick Bommarito

6   **Re/Envisioning Birth Work: Community-Based Doula
    Training for Low-Income and Previously Incarcerated
    Women in the United States**   85
    Rebecca L. Bakal and Monica R. McLemore

7   **Sustainable Metrics: Using Measurement-Based Quality
    Improvement to Improve Maternity Practice While
    Avoiding Frustration and Pitfalls**   99
    Kathleen H. Pine and Christine H. Morton

8   **Unsustainable Surrogacy Practices: What We Can
    Learn from a Comparative Assessment**   115
    Elly Teman and Zsuzsa Berend

Part II   Sustainable Maternity Solutions in Latin America

9   Childbirth in Chile: Winds of Change 131
     Michelle Sadler, Gonzalo Leiva, and Ricardo Gómez

10   Humanizing Care at the Maternity Hospital Estela
     de Carlotto in Buenos Aires: Providers Relearning Their Roles 145
     Celeste Jerez

11   Luna Maya Birth Centers in Mexico: A Network
     for Femifocal Care 157
     Cristina Alonso, J. M. López, Alison Lucas-Danch, and Janell Tryon

12   Reconstructing Referrals: Overcoming Barriers
     to Quality Obstetric Care for Maya Women
     in Guatemala Through Care Navigation 171
     Kirsten Austad, Anita Chary, Jessica Hawkins, Boris Martinez,
     and Peter Rohloff

**Part III   Sustainable Maternity Solutions
             in Low- and Middle-Income Countries**

13   A Sustainable Model of Assessing Maternal Health
     Needs and Improving Quality of Care During
     and After Pregnancy.. 187
     Mary McCauley and Nynke van den Broek

14   Sustainable Maternal and Newborn Care in India:
     A Case Study from Ladakh 197
     Kim Gutschow, Padma Dolma, and Spalchen Gonbo

15   Giving Birth at Home in Resource-Scarce Regions of India:
     An Argument for Making the Women-Centric Approach
     of the Traditional Dais Sustainable 217
     Bijoya Roy, Imrana Qadeer, Mira Sadgopal, Janet Chawla,
     and Sandhya Gautam

16   It Takes More Than a Village: Building a Network
     of Safety in Nepal's Mountain Communities 233
     Vincanne Adams, Sienna R. Craig, Arlene Samen,
     and Surya Bhatta

17   Tranquil Birth: Revising Risk to Sustain
     Spontaneous Vaginal Birth.................................. 249
     Kathleen Lorne McDougall

18   Sustainable Birth Care in Disaster Zones
     and During Pandemics: Low-Tech, Skilled Touch............... 261
     Robbie Davis-Floyd, Robin Lim, Vicki Penwell, and Tsipy Ivry

**19   Sustainable Newborn Care: Helping Babies Breathe
     and Essential Newborn Care** 277
     Chiamaka Aneji and George Little

20   Conclusion: Sustainable Maternity Care in Disruptive Times 295
     Kim Gutschow, Robbie Davis-Floyd, and Betty-Anne Daviss

Correction to: Introduction: Sustainable Birth in Disruptive Times C1

Index 309

About the Editors and Contributors

Editors

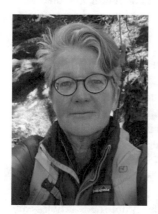

Kim Gutschow, PhD, is a Lecturer in Anthropology and Religion and affiliated with Public Health, Asian Studies, and Women's, Gender, and Sexuality Studies at Williams College, in Williamstown, Massachusetts, where she has taught since 2003. Since 1989, she has published over 35 articles on maternity care, maternal death reviews, and counting maternal mortality in India and the USA, as well as on the gender dynamics and discourses of Buddhist monasticism, Tibetan medicine, community-based irrigation, and land use practices in the Indian Himalayas. She is the author of *Being a Buddhist Nun: The Struggle for Enlightenment in the Himalayas* (Harvard 2004) which won the Sharon Stephens Prize for best ethnography (2005). Her collaborative research projects with Ladakhi teams have received several awards including a Humboldt Research Fellowship for Experienced Researchers (2009) for *Birth: From Home to Hospital and Back Home Again*; a National Geographic Award (2019) for "Climate Change Adaptation: By the People & For the People"; as well as a postdoc at the Harvard Society of Fellows (1997–2000) for research on gender, social power, and birth in the Indian Himalayas. She raised $100,000 for Zangskari women and nuns through the Zanskar Project from 1991 to 2015 (https://gadenrelief.org/project/zangskar-project/) .

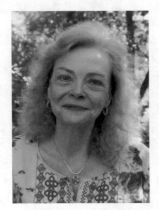

Robbie Davis-Floyd, PhD, Senior Research Fellow, Department of Anthropology, University of Texas at Austin, and Fellow of the Society for Applied Anthropology, is a well-known medical anthropologist, midwifery and doula advocate, and international speaker and researcher in transformational models in maternity care. She is author of over 80 journal articles and 24 encyclopedia entries, and of *Birth as an American Rite of Passage* (1992, 2003) and *Ways of Knowing about Birth: Mothers, Midwives, Medicine, and Birth Activism* (2018); coauthor of *The Power of Ritual* (2016); and lead editor of 13 collections, including the award-winning volumes *Childbirth and Authoritative Knowledge* (1997) and *Cyborg Babies* (1998), and the "seminal" *Birth Models That Work* (2009). Her most recent collection, coedited with Melissa Cheyney, is *Birth in Eight Cultures* (2019). *Birthing Models on the Human Rights Frontier: Speaking Truth to Power*, coedited with Betty-Anne Daviss, is in press. As a Board Member of the International MotherBaby Childbirth Organization, Robbie served as lead editor for the "International Childbirth Initiative: 12 Steps to Safe and Respectful MotherBaby-Family Maternity Care" (a joint IMBCO/FIGO global initiative). She presently serves as lead editor for a Routledge series called "Social Science Perspectives on Childbirth and Reproduction" and as senior advisor to the Council on Anthropology and Reproduction. Many of her published articles are freely available on her website: www.davis-floyd.com.

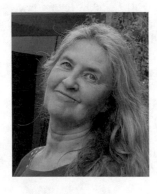

Betty-Anne Daviss, MA, BMJ, RM (Registered Midwife), has served as a midwife for 45 years, practicing in various countries on six continents, and as a researcher in the social sciences and clinical epidemiology for over 25 years. She is an Adjunct Professor in Gender and Women's Studies at Carleton University, Ottawa, Ontario, Canada, and has taught since the 1980s on reproductive issues and the politics of gender and health, while working towards midwifery legislation in North America and abroad. She coauthored the large prospective home birth study of Certified Professional Midwives in North America published in the BMJ (2005) that continues to be accessed 500–800 times a month and the World Report on Postpartum

Hemorrhage when she worked for the International Federation of Gynecology and Obstetrics (FIGO) (Lalonde et al. 2006), which continues to be used with updates, and was the co-principal investigator and principal writer for the Frankfurt study comparing vaginal breeches born with the mothers on their backs versus in upright positions (Louwen et al. 2017). The only midwife in Canada in the last two decades to have achieved official hospital privileges to attend breech births without a transfer to obstetrics, Betty-Anne has been involved with over 170 planned vaginal breech births, and provided workshops, rounds, and/or plenaries on vaginal breech in Europe, Africa, North and South America, China, India, Australia, and Turkey. She has testified for 10 midwifery hearings/court cases and 11 state and 3 provincial legislative processes. Some of her published articles are freely available on her website: www.understandingbirthbetter.com.

Contributors

Vincanne Adams, PhD, is professor in the Department of Anthropology, History, and Social Medicine and the joint Program in Medical Anthropology at the University of California, San Francisco. She serves as editor of the journal *Medical Anthropology Quarterly* and is the author of *Markets of Sorrow, Labors of Faith*; *Sex in Development*; *Metrics*; and other books. She teaches and conducts research on several topics, including safe motherhood in Tibet, Nepal, and the USA.

Cristina Alonso, MPH, CPM, founded the Luna Maya birth center in Chiapas in 2004 and opened the second Luna Maya birth center in Mexico City in 2014. She was a founding member and served as president of the Mexican Midwifery Association, and has served on several birth and midwifery boards including the Midwives Alliance of North American and Human Rights in Childbirth. In 2018 she founded the Mexican Network of Birth Centers and published the book *Open a Midwifery Center* in Spanish. This book was later adapted, translated, and published for a global audience in 2020. Author of several articles on midwifery in Mexico, she is currently a Doctor of Public Health candidate at Harvard University.

Chiamaka Aneji, PhD, is an Associate Professor of Pediatrics in the Division of Neonatal-Perinatal Medicine, McGovern Medical School, at the University of Texas Health Science Center at Houston. She is a master trainer of the Helping Babies Survive program and a Fellow of the American Academy of Pediatrics. Her academic career focuses on medical education and global health with a focus on Africa and quality improvement in health care. She is a recognized master educator and has taught Helping Babies Survive courses in North America, Nigeria, and Haiti.

Kirsten Austad, MD, MPH, Center for Research in Indigenous Health, Wuqu' Kawoq | Maya Health Alliance, Tecpán, Guatemala, is an Assistant Professor at Boston University School of Medicine. She is a family medicine physician and public health researcher with field experience in the Dominican Republic, Guatemala, Ghana, and Lesotho. She completed her medical education at Harvard Medical School, her residency at Boston Medical Center, and her fellowship training at the Edmond J. Safra Center for Ethics and the Global Women's Health Fellowship at Harvard University. Since 2013, she has directed comprehensive women's health programming for the Maya Health Alliance and Friendship Bridge—nongovernmental organizations in Guatemala.

Rebecca L. Bakal, MPH, is a community health professional based in Chicago, Illinois. She is currently Program Manager of Health Education at the Jewish United Fund. In her research and practice, she examines community health education and peer support as tools to improve health equity. She has presented her work nationally and is currently finalizing a health education curriculum on genetics for international distribution. She also practices as a full-spectrum doula.

Zsuzsa Berend, PhD, Academic Administrator, Department of Sociology, University of California, Los Angeles, has been teaching sociology at UCLA since 1996 and is the academic administrator of the departmental Honors Program. Her earlier research was in the field of historical sociology. Her most recent research was an ethnographic study of a large public surrogacy information and support forum. She has published articles in *Medical Anthropology Quarterly*, *Sociological Forum*, *Anthropology and Medicine*, and *American Anthropologist*. Her book, *The Online World of Surrogacy*, was published in 2016 by Berghahn Books.

Surya Bhatta is the Executive Director of One Heart Worldwide, based in Kathmandu, Nepal. He is a public health professional and health development practitioner who has been trained in Nepal and the USA. He earned his master's in Healthcare Delivery Science from a joint program at Dartmouth's Geisel School of Medicine and the Tuck School of Business.

Rachael Kulick Bommarito, PhD, studies direct entry midwifery and planned home birth in high-income countries. She is an Accreditation Coordinator at the Midwifery Education Accreditation Council (MEAC). MEAC creates standards and criteria for the education of midwives in the USA and is a federally approved accreditation agency.

Anita Chary, MD, PhD, Center for Research in Indigenous Health, Wuqu' Kawoq–Maya Health Alliance, Tecpán, Guatemala, is an emergency physician at Massachusetts General Hospital and Brigham and Women's Hospital. She is chief resident at the Harvard Affiliated Emergency Medicine Residency and a clinical fellow at Harvard Medical School. Dr. Chary is also an anthropologist whose research focuses on health disparities and health systems development in low-resource settings. She has worked with Maya Health Alliance, a nongovernmental organization in Guatemala, since 2008 on child nutrition, women's health, and chronic disease programs.

Janet Chawla, BA, MA, is an activist, childbirth educator, scholar, and founder-director of the NGO MATRIKA (www.matrika-india.org), a trust for research and advocacy on traditional midwifery and noninvasive birth methods. She researches, writes, and lectures on traditional midwives (*dais*) and indigenous body knowledge. MATRIKA's data on rituals, birth songs, notions of goddess and demoness, ghosts and ancestors span the gaps between medicine, religion, and gender. Chawla taught classes to prepare women and couples for natural childbirth for 25 years in Delhi and meanwhile earned an MA in Religious Studies (1985) focusing on the role of the *dai* as a ritual practitioner. She lectures and writes on the religio-cultural and ethnomedical aspects of dais' traditions. She is author and editor of the book *Birth and Birth Givers: The Power Behind the Shame* (2006). She has taken part in the JEEVA initiative since its inception in 2007 and lives in New Delhi, India.

Sienna R. Craig, PhD, is Associate Professor in the Department of Anthropology at Dartmouth College in Hanover, New Hampshire, where she teaches and conducts research on medical anthropology, global health, and migration and social change, with a focus on Tibetan and Himalayan communities. She is author of *Healing Elements: Efficacy and the Social Ecologies of Tibetan Medicine* and coeditor of *Medicine Between Science and Religion: Explorations on Tibetan Grounds*, among other books and articles.

Elizabeth Davis, CPM, BA, has been a midwife, international educator, consultant, and reproductive health-care specialist for over 40 years and is the author of six books on topics of midwifery, sexuality, and female psychology (see https://elizabethdavis.com for details). She served as Regional Representative and Education Committee Chair for the Midwives Alliance of North America, as President of the Midwifery Education Accreditation Council, and as midwife consultant to the State of California's Alternative Birthing Methods Study. She received the Brazen Woman Award from the California Association of Midwives and a Lifetime Achievement Award from Midwifery Today. She is cofounder of the US-accredited National Midwifery Institute and author/instructor of Heart & Hands Coursework (see https://nationalmidwiferyinstitute.com).

Padma Dolma, DNB, MD, MBBS, is Chief Obstetrician at Sonam Norbu Memorial Hospital (SNMH) in Leh, Ladakh, India, where she has worked since 2005. She has conducted research on maternal and newborn health in Ladakh since 2006, including ongoing collaborations with researchers from the University College London and Rochester University on high-altitude pregnancy outcomes, newborn and pediatric survival rates, and perinatal health. She has worked with Kim Gutschow since 2006, and they have jointly presented their research on birth outcomes and maternal survival in Ladakh at international conferences in Rome (2007), Leh, Ladakh, India (2011), and Heidelberg, Germany (2012), as well as coauthored a chapter in *Global Health: A Challenge for Interdisciplinary Research* (2012) called "Global Policies and Local Implementation: Maternal Mortality in Rural India."

Helen Dresner Barnes, MSc, RM, BMedSci, Lecturer in Midwifery, University of Bradford, West Yorkshire, UK, practiced in an award-winning caseload midwifery team for 15 years before moving on to the University of Bradford as a Midwifery Lecturer. She has published articles in AIMS, *Midwifery Matters, The Practising Midwife, Essentially MIDIRS*, and the *Journal of Child Language*. For the last 10 years, Helen has focused on developing knowledge and clinical skills in breech, organizing two successful international breech conferences in the UK in 2014 and 2017. In 2016, her team won a national award from the UK Royal College of Midwives for their collaborative, multidisciplinary breech service.

Bria Dunham, PhD, MPH, CPH, Department of Health Sciences, Boston University, Boston, Massachusetts, USA, is a Clinical Assistant Professor and Program Director of Health Science at Boston University and an Affiliate Faculty in Women's, Gender, and Sexuality Studies. Her scholarly work integrates evolutionary and humanized understandings of childbirth with the aim of improving psychosocial outcomes for pregnant persons.

Sandhya Gautam, MA, is Project Coordinator, JEEVA Project, and also serves as Consultant, Centre for Health and Social Justice New Delhi, India. She worked with the grassroots-level organization in Himachal Pradesh (1994–2007) on Women's Reproductive Health and Rights, and presently she is with the Centre for Health and Social Justice, New Delhi. She coordinates the National Alliance for Maternal Health and Human Rights (NAMHHR) and is a member of CommonHealth—a network working on maternal health, neonatal health, and safe abortion issues. She is one of the JEEVA Shepherds, and since 2008 she has supervised the JEEVA Research Project as Project Coordinator. She is from Nahan in the Sirmaur District of Himachal Pradesh.

Ricardo Gómez, MD, is a Chilean obstetrician, father, university teacher, researcher, and social communicator in educational platforms. He directs the Center for Perinatal Diagnosis and Research (Pontificia Universidad Católica de Chile) at La Florida Hospital and is Head of Maternal Fetal Medicine and Women's Ultrasound in Santa María Clinic, Santiago, Chile.

Spalchen Gonbo, MD, MBBS, DCH, is the Chief Pediatrician at Sonam Norbu Memorial Hospital (SNMH) in India where he has worked since 2005. He has an MBBS in Pediatrics and Neonatology from Jammu Medical College, has received advanced training in newborn resuscitation at AIMMS since 2009, and has collaborated with researchers from Rochester University on newborn survival and neonatal outcomes at SNMH since 2009. Together with Dr. Padma, he has been responsible for developing the SNCU (Special Newborn Care Unit) at Leh's Sonam Norbu Memorial Hospital since 2006.

Sara Hall, MSN, WHNP-BC, is a Women's Health Nurse Practitioner at a private family planning clinic in Massachusetts. Her scholarly and clinical interests include contraception counseling, normal physiologic childbirth, breastfeeding, trauma-informed care, and promotion of bodily autonomy in health care.

Jessica Hawkins, BA, is a medical student at the University of California, Berkeley–University of California, San Francisco Joint Medical Program. She has worked with the Maya Health Alliance, a nongovernmental organization in Guatemala, on health systems research and women's health programs since 2016. She is affiliated with the Center for Research in Indigenous Health, Wuqu' Kawoq–Maya Health Alliance, Tecpán, Guatemala.

Anita Hedditch is a midwife and Breech Team Lead at Oxford Radcliffe Hospitals NHS Foundation Trust, Oxford, England. As an intrapartum midwife for 26 years, Hedditch performs and teaches ECV (extra cephalic version) and has developed a midwifery team that supports breech birth, focusing on upright positions and collaborative care with obstetricians. The team members work to local guidelines that have been developed from expert training and local experience and collect detailed information of each birth, which is pooled to inform safety and for ongoing learning. Her role has provided opportunities to speak at conferences and teach within the UK setting and abroad. She has also supported an obstetric unit in Germany in breech birth provision and is an assessor in their yearly mandatory training.

Tsipy Ivry, MA, BSc, PhD, is senior lecturer and chair of the graduate program in medical and psychological anthropology in the Anthropology Department, University of Haifa, Israel. She is author of a comparative ethnography, *Embodying Culture: Pregnancy in Japan and Israel* (2010). Since 2006, she has studied the intersections of religion and reproductive biomedicine, particularly related to rabbinically mediated assisted conception and post-diagnostic decisions. Her most recent work explores pregnancy and childbirth following the March 11, 2011, disasters in Eastern Japan. Her research is funded by Israeli Science Foundation grants and recently by a Japan Foundation fellowship.

Celeste Jerez, BA, PhD, is Professor in Social Anthropology at the University of Buenos Aires (UBA), Argentina. Her dissertation was on childbirth activism against obstetric violence in Buenos Aires (2015). She is also a PhD Fellow in Anthropology, with a workplace at the Research Institute for Gender Studies, School of Philosophy and Liberal Arts, UBA. She is part of a teaching team on Feminist Anthropology (UBA) and a research project affiliated with the groups "Gender and Emotions in Political Participation" (UBACyT Project), "Gender and Public Policies program"

(IESCODE–UNPAZ), and "Gender, (In)Equalities and Rights in Tension" (CLACSO Working Group). She has published articles in national and international journals. Her current research topic addresses feminist anthropology, emotions, health providers, and attention to sexual and reproductive health in the Buenos Aires suburbs.

Vijaya Krishnan, CPM, DPT, LCCE, FACCE, is a Certified Professional Midwife and the cofounder of The Sanctum, Natural Birth Center in Hyderabad, India, which has pioneered a unique Collaborative Model of Care. With a doctorate in physical therapy, she has also created a wide array of wellness programs for women throughout their reproductive cycle. She is the Program Director for the Healthy Mother Lamaze Accredited Childbirth Educator Program, which trains Lamaze educators all over India. She has been awarded the "Lifetime Achievement Award for Service to MotherBaby" by Midwifery Today.

Gonzalo Leiva is a Chilean midwife who holds a master's in Health Administration. He works at the Center for Perinatal Diagnosis and Research, Faculty of Medicine, Pontificia Universidad Católica de Chile, and in the maternity unit of La Florida Hospital in the city of Santiago. This maternity unit has implemented the successful "Safe Model of Personalized Childbirth" which is recognized as a pillar and example of safe delivery and respectful care within the country. He is an activist on respectful birth and a founding member and director of the Chilean Observatory of Obstetric Violence.

Robin Lim, CPM, is a Filipino American midwife, mother, grandmother, author, and founder and Executive Board Director of *Yayasan Bumi Sehat*, a nonprofit organization in Indonesia. Lim also serves on the board of Bumi–Wadah, Philippines. Her passion is Human Rights in Childbirth. She constructed the Bumi Sehat birth and health-care center in Ubud, Bali, which has recently moved into a new building built with the funds from her 2011 CNN Hero of the Year Award. Her work has also taken her into the heart of disaster zones following earthquakes in Indonesia, Haiti, and Nepal; the super typhoon Haiyan in the Philippines; the volcanic eruptions in Bali; and the tsunami that devastated Aceh, where Bumi Sehat still supports a community health clinic and birth center. Bumi Sehat has also completed the construction of the Angel Hiromi Childbirth Center in Sentani, Papua. http://iburobin.com.

George Little, MD, is Active Emeritus Professor of Pediatrics and of Obstetrics and Gynecology, Geisel School of Medicine at Dartmouth in Hanover, New Hampshire. He is Emeritus Chair of Maternal and Child Health (MCH) at the Dartmouth–Hitchcock Medical Center, a Fellow of the American Academy of Pediatrics from which he received the Virginia Apgar Award, and an Honorary Fellow of the American College of Obstetrics and Gynecology. His academic career focuses on clinical and systems neonatology, including a global focus that emphasizes Africa, the Middle East, and the Balkans. He is a recognized educator and author and is coeditor of *Religion and Ethics in the Neonatal Intensive Care Unit* (Oxford 2019).

J. M. López, PhD, is a medical anthropologist specializing in sexual, reproductive, and maternal health matters and the design and ethics of collaborative ethnography. They are a Lecturer in Society and Health at the School of Pharmacy and Medical Sciences, University of Bradford, Bradford, UK. Their broader research interests lie in family life, intimate relationships, and life course in societies or populations affected by violence and/or conflict. Dr López's research region is principally, though not exclusive to, Mexico and the UK.

Alison Lucas-Danch, MPH, MSW, is a trained infant–parent psychotherapist who has specialized specifically in reproductive mental health care. Her research has focused on improving perinatal health equity within systems-level program planning and evaluation. Recently, she has worked in the 0–3-year field, again with the lens of reducing disparities in pregnancy and early childhood, with the overall goal of promoting equitable beginnings of life for each child.

Boris Martinez, MD, is a resident physician in the Department of Internal Medicine at Saint Peter's University Hospital in New Brunswick, New Jersey. He has extensive experience as a Kaqchikel Maya-, Spanish-, and English-speaking physician in underserved communities in his native Guatemala and New Jersey. Dr. Martínez has spearheaded community-based research in nutrition, early childhood development, maternal health, and health systems with Maya Health Alliance, a nongovernmental organization in Guatemala, since 2014. He is affiliated with the Center for Research in Indigenous Health, Wuqu' Kawooq | Maya Health Alliance, Tecpán, Guatemala.

Monica R. McLemore, PhD, MPH, RN, FAAN, School of Nursing, University of California, San Francisco (UCSF), is a tenured associate professor in the Family Health Care Nursing Department, an affiliated scientist with Advancing New Standards in Reproductive Health, and a member of the Bixby Center for Global Reproductive Health. She retired from clinical practice as a public health and staff nurse after a 28-year clinical nursing career. Her research program is focused on understanding reproductive health and justice. She has published 56 peer-reviewed articles and various Op-Eds and commentaries. She is the recipient of numerous awards and was inducted into the American Academy of Nursing in October, 2019.

Mary McCauley, BScMedSci, MBChB, MRCOG, PhD, is Academic Clinical Lecturer, Centre of Maternal and Newborn Health, Liverpool School of Tropical Medicine, and obstetrician and gynecologist at Liverpool Women's Hospital, UK. She specializes in implementation research to improve health outcomes during and after pregnancy for mothers and babies living in low-resource settings.

Kathleen Lorne McDougall, PhD, is an independent scholar. Her birth study was completed while she was a member of the Anthropology of the First 1000 Days research cluster at the University of Cape Town, South Africa. She was a postdoctoral fellow in Anthropology at the University of Cape Town and is also a graduate of the University of Cape Town.

Christine H. Morton, PhD, is a medical sociologist at Stanford University School of Medicine in California, whose qualitative and mixed-methods research on maternal and neonatal health has informed clinical quality improvement practices and policies in California and the USA. She is the author of *Birth Ambassadors: Doulas and the Re-Emergence of Woman-Supported Childbirth in America* (2014) and founder of ReproNetwork.org in 1998—an international listserv with over 600 subscribers, mostly social scientists and medical practitioners interested in reproductive/maternal practices, policies, and ideologies.

Vicki Penwell, CPM, LM, MS, MA, is the founder and Executive Director of Mercy In Action Vineyard, Inc., responsible for the safe delivery of more than 15,500 births in the Philippines since 1991, at no cost to the parents, and with outcomes four times better than the Philippines national average. She also serves as Executive Director of the Mercy In Action College of Midwifery, a 4-year Bachelor of Science midwifery college accredited by MEAC in the USA. Vicki holds a master's degree in Midwifery and another master's degree in Intercultural Studies from the Philippines. Vicki lives with her husband of 41 years in Olongapo, Philippines, where she and her team care for the poorest of the poor. She continues to travel and teach midwifery around the world, as well as to attend births and respond to disasters as needed.

Kathleen H. Pine, PhD, is an Assistant Professor in the College of Health Solutions at Arizona State University in Phoenix. Her research, much of which examines health information technology and childbirth and data practices in health care, bridges human-centered computing, organization studies, and science and technology studies. Her research has been published in venues including the *Academy of Management Journal*, ACM CHI, PACMHCI, and the *International Journal of Medical Informatics*.

Imrana Qadeer, PhD, is a well-known public health expert. She is a Distinguished Professor with the Council for Social Development, New Delhi, India. For 35 years she served as Professor at the Centre for Social Medicine and Community Health (CSMCH), Jawaharlal Nehru University, New Delhi, and was a JP Naik Fellow at the CWDS. She has also served as lead editor for four collections, the latest of which is *Universalising Healthcare in India: From Care to Coverage*. She is currently a member of the ICMR's Scientific Advisory Board and also worked with the Ministry of Health and Family Welfare, the Planning Commission, Population Commission, and the advisory and monitoring bodies for the National Rural Health Mission. She is part of the JEEVA Collective that opposes the banning of *dais*' work in India and advocates for their recognition as community-level maternity and new-born care providers.

Peter Rohloff, MD, PhD, is an Assistant Professor in the Department of Global Health Equity at Brigham and Women's Hospital and at Harvard Medical School in Boston, Massachusetts. Dr. Rohloff is an internist, pediatrician, and global health researcher with expertise in noncommunicable and chronic disease program development, childhood undernutrition, health disparities in indigenous populations, pediatric disabilities and rare diseases in developing countries, and Mayan languages and culture. He completed his medical education and graduate studies in parasitology at the University of Illinois in Urbana–Champaign and his residency in internal medicine and pediatrics at Brigham and Women's Hospital and Boston Children's Hospital. He founded the nongovernmental organization Maya Health Alliance in Guatemala in 2006 and serves as the organization's Chief Medical Officer. He is affiliated with the Center for Research in Indigenous Health, Wuqu' Kawoq–Maya Health Alliance, Tecpán, Guatemala.

Bijoya Roy, PhD, is Assistant Professor, Public Health and Gender Studies, Centre for Women's Development Studies, New Delhi, India, with an interdisciplinary background in Food and Nutrition, Social Work, and Public Health. Her research, teaching, and writing include public–private partnerships in health care, commercialization of health care, childbirth practices and medicalization, midwifery practices, and women's health-care workforce and research methodology. She served as the editor of the *Indian Journal of Gender Studies'* Special Issue on *Gender and Commercialisation of Health Care* and in 2020 was selected as Shepherd to the JEEVA Collective (Birthing Study Collective). She currently serves as member for the Institutional Ethics Committee, Public Health Resource Network, New Delhi.

Mira Sadgopal, MD, MBBS, worked as a doctor and rural development worker in Madhya Pradesh, India (1974–1989), where she related with *dais* among village women. After joining the Medico Friend Circle, she became active in the women's health movement. In 1986 she cofounded the Lok Swasthya Parampara Samvardhan Samithi (LSPSS). In 1992 she was elected Ashoka Fellow for work in Fertility Awareness Education. In 1999 she cofounded the Tathapi Trust for Women and Health Resource Development (www.tathapi.org) in Pune. She founded the JEEVA initiative in 2007. She lives in Nandurbar, Maharashtra, India, and serves as Principal Investigator, JEEVA Project, and health activist, Managing Trustee, Tathapi Trust, Pune, India.

Michelle Sadler, PhD, is a Chilean medical anthropologist who currently works at the Faculty of Liberal Arts, Universidad Adolfo Ibáñez, Chile. She is director of the Chilean Observatory of Obstetric Violence and member of the Medical Anthropology Research Center at Universitat Rovira i Virgili, Tarragona, Spain. She has 20 years of experience researching childbirth models in Chile, has assessed policies towards respectful maternity care, and has led civil society organizations that seek to promote change in maternity-related issues.

Arlene Samen is founder and President of One Heart Worldwide. She has been a nurse practitioner in maternal fetal medicine for over three decades. In 1997, she met His Holiness the Dalai Lama, who asked her to take her expertise and help women and children dying in childbirth in Tibet. Since that time, she has dedicated her life to serving pregnant women living in remote parts of the world. She has received many awards, including being named a CNN Hero, a Ranier Arnhold Fellow through the Mulago Foundation, and a participant in the Skoll World Forum.

Elly Teman, PhD, is a senior lecturer in cultural and medical anthropology at the Department of Behavioral Sciences at Ruppin Academic Center in Israel. Her research in the anthropology of reproduction has focused on women's experiences of surrogacy and prenatal testing. Elly is the award-winning author of an ethnography on gestational surrogacy in Israel entitled *Birthing a Mother: The Surrogate Body and the Pregnant Self* (2010). Her publications have appeared in *Social Science and Medicine*, *Medical Anthropology Quarterly*, *Culture, Medicine and Psychiatry*, and elsewhere. These publications include articles on surrogacy policy, on the experiences of gestational surrogates and intended mothers, and on religious Jewish women's reproductive lives.

Janell Tryon received her MPH in Health and Social Behavior from the University of California, Berkeley, and is a first-year doctoral student with the Department of English at the University of Massachusetts, Amherst. She has worked as a community-based researcher for NYC's Department of Health and Mental Hygiene, the San Francisco Community Health Center, and the San Francisco Department of Public Health, advocating for people living with HIV, people who use drugs, and people experiencing homelessness. Janell has also worked in the field of reproductive justice and conducted research at Luna Maya Birth Center in Chiapas, Mexico, during which time she coauthored the work presented in this volume.

Nynke van den Broek, PhD, FRCOG, DTM&H, MBBS, Centre for Maternal and Newborn Health, Liverpool School of Tropical Medicine, Liverpool, UK, is an Obstetrician-Gynaecologist trained in Tropical Medicine with recognized international expertise in global health and development. Working through effective links with governments and international partners to promote health of vulnerable populations in low- and middle-income settings, Nynke has designed, sourced funding for, and implemented programs that aim to improve access to, availability, and quality of health care for women and children through high-quality research and technical assistance.

List of Acronyms

AAP	American Academy of Pediatrics
ANM	Auxiliary Nurse Midwife
ACOG	American College of Obstetrics and Gynecology
BEmOC	Basic Emergency Obstetric Care
CDC	Centers for Disease Control and Prevention
CEmOC	Comprehensive Emergency Obstetric Care
CPAP	Continuous Positive Airway Pressure
CPMs	Certified Professional Midwives
EFM	Electronic Fetal Monitoring
EMDR	Eye Movement Desensitization and Reprocessing
EmOC	Emergency Obstetric Care
ENC	Essential Newborn Care
ECEB	Essential Care for Every Baby
ECSB	Essential Care for Small Babies
FIGO	International Federation of Gynecology and Obstetrics
GDA	Global Development Alliance
HBB	Helping Babies Breathe
HBS	Home Birth Summit
HIC	High-Income Countries
ICI	International Childbirth Initiative
ILCOR	International Liaison Committee on Resuscitation
KMC	Kangaroo Mother Care
LBW	Low Birthweight
LMIC	Low- and Middle-Income Countries
MAWS	Midwives Alliance of Washington State
MEAC	Midwifery Education Accreditation Council
MMR	Maternal Mortality Ratio (maternal deaths/100,000 live births)
NOS	Network of Safety
NR	Neonatal Resuscitation
NMR	Neonatal Mortality Ratio (neonatal deaths/1000 live births)
NRP	Neonatal Resuscitation Program

OOH	Out-of-Hospital
PPV	Positive Pressure Ventilation
QI	Quality Improvement
RART	Right Amount at the Right Time
SC	Scheduled Caste
SDG	Sustainable Development Goals
SGA	Small for Gestational Age
SSC	Skin-to-Skin Care
ST	Scheduled Tribe
TLTL	Too Little Too Late
TMTS	To Much Too Soon
WHO	World Health Organization

Chapter 1
Introduction: Sustainable Birth in Disruptive Times

Kim Gutschow and Robbie Davis-Floyd

Our volume addresses the ongoing crisis in maternity care in language that calls to mind a brief manifesto on sexual and reproductive health and justice in these disruptive times:

> Only when public health responses to COVID-19 leverage intersectional, human-rights centered frameworks, transdisciplinary science-driven theories and methods, and community-driven approaches, will they sufficiently prevent complex health and social adversities for women, girls, and vulnerable populations. (Hall et al. 2020: 1176)

While this statement was composed in response to the raging COVID-19 pandemic, it applies as much to our volume. Our volume is *intersectional*, for we illustrate how different social hierarchies—of wealth, sexism, racism—intersect to produce suffering and harm for women, newborns, and providers across the globe. We adopt a *human rights framework* as every chapter shows, implicitly or explicitly, that women's rights are human rights, that marginalized communities suffer the most when human rights are denied, or that human rights in healthcare are on a collision course with the privatization of health care. Our volume is *transdisciplinary* because our 50 authors include a range of researchers with clinical, academic, and policy expertise, including midwives, nurses, obstetricians, pediatricians, neonatologists, medical anthropologists, sociologists, public health researchers, social workers, activists, and policy makers. Our volume is *science-driven*, as it builds upon and reflects the recent scientific consensus on maternal and newborn health that we outline below.

The original version of this chapter was revised. The correction to this chapter is available at https://doi.org/10.1007/978-3-030-54775-2_21

K. Gutschow (✉)
Department of Anthropology and Religion, Williams College, Williamstown, MA, USA
e-mail: Kim.Gutschow@williams.edu

R. Davis-Floyd
Department of Anthropology, University of Texas Austin, Austin, TX, USA
e-mail: davis-floyd@outlook.com

Last but not least, our approach is *community-driven*, as we provide models of birth or maternity care that are based in local and participatory knowledges and practices.

The COVID-19 crisis reveals preexisting dysfunctionalities in maternity care that we address. Even more importantly, the disruptions of COVID-19 offer a turning point where practices can be shifted in dramatic ways that address long-standing problems and concerns. We know that hospitals are major sites of contagion, and yet for nearly 50 years, global health experts have advocated for hospital-based births across the world rather than advocating for a mix of sites including hospitals, maternity care clinics, freestanding birth centers, and home births. Similarly, the broad push for obstetric care in the twentieth century (Davis-Floyd and Cheney 2019; Devries et al. 2001; Berry 2010, Wendland 2010) has systematically sidelined midwives. Yet the recognition that midwifery care can avert 80% of the maternal and newborn deaths and stillbirths across the globe (Homer 2014) with higher-quality care and lower cost than existing obstetric models of care deserves our attention in this era of scarcity and disruption.

It is now obvious that a more decentralized approach to birth—involving freestanding birth centers or primary care clinics, home settings, and midwifery care for low-risk women with access to higher level facilities where needed—produces better outcomes and is more cost effective and woman-centered. In large world regions, such as sub-Saharan Africa and South Asia, only 57% and 72% of all births, respectively, are facility based. In most countries, there are large rural-urban and wealth disparities in maternal outcomes that midwifery care can address more sustainably than obstetric care, given the shortage of obstetricians and the high costs of training them and having them unnecessarily attend low-risk births (Homer 2014; UNICEF 2020).

Across the globe, in high-income countries (HIC) as well as low- and middle-income countries (LMIC), training midwives and promoting out-of-hospital (OOH) births at freestanding birth clinics or at home is more sustainable and feasible than hiring obstetricians and building costly hospitals. In sub-Saharan Africa alone, it was estimated that 300,000 more midwives would be needed by 2035 just to achieve 75% skilled attendance at birth (Hoope-Bender et al. 2014). This volume emphasizes innovative, resilient, and sustainable models of maternity care that can flourish amidst scarcity and disruption. It overturns conventional policies about maternity care that have become as pervasive as they are ineffective. It considers why lean, flexible midwifery-based models of care are needed now more than ever before.

1.1   Sustainability and Disruption

We privilege *sustainability* and *disruption* to highlight two rather different but coexisting social trends. We define *sustainable* as characterized by improving outcomes for mothers and newborns while lowering costs in human and financial terms. In accord with the focus on sustainability reflected in the Sustainable Development Goals (SDGs), we understand as sustainable *those solutions that can be scaled up or across similar settings while adapting to local cultural contexts in ways that preserve an ecological balance between mothers, newborns, families, and providers.* Our order of importance is intentional: mothers' and newborns' rights and health come first, followed by the health and needs of families and providers (see our Appendix on the foundational principles of the International Childbirth Initiative or ICI). Many of our essays focus on providers' rights and protocols, as we recognize that most healthcare settings privilege the authority of providers over mothers or their families (Davis-Floyd 2018). The maternity care models described in this volume are sustainable because they respond to and work with the ongoing social disruptions caused by shifting and intersectional dynamics of income, gender, sex, race, and power, as well as climate change, political conflict, and migration in many locations.

Each chapter in our volume explicitly addresses *sustainability* via a different paradigm or model of care. Sustainability can mean the ability to be scaled up or across a variety of settings from home to hospital as in our chapters on Nepal, India, Guatemala, or Mexico or across different cultural contexts such as in our chapters on Nepal, South Africa, and the United States. Sustainability should mean holistic and humanistic care that centers women's needs and agency while mitigating provider burnout. Sustainability can imply lean and flexible maternity care that can be set up or shifted quickly when disasters or pandemics destroy or disable healthcare institutions as illustrated in Chap. 19 and during the COVID-19 pandemic (Davis-Floyd et al. 2020). Sustainability can mean adapting care so that midwives and obstetricians collaborate rather than compete, as demonstrated in Chap. 3 on sustainable breech care, Chap. 4 on sustainable transfers of care in the United States, Chaps. 5 and 14 on midwives and obstetricians collaborating in the Netherlands and India, and Chaps. 9 and 10 that describe innovative hospitals incorporating humanistic care and midwifery care in Chile and Argentina.

Sustainability should mean adopting practices that conserve costs, eliminate interventions, reduce redundancies in care, and recognize the knowledge and skill of midwives in supporting women's health and rights. Sustainability can mean a model of doula care created by and for women of color that reduces interventions, helps women of color combat racism in hospitals, and provides employment to previously incarcerated women and women of color as illustrated in our chapter on innovative models of doula care in California, USA. Sustainability can mean improving provider skills or shifting provider practices through stakeholder participation and input, as illustrated in our chapters on India, the United States, South Africa, Argentina, and Guatemala. Sustainability can mean metrics that slowly shift maternity care in the United States towards evidence-based practices, thereby reducing iatrogenic harm and cutting costs in the United States, which has some of the highest maternity care costs and some of the worst maternal and neonatal outcomes in high-income countries (HIC) (WHO et al. 2015; UNICEF 2019). Sustainability can mean overcoming discrimination against indigenous women, women of color, and low-caste women via the provision of compassionate, skilled, and community-based care—as illustrated in our chapters on the United States, India, Mexico, Guatemala, South Africa, Nepal, Indonesia, and the Philippines. Sustainability can mean a femifocal model of care that emphasizes reproductive rights, women's and family's joint needs, and continuity of care throughout the lifetime, as described in our chapter on Mexico, but echoed in many other chapters in our book.

We highlight *disruption* to signal that our models may disrupt the status quo or conventional balance of power between obstetricians and midwives, providers and childbearers, or hospital and home birth settings. The models of birth we describe disrupt or aim to mitigate growing health inequities, inaccessible or low-quality care, and other dysfunctionalities that produce excess maternal and neonatal deaths today. Our volume attends to how birth providers, mothers, and community members are disrupting conventional birth models that have never been optimal by collaborating on new practices, protocols, or ways of thinking. Every chapter in this volume responds to the systemic forces of poverty, marginalization, racism, or sexism. Our case studies adapt practices of maternity care to a fractured global landscape of rising scarcity, social inequality, and personal fragility that was only heightened by the COVID-19 pandemic or the Ebola epidemic of 2013–2015 (Davis-Floyd, Gutschow, and Schwartz 2020; Strong and Schwartz 2019; Strong and Schwartz 2016).

The birth models we explore aim to disrupt the unproductive binaries that pit people against one another instead of promoting their collaboration—providers versus patients, obstetricians versus midwives, home versus hospital providers, the state versus its citizens, public versus private healthcare, and high-resource versus low-resource communities. We present innovative birth practices, policies, and metrics that disrupt the institutional inertia that has perpetuated a landscape of shortages—of skilled providers, of evidence-based practices, or of humanized and compassionate care. Our chapters illustrate disruptive conflicts or situations yet move towards a sustainable consensus. They describe how ineffective practices are disrupted or abandoned in search of improved care that benefits and empowers women as well as providers. They privilege evidence-based solutions that disrupt outmoded medical traditions and bureaucratic hierarchies that have obstructed progress in reducing maternal and neonatal mortality and morbidity.

Our volume presents a range of community-based solutions, each adapted to specific local constraints and contexts, in order to illustrate diverse approaches to the unifying goal of improved maternal and newborn outcomes and experiences. Our volume showcases innovations that have spread from the Global South to the Global North, such as the movements against obstetric violence and abusive care that began in Latin America and have spread across the globe (Sadler et al. 2016; Bohren et al. 2015). We also address birth models that work in widely different countries, such as task shifting among midwives and obstetricians in the Netherlands, the United Kingdom, Canada, South Africa, India, Indonesia, and disaster settings. Our chapters foreground models of care that honor women's agency and collaboration with providers and those that show collaboration among providers within existing hierarchies of institutional care. We illustrate cooperation among doulas, mothers, and communities in India and the United States and between community midwives and hospital-based midwives in the United States, the Netherlands, Canada, and South Africa. Our chapters explicitly address the need for continuity of care between home and hospital settings or among a variety of providers such as midwives, both professional and traditional, obstetricians, nurses, and doulas.

Our birth models illustrate innovative and collaborative paradigms of maternity care that aim to center mothers, newborns, and providers in more humanized exchanges with each other. These birth models offer sustainable solutions that attend to the normal physiology of labor/delivery but also recognize obstetric emergencies while focusing on continuity of care between home and hospital, community and provider, and mother and newborn. We build on a growing awareness of the importance of compassionate care for the social and psychological well-being of mothers, families, and providers in communities shaped by the structural violence of poverty, racism, and sexism. Our volume describes the skill-building and communication required to create and manage collaborative models of care in ways that change behavior and outcomes.

We are interested in *both the margins and the centers of birth work*. We foreground women who have been most marginalized by conventional obstetrics— including low-income, indigenous, low-caste, and previously incarcerated women. We demonstrate the value of including community-based health workers, patient advocates, midwives, or doulas who can advocate and empower clients whose voices and agency have long been discounted by obstetric models of care. By putting midwifery care at the center of our analysis, we celebrate the holistic care that has been neglected within facilities and communities across the globe while enhancing their ability to help vulnerable mothers and their communities. We empower providers whose voices have long been discounted by medical hierarchies when we foreground midwives, nurses, dai (traditional Indian midwives), and doulas within care practices that respect their experiences as family members, community members, and workers. In short, we see the soul of midwifery as caring for others—an attitude and practice that has long been neglected in healthcare in the United States (Kleinman 2019).

We emphasize the agency and human rights of women when we illustrate how midwifery models of care can empower women and ensure birth safety even in the most remote or marginalized settings. We do not expect to overturn social and health inequalities overnight. But we do provide models that explicitly target discrimination or denial of access for the most vulnerable—usually women, newborns, and their families. When women step into healthcare facilities, they are already entering a space where their voices count less and their knowledges are less authoritative than those of the providers (Davis-Floyd and Cheney 2019; Davis-Floyd and Sargent 1997). Both the Ebola epidemic of 2013–2015 (Strong and Schwartz 2019; Strong and Schwartz 2016) and the COVID-19 crisis (Davis-Floyd et al. 2020) illustrated ways that disruptive times can make pregnant women even more vulnerable to discrimination by medical authorities, who may suspect them or their families as vectors of contagion or limit their ability to self-advocate given their need for care as well as scarcity of resources for all.

Put another way, *rather than seeking a single recipe for success,* we identify the *key ingredients that make birth sustainable and adaptable in disruptive times.* Our volume promotes a variety of models of care in which both providers and mothers collaborate to improve outcomes and change their practices and prejudices about each other. We highlight ongoing debates over what kinds of care are most and least appropriate for improving maternal and neonatal health in communities that face high degrees of vulnerability and socioeconomic inequality. We describe models of care that can be scaled up across similar settings while offering lessons that can be applied in very different landscapes of maternity care elsewhere.

We would like to add a brief note on language. Our volume represents 50 authors describing models of birth in more than 18 countries, working with a wide range of populations, languages, and cultures. We respect the diversity of terms used to describe childbearers, mothers, and providers, by not seeking to impose uniform terms on our individual authors or within this volume. We appreciate the efforts to reduce marginalization and increase inclusivity by using nonbinary terms but also note that women are still denied voice and human rights across many parts of the globe. As such, we do not wish to abandon the term woman just yet.

1.2   Evidence-Based Consensus on Maternal and Newborn Health

We build on current efforts to correct previous gaps in knowledge and care provision that have privileged obstetric over midwifery care while producing excess morbidities and higher costs for low-risk women without significant benefit in maternal or neonatal outcomes. We build on a long-standing focus on "birth models that work" (Davis-Floyd et al. 2009), arguing that to understand successful models is more critical than mounting another extensive critique of birth models that produce iatrogenic harm due to lack of access, lack of high-quality care, or an overly technocratic approach (Davis-Floyd 2018). Instead, we briefly summarize a consensus around safe, respectful birth care that has shaped our findings in this volume. This consensus is articulated in a set of documents that summarize decades of research and practice within maternal and neonatal health:

- The *Lancet* series on Maternal Health 1–6 (September 2016)
- The *Lancet* series on Midwifery 1–4 (June 2014)
- The *Lancet* series on Every Newborn 1–5 (May 2014)
- The *International Childbirth Initiative (ICI): 12 Steps to Safe and Respectful MotherBaby-Family Maternity Care*

This introduction briefly describes the key principles that emerge from this consensus to illustrate the key features of sustainable models of childbirth. Rather than summarize the extensive research and findings here, we refer readers to several valuable lists:

- The 78 essential interventions in maternity care *recommended for use* and the 37 interventions in maternity care *not recommended for use* (Miller et al. 2016)

- The 72 out of 122 effective practices that fall within the midwifery scope of care (Renfrew et al. 2014) and that, if applied, could prevent 80% of global maternal and neonatal deaths (Homer 2014)
- The 20 critical interventions for newborn care (Bhutta et al. 2014)

All of these interventions have proven benefit for maternal and neonatal outcomes, yet many are still underused or inaccessible to the 140 million women who give birth every year. Despite extensive research and implementation efforts, we still have routine procedures and obstetric models of maternity care across the globe that produce known harm or little benefit for mothers and newborns. This volume calls for more sustainable models of maternity care that disrupt the previous failures of poor access, poor-quality care, and/or harmful experiences for mothers, newborns, and providers.

1.3 How the Models in This Volume Promote Maternal Health

The true engine of change in maternal health will not be the formal clinical guidelines, polished training curricula, model laws, or patient rights charters we produce. The engine will be the determination of people at the front lines of health systems—patients, providers, and managers—to find or take the power to transform their lived reality. (Freedman 2016: 2069)

Most of the chapters in our volume illustrate this claim, by showing how providers, mothers, and activists have transformed the landscape of maternity care within their region to make it more holistic, humane, and responsive to their needs. We asked our 50 contributors to describe sustainable models of birth that might solve what Freedman (2016: 2068, our emphasis) terms a *"a dangerous disconnect between the way the global health community has framed problems, proposed strategies, and pushed solutions, and the lived experience of people and providers."* Our volume very much follows the lived experiences of providers and families while addressing gaps in access and quality of care. Further, we attempt a "radical reappraisal" of maternal health priorities and strategies that *Lancet* editor Richard Horton (2016: 2068) calls for in this disruptive era of global pandemics, the climate crisis, and increasing scarcity.

Let us briefly review the four major drivers that influence current patterns of maternal mortality and morbidity (Graham et al. 2016):

1. Demographic transitions from high to low fertility and high to low mortality that still leave a high unmet need for contraception, especially in fragile settings
2. Epidemiological transitions from infectious diseases to chronic and noncommunicable diseases that influence an obstetric transition in which a declining proportion of maternal deaths are due to direct obstetric causes (i.e., postpartum hemorrhage, hypertension, sepsis, abortion, obstructed labor) while indirect

causes of maternal mortality (i.e., preexisting medical conditions, poverty, poor nutrition) are on the rise
3. Socioeconomic transitions including rising inequality, increased proportions of women in the workforce, and political disruptions that influence later childbearing and more chronic diseases, as noted above
4. Environmental transitions of climate change, environmental degradation, natural and human-made disasters, and migrations that place a greater burden on women and marginalized communities

These four shifts have produced a "grand divergence" in maternal mortality whereby the most vulnerable groups of women have been left behind (Graham and Hussein 2006). Our volume illustrates how marginalized women continue to be vulnerable to maternal mortality and morbidity and how their voices are often neglected in clinical protocols or policy frameworks. Our chapters present innovative approaches to maternity care that directly address unequal access or discrimination on the basis of race, language, ethnicity, and gender. We describe models of care that make it easier for indigenous women, women of color, and low-income women to access and afford care in India, Indonesia, the Philippines, South Africa, Nepal, Mexico, United States, Guatemala, Argentina, Germany, United Kingdom, Japan, Canada, Chile, the Netherlands, Israel, and Denmark. We just ranked our case countries according to total maternal deaths, from greatest to least, in 2017 (WHO et al. 2019). Each of our 50 contributors was asked to identify successful and sustainable models of maternity care from around the globe that promote best practices and evidence-based care.

We address the growing consensus that obstetric models alone often provide care that is either "too much too soon" (TMTS) or "too little too late" (TLTL), as Miller et al. (2016) so vividly argue. The push to provide care across thinly populated world regions with low infrastructure led to the spread of obstetric models of care without the skills to prevent overuse of interventions that cause iatrogenic harm. Given the widespread technocratic models of care that view birth as a pathology and mothers as patients whose pregnancies, labors, or deliveries require management and intervention, it is no accident that over-medicalization resulted (Davis-Floyd 2003, 2018; Wagner 2004; Davis-Floyd and Cheney 2019). Instead of TMTS or TLTL, we recommend RART maternity care, or the "right amount at the right time" (Davis-Floyd and Cheney 2019).

We will not list the 78 evidence-based interventions recommended during antepartum, intrapartum, and postpartum care, but we will dwell briefly on the 37 common interventions that are *not recommended* because they are so pervasive, despite the fact that they produce more harm than benefit, as Miller et al. (2016) remind us. We believe that every reader of this volume needs to be reminded that these interventions are not recommended yet a sizeable fraction of the 140 million women who give birth each year will suffer them, due to provider ignorance, disregard, or disrespect.

For *antenatal care*, the list of contraindicated interventions includes routine 24-week ultrasounds, many routine screening tests including for preterm pregnancy,

placental growth factor, gestational diabetes, Doppler velocimetry for uteroplacen-
tal circulation, and tests for bacterial vaginosis, chlamydia trachomatis, cytomega-
lovirus, periodontal disease, and for anti-A and anti-B antibodies in low-risk,
asymptomatic women. Most tellingly, routine involvement of obstetricians or gynecologists during pregnancy is *not recommended* for improved perinatal results
(Miller et al. 2016). As we see in our chapters on Latin America, the United States,
and other high-resource countries, obstetricians still attend many pregnancies, and
many of these routine screenings are applied to low-risk women with high costs but
little benefit.

For *intrapartum care*, the interventions to be avoided include routine speculum
exams, routine cardiotocography, routine fetal pulse oximetry, routine amniotomies, and routine oxytocin augmentation (Miller et al. 2016). Obstetrician and
Professor of Maternal-Fetal Medicine at Harvard Michael Greene (2006) directly
referenced the way that technocratic obstetrics was hoping for a deus ex machina
(the title of his essay) from the recently adopted intervention of fetal pulse oximetry
(which measures fetal oxygen levels during labor via a cap placed on the fetal scalp)
that would replace the older, ineffective technology of electronic fetal monitoring
(EFM). In an opinion piece for the *New England Journal of Medicine* that was
widely picked up by the *New York Times* and other news sources across the United
States, Greene argued (2006: 2248) against fetal pulse oximetry, doubting its ability
to "mitigate the unintended and undesirable consequences of our last ineffective,
but nonetheless persistent technological innovation." In an interview I conducted
shortly after his opinion piece was published, Greene implied that continuous EFM
was a cost-saving protocol that contributed to an unfortunate rise in cesareans with
little disregard for the maternal morbidity this involved.[1]

As Gutschow, Dolma, and Gonbo describe in Chap. 14, the use of EFM has
directly led to a rising cesarean rate at the award-winning hospital in Leh, India,
where the maternal mortality ratio (MMR, maternal deaths/100,000 live births) over
the past 20 years has been lower than Argentina's and only a fraction of the all-India
MMR for the same period (Gutschow and Dolma 2012, Gutschow 2011). Yet, unlike
many public and private hospitals across India and the globe, where rising cesarean
rates that remain under 30% are ignored, the team of obstetricians engaged in collaborative and concerted efforts to identify provider-related bias and address their
cesarean rate and improve maternity care overall.

For *postpartum care*, routine palpation of the uterus in the absence of bleeding,
routine antibiotics for low-risk women, aspirin for thromboprophylaxis, and vitamin A supplementation are not recommended. Despite significant evidence that all
of these interventions cause harm or have little or no maternal or perinatal benefit,
they are prevalent throughout low-, middle-, and high-income countries, while the
guidelines around their use remain confusing (Miller et al. 2016).

---

[1] Gutschow interviewed Greene December 2006 about the overuse of EFM and other interventions
in obstetrics. He acknowledged the predicament of reducing continuous EFM for women in labor
with intermittent auscultation given the shortage of labor/delivery nurses, whose labor is more
expensive than machines.

Our chapters illustrate some of the efforts to curtail the most dramatic examples of overused interventions that cause iatrogenic harm such as cesareans, labor induction, and labor augmentation in Latinx countries, India, and South Africa. Their overuse is not consistent but can vary considerably among countries, regions, individual facilities, or even providers. For instance, a single facility or region may have TMTS care for wealthy or elite women in the form of too many augmentations, inductions, and/or cesareans, even as marginalized women may be denied access to lifesaving care and treatment—as evidenced in our chapters on Guatemala, South Africa, India, and the United States. Our chapter on the *dais* (traditional midwives) of India indicates that tribal and Dalit women may be denied cesareans or other lifesaving interventions, even as they receive routine amniotomies or episiotomies that provide little or no benefit at the same facilities. Our chapter on Guatemala shows that indigenous women often do not receive timely care, as they are made to wait outside facilities or denied entrance even when presenting with life-threatening complications such as severe eclampsia. Our chapters on Mexico, Argentina, and Chile demonstrate that many women are treated with disrespect and abuse and/or are subjected to unnecessary cesareans and other interventions when they are deprived of midwifery care.

We cannot cover every country or every failure of care in this volume. But we do aim to build on existing knowledges, provide ways to correct past mistakes, and move beyond the bureaucratic inertias that have left so many women and newborns without adequate care.

1.4 How Our Volume Promotes the Midwifery Model of Care and Supports Marginalized Groups

> Governments and policy makers can no longer pretend to provide life-saving care, using phrases such as skilled birth attendant and EmOC [Emergency Obstetric Care] to mask poor quality; skill and emergency care need to actually be provided, adequate numbers and training of staff should be ensured, capability and basic infrastructure of facilities should be improved, timely referral should be ensured where necessary, and women should get appropriate high quality content of care. (Campbell et al. 2016: 2203)

The state of affairs that Campbell et al. (2016) document across the globe is reflected in our volume as well. The policy of simply counting percentage of births in facilities or percentage taking place with a skilled birth attendant has proven unreliable at best and disastrous at worst, as there are too many places in the world where facilities lack skilled providers, essential medicines, proper protocols, or even the basic infrastructure of electricity and water. Our volume addresses these gaps by highlighting models that do include providers and community members in the design of and decision-making about their innovative models of care. For example, Chap. 11 and Chap. 16 describe new models that provide continuity of care between community and clinics, as well as between families, communities, and midwives in Mexico and Nepal, respectively. Our volume addresses the problems of marginalization, referral, and collaboration between midwives and obstetricians, and other challenges that lurk under the surface of the more pervasive gaps in care identified by this and other global surveys. Chapter 12 and Chap. 15 describe systems that help indigenous women self-advocate and improve their access to care in countries where they often receive suboptimal care or are denied access to facilities such as Guatemala and India.

We know that a more universal application of the midwifery model of care could avert more than 80% of the world's maternal deaths, newborn deaths, and stillbirths (Homer 2014). Even in high-income countries, skilled and compassionate midwifery care could reduce maternal deaths by 30%, a considerable feat given how low maternal mortality ratios already are in those countries (Shaw et al. 2016). This news should not be surprising, given the known iatrogenic harm and excess deaths produced by over-medicalized obstetric models of care in high-income countries (Koblinsky et al. 2016). Further, we know that many of the recommended interventions to improve maternal and neonatal outcomes lie within the midwifery scope of care (Renfrew et al. 2014; Hoope-Bender et al. 2014).

Yet midwives have been sidelined in the United States—which has the worst maternal outcomes in the OECD—as well as in India and Brazil, where cesareans in private facilities have risen to shocking levels and maternal mortality has not declined as rapidly as hoped (Renfrew et al. 2014). Three middle-income countries—India, China, and Brazil—which collectively account for one-third of the world's births, have largely ignored midwifery care while promoting a culture of intervention and obstetric models of birth (Renfrew et al. 2014). More than 15 years of evidence-based studies proving the safety of planned, midwife-attended out-of-hospital births in North America (Cheney et al. 2014; Daviss and Johnson 2005) have made little impact on obstetric hegemony and dominance. Even as COVID-19 prompted women in the United States to seek out-of-hospital (OOH) births and some public hospitals in New York turned women away, ACOG failed to advocate for the safety of OOH births (Davis-Floyd et al. 2020).

We have two chapters on India, where an annual 27 million births and 35,000 maternal deaths account for one-fifth and one-eighth of the world's births and maternal deaths, respectively (WHO et al. 2019). Both chapters illustrate high-quality models of care in rural India that promote reproductive rights, women's agency, and experiences and integrate midwifery models of care in ways that promote excellent maternal and neonatal outcomes within indigenous communities who fall under designations known as Scheduled Tribe (ST) or Scheduled Caste (SC). Although these populations often have some of the worst maternal and newborn outcomes in India due to lack of access to care, one of our chapters on India illustrates highly humanistic community-based traditional midwives known as *dais* who produce *better outcomes* than regional or national averages. Our other chapter on Ladakh, India, highlights a humanistic hospital providing optimal care that has received India-wide recognition for its outstanding care in a remote mountain region where 90% of the population has ST status. Other chapters in our volume also highlight sustainable, scalable, community-based models of midwifery care that privilege the agency of marginalized or indigenous communities while providing excellent outcomes in some of the most remote districts of Nepal, Guatemala, and Mexico.

We build on the awareness that the push towards facility-based birth and skilled birth attendance has often not focused on quality of care. The WHO (2006) has defined "quality of care" as care that is "safe, effective, timely, efficient, equitable, and people-centered." Each of these terms can be further broken down to promote a multidimensional concept that is carried out within a healthcare system through service delivery, health workforce, information, medical products, vaccines, technologies, financing, and leadership/governance. Our chapters illustrate that improving quality will require addressing two "blind spots" in global maternal health policy and practice (Van Leberghe et al. 2014; Miller et al. 2016):

- Quality care means skilled, respectful, and person-centered care.
- Understanding and mitigating over-medicalization must become a key priority.

Our models go further in illustrating how collaborations among communities, providers, activists, and policy makers directly harness women's agency, authority, and empowerment within the realm of maternity care. We recognize that women's birth experiences, including medically induced traumas, can stay with them for a very long time (Gutschow 2016a; Gutschow 2011, Davis-Floyd 2018; Davis-Floyd and Cheney 2019; Strong and Schwartz 2019).

Our volume builds upon the key finding that for many middle- and low-income countries, "care led mostly by obstetricians without the balance that midwives bring to the health system might reduce mortality and morbidity but might also reduce quality and increase cost" (Renfrew et al. 2014: 1140). We argue that in both middle- and high-income settings, care by obstetricians alone has at times increased mortality and morbidity, as well as cost, at the expense of quality and woman-centered care. We also know that unnecessary interventions in maternity care cost the United States $18 billion each year (Conrad et al. 2010).

As Davis-Floyd et al. (2020) have shown, US maternity care providers responded to the COVID-19 crisis with radical shifts. Some hospital-based providers became more willing to acknowledge the safety of out-of-hospital births as clients inundated birth centers and OOH midwives with requests to transfer their care. Further, New York's governor Cuomo issued executive orders to allow licensed home birth midwives from other states and Canada to practice in New York State, in order to increase OOH birthing options. Our volume demonstrates that *when midwives, doulas, and birth activists work together with communities, they can create sustainable solutions* that disrupt the dominant models of obstetric care that contribute to excess mortality, morbidity, and costs.

1.5 How We Promote Newborn Health and Survival

Our chapters on India, Nepal, and Guatemala each illustrate how universal rollout of essential newborn care (ENC) needs to intersect with improved maternal care, as there are interactive effects between maternal and neonatal complications. In many low-resource settings, there may be only one (or no) skilled provider who can attend to both newborn and maternal emergencies, which causes delay or gaps in care. While ENC provision costs little, it requires training, motivation, and knowledge transfer to be systematically and universally applied across the developing world. Yet coverage is often lacking in the high mortality settings where ENC is needed most. In South Asia, less than 5% of all facility-based births have access to neonatal intensive care.

Globally in 2018, there were 2.5 million neonatal deaths and 2.6 million stillbirths (UNICEF 2019). The relationship between maternal deaths and neonatal deaths relates to cause and timing. Around 40% of all neonatal deaths, 40% of stillbirths, and 46% of maternal deaths occur during labor, delivery, or the first day of newborn life (Lawn et al. 2014). Half of all stillbirths occur intrapartum and are closely related to early neonatal deaths (Lawn et al. 2014). In 2018, the three leading causes of neonatal mortality—preterm birth complications (35%), intrapartum-related complications (24%), and sepsis (15%)—accounted for three-quarters of all newborn deaths (UNICEF 2019). The remaining quarter of newborn deaths were caused by congenital abnormalities (11%), pneumonia (6%), tetanus and diarrhea (1%), and other factors (7%), including iatrogenic factors related to poor newborn care (UNICEF 2019). Around three-fourths of newborn deaths occur in the first week of life. High-quality care during labor, delivery, and the immediate postpartum period is likely to have a triple return in reducing maternal deaths, neonatal deaths, and stillbirths (Tuncalp et al. 2015). Our chapters on India, Nepal, Argentina, Chile, Mexico, the Netherlands, and disaster settings each describe midwifery models of care that promote optimal maternal and newborn outcomes, including routine or basic intrapartum care, newborn resuscitation, essential newborn care, and breastfeeding.

Neonatal deaths (during the first 28 days of life) account for almost half (47%) of all under-five child deaths globally (UNICEF 2019). The share of under-five deaths that occur in the neonatal period varies: for South Asia it is 62%, for Europe and North American it is 54%, and for sub-Saharan Africa it is 36%. Survival hardly guarantees good health for the most vulnerable newborns. Besides mortality, each year roughly 19 million newborns develop life-threatening conditions that have long-term sequelae, including intrapartum-related brain injuries, severe sepsis, and pathological jaundice (Lawn et al. 2014).

In 2010, of the 15 million babies born preterm—before 37 weeks—more than one million died of preterm birth complications and another million died of causes where preterm birth is a risk factor, such as neonatal sepsis or intraventricular hemorrhage (Lawn et al. 2014). Of the 13 million preterm babies who survived, 4.4% will have mild neurodevelopmental impairment, and 2.7% will have severe impairment, often for life (Lawn et al. 2014).The long-term effects of being born preterm or small for gestational age (SGA) are still being quantified but include high risk of insulin resistance, greater glucose intolerance, hypertension, obesity, and other non-communicable diseases (Lawn et al. 2014). Chapter 14 on Ladakh, India, and Chap. 19 on Helping Babies Breathe explicitly discuss low-tech and low-cost training in newborn resuscitation and essential care for preterm, small, or sick newborns that have saved millions of lives since their rollout in the past decade.

Being born SGA—defined as under 10% of the normal birth weight for a particular gestational age and sex—adds a further risk of mortality. There are roughly 20 million babies born each year with low birth weight, either because they are preterm or SGA (Lawn et al. 2014). In South Asia alone, 40% of all births are SGA. Preterm SGA babies are 15 times as likely to die, and SGA babies born at term are nearly twice as likely to die as babies born average for gestational age (Lawn et al. 2014). Roughly 800,000 neonatal deaths are due to SGA, and another 800,000 neonatal deaths are due to suboptimal breastfeeding (Lawn et al. 2014). Statistically, male babies have a higher biological risk of life-threatening neonatal complications such as prematurity, severe sepsis, and intrapartum-related encephalopathy. Yet in countries like India where female newborns receive less or suboptimal care, this advantage for female survival is cancelled out, and newborn survival is higher for males than for females (Lawn et al. 2014; Darmstadt et al. 2015).

Rates of prematurity are increasing in both high- and low-resource countries and ranged from an average of 5% across high-income countries (HIC) to 25% in low- and middle-income countries (LMIC) in 2010 (Simmons et al. 2010). The causes of preterm birth include a range of preconception risk factors such as birth spacing, maternal diet, maternal malnutrition, genetic and epigenetic factors, as well as the poor management of maternal risk factors such as diabetes, anemia, hypertension, obesity, smoking, urinary tract infections, HIV and other STDs, and poor mental health (WHO 2012; Blencowe et al. 2012). They also include a range of pregnancy-related complications such as multiple pregnancies, young or advanced maternal age, and the use of artificial reproductive technologies (WHO 2012).

As we discuss in Chaps. 14 and 19, the total costs of providing essential newborn care (ENC) are remarkably low and the survival benefits unquestionable, even as universal implementation is ignored in many low- and middle-income countries (LMIC). ENC is defined as immediate drying and stimulation of newborns, skin-to-skin care—often called kangaroo mother care (KMC)—hygienic cord care, delayed cord cutting, hand washing, immediate breastfeeding, vitamin K prophylaxis, and neonatal resuscitation for babies not breathing at birth (Lawn et al. 2014; St. Clair et al. 2014). Studies have shown that proper cord care can reduce neonatal mortality by 23%, that early breastfeeding reduces neonatal deaths by 44%, and that skin-to-skin care can reduce 20% of neonatal deaths caused by preterm complications in low-resource settings (Bhutta et al. 2014). The newborn resuscitation training that we explore in our chapter on Ladakh, India has been proven to reduce intrapartum-related neonatal deaths by 30% and early neonatal deaths by 38% (Bhutta et al. 2014) across the globe.

Our chapters on India, Nepal, and Guatemala each illustrate how the universal rollout of ENC needs to intersect with improved maternal care, as there are interactive effects between maternal and neonatal complications. In many low-resource settings, there may be only one (or no) skilled provider who can attend to both newborn and maternal emergencies, which causes delay or gaps in care. While ENC provision costs little, it requires training, motivation, and knowledge transfer to be systematically and universally applied across the developing world. Yet coverage is often lacking in the high mortality settings where ENC is needed most. In South Asia, less than 5% of all facility-based births have access to neonatal intensive care.

1.6 Counting Maternal and Neonatal Mortality in Our Case Countries

Maternal and neonatal mortality have long been used to index the quality of maternal and neonatal health in given countries, as well as to express the magnitude of the problem to policy makers and the public. Indeed, maternal deaths are often thought of as representing a canary in a coal mine in terms of recognizing how well health systems are functioning (Declerqc and Shah 2018). Put differently, if 295,000 women across the globe are still dying each year (WHO et al. 2019) from an ordinary physiologic process—childbirth—because of complications that are mostly treatable and/or preventable, something must be terribly wrong. Our volume explores the structural violence of poverty, sexism, racism, and other social factors that contribute to these maternal deaths.[2] Before we discuss the maternal and neonatal mortality in our case countries, let us briefly discuss the counting of deaths, a topic that has only grown in significance during the COVID-19 pandemic.

> The state of maternal mortality in the world today—mostly underestimated and mostly avoidable—is clear evidence that *what you count is what you do.* (Graham and Hussein 2006: 235, emphasis theirs)

Critically, the very countries and regions that produce the most maternal deaths also have the least reliable methods of counting those deaths, because those same countries also tend to have the weakest civil registration systems (Byass and Graham 2011; Gutschow 2016b). Whether it is maternal deaths or deaths from COVID-19, counting matters because governments and policy makers need to agree if deaths are rising (and policies may be failing) or if the deaths are falling (and policies perhaps succeeding) in a specific country, region, or city (Gutschow 2016b). Further, mortality estimates need to be contextualized with "bottom-up, community-based research" (Byass and Graham 2011: 1120), as our volume illustrates. As COVID-19 has shown, estimates of mortality themselves constitute a public health intervention with real and measurable effects. In maternal healthcare as in pandemics, to count deaths is to intervene in the policy realm where decisions are made (Gutschow 2016b). If a city, state, or the CDC undercounts maternal deaths or COVID-19 deaths and makes policies assuming deaths are declining when they are actually rising, then the initial act of undercounting is an intervention that forms the basis for future interventions that may not have their intended effects. In sum, inaccurate counting can lead to failed policies (Gutschow 2016a, b).

---

[2] The WHO (2019: 10) defines a maternal death as "the death of a woman while pregnant or within 42 days of termination of pregnancy, irrespective of the duration and site of the pregnancy, from any cause related to aggravated by the pregnancy or its management but not from unintentional or incidental causes." It also defines a late maternal death as "direct or indirect maternal deaths occurring from 42 days to 1 year after termination of pregnancy." Gutschow (2016b) discusses the salient issues surrounding these definitions and arguments for the more recent term, late maternal death.

Further, mortality averages—at global, country, or even regional levels—obscure further inequalities within those averages, which must be identified and named. Thus, the gaps in maternal mortality ratios and in skilled attendance at birth between the richest and poorest nations are as important as the gaps within a single country between the upper wealth quintile and the poorest wealth quintile. These in-country inequities are discussed in our volume and should be kept in mind as we turn to mortalities in our case countries. We consider the latest WHO estimates of annual maternal deaths and neonatal deaths (Figs. 1.1 and 1.3) across our case countries, as well as maternal mortality ratios (MMR, maternal deaths/100,000 live births) and neonatal mortality ratios (NMR, neonatal deaths/1000 live births) (Figs. 1.2 and 1.4). Total maternal deaths and MMR are directly influenced by a country's total fertility rate (TFR), population size, and maternal mortality ratio. The log scales we provide illustrate the wide range of total annual maternal and neonatal deaths across our case countries (see Figs. 1.1 and 1.3).

Both India and the United States are outliers with outsized shares of maternal and neonatal deaths. India, with its 1.28 billion people, 27 million births, 35,000 maternal deaths, and 549,000 neonatal deaths per year (Figs. 1.1 and 1.3), is home to 17% of the world's population, 20% of the world's live births, 15% of its maternal deaths, and 27% of its neonatal deaths (WHO et al. 2019; UNICEF 2019). With its 750 maternal deaths, the United States had 14 times the maternal deaths of Japan in 2017, yet only triple the population (Fig. 1.1). With an MMR of 19, the United States ranks first in MMR in the OECD and roughly 3–7 times the MMR of our other high-income case countries like Israel, Japan, Germany, the Netherlands, Denmark, and Canada (Fig. 1.2). Further, unlike almost every high-income country where maternal mortality decreased between 2000 and 2017, in the United States *the maternal mortality ratio increased by 58%* (WHO et al. 2019).

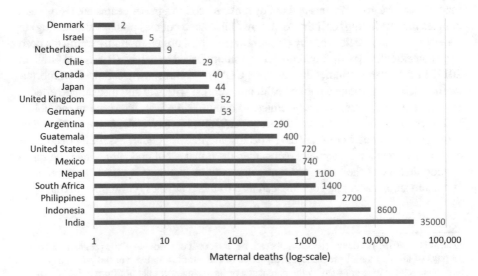

Fig. 1.1 Total maternal deaths in 2017 in our case countries. (Data from WHO 2019)

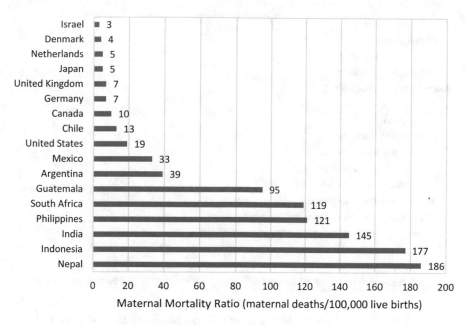

Fig. 1.2 Maternal mortality ratios (MMR) in 2017 in our case countries. (Data from WHO 2019)

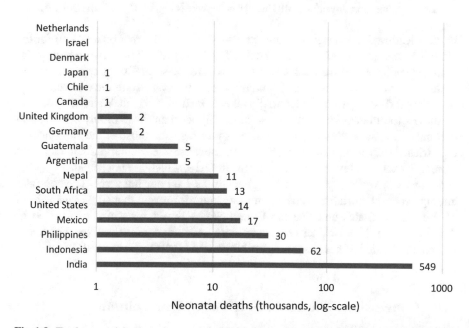

Fig. 1.3 Total neonatal deaths in thousands in 2018 in our case countries. (Data from UNICEF 2019)

Because the United States and India represent such outsized proportions of the global burden of maternal and newborn deaths (Figs. 1.1 and 1.3), they have been the focus of scrutiny and critique of their maternity care (Gutschow 2016b). Each has faced accusations of human rights abuses in their poor maternity care from the

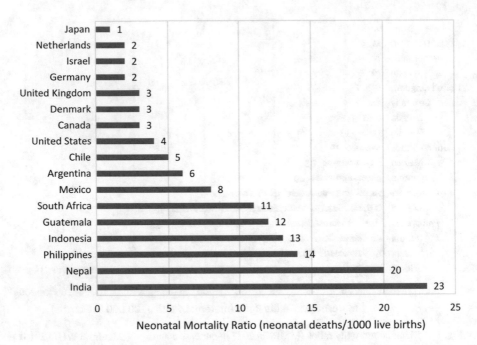

Fig. 1.4 Neonatal mortality ratio (NMR) in 2018 in our case countries. (Data from UNICEF 2019)

world's leading human rights organizations—Amnesty International (2010) for the United States and Human Rights Watch (2009) for India. These two reports offer scathing testimony of the denial of access to care, poor quality of care, as well as systemic inequities in outcomes within these countries and systemic undercounting of maternal deaths (Amnesty International 2010; Human Rights Watch 2009).

India's total newborn deaths are so much higher than those of any other nation that only a log scale could accommodate its numbers and those of the high-income countries (HIC) in our volume (Fig. 1.3). Because the Netherlands, Israel, and Denmark each had fewer than 1000 deaths in 2018, which are not rounded up, they show up as 0, while Japan and Chile show up as 1 on our log scale. The contrasts among neonatal mortality ratios in our case countries reveal that Chile ranks ahead of the United States and that the United States is not far ahead of Mexico or Argentina (Fig. 1.3). Besides producing more newborn deaths than Nepal or South Africa, the United States has far higher NMR and MMR than other HIC.

1.7 Conclusion: The Three Sections of Our Volume

The first section of our volume focuses on high-income countries (HIC) that illustrate the remaining challenges of building more inclusive, holistic, and collaborative models of care that transcend ongoing disparities and hierarchies. The chapter by Davis explains why and how holistic models of midwifery care and education enable the collaboration and agency of both mother and midwife far more effectively than technocratic models of education or care. Daviss, Hedditch, Krishnan, and Barnes explore new models of upright breech delivery that involve cooperation and collaboration between midwives and obstetricians skilled in the knowledge of physiologic birth. Dunham and Hall's chapter on sustainable transfers of care from home to hospital argues for improving collaborations between transferring and receiving providers, as well as for continuity of care and support personnel where possible, so as to avoid unnecessary duplication of care and unnecessary interventions. Bommarito explores the remarkable flexibility and collaboration achieved between midwives and obstetricians in the Netherlands that effectively maintains their well-integrated maternity care system. Bakal and McLemore show that doulas working among women of color, some previously incarcerated, can empower their clients and each other to begin to counter the systemic racism in maternity care in the United States. Pine and Morton argue that improved metrics for measuring the quality of maternity care can be used to improve maternal outcomes across the United States. Teman and Berend show how lessons from sustainable surrogacy in Israel might apply to the US context. Each of these chapters extends the lessons learned about how to promote woman-centered care and improve metrics on maternal outcome accountability and counting (Shaw et al. 2016; Gutschow 2016a, b).

Our second section on Latin American countries privileges a variety of radical solutions to a pattern of obstetric violence, disrespectful care, and overly medicalized care that does not provide equal access for indigenous or low-income women. Sadler, Leiva, and Gomez illustrate how the movement towards humanized childbirth and against obstetric violence in Latin America influenced Chile's slow shift towards woman-centered, compassionate care. Jerez shows how activists and providers in Buenos Aires, Argentina are making radical changes in maternity wards to humanize birth, advocate for reproductive rights, and promote gender and sexual diversity, as well as to overcome gender-based violence. Alonso, Lopez, Lucas-Danch, and Tryon illustrate a "femifocal" model in Mexico that offers humanized, high-quality continuity of care across the life cycle that includes well-woman care, gynecological care, and alternative therapies. Austad, Chary, Hawkins, Martinez, and Rohloff show how trained patient advocates can help indigenous clients and their midwives negotiate for improved care at Guatemalan institutions where they often have been denied access or given substandard care.

Our third section addresses maternal and newborn care in low- and middle-income countries (LMIC). Macauley and van den Broek argue that global efforts to improve maternal care quality must include the use of midwifery models of care and quality audits to improve accountability in providing emergency obstetric care in rural and low-income settings. Aneji and Little explore the development of three sustainable, low-tech curricula: Helping Babies Breathe (HBB), Essential Care for Every Baby (ECEB), and Essential Care for Small Babies (ECSB); these programs are addressing the main causes of neonatal mortality in low-resource settings. Gutschow, Dolma, and Gonbo illustrate how two female obstetricians and one pediatrician in a remote Himalayan region of India have overseen 40 years of remarkable maternal and newborn outcomes—including the creation of the region's most advanced special newborn care unit—at a humanistic and award-winning public hospital. Roy, Qadeer, Chawla, Sadgopal, and Gautam show how dais in four Indian districts provide skilled, high-quality, responsive, and culturally safe humanized care to mothers and newborns that contrasts sharply with the poor-quality, often abusive care that regional facilities provide. Adams, Craig, Samen, and Bhatta describe a network of safety model that integrates maternal and newborn care while staying responsive to local community needs, cultural practices, and differing Hindu and Buddhist beliefs within the Nepal Himalayas. MacDougall traces how a midwifery model of care can transcend both public/private and Black/White binaries within the landscape of maternity care in post-apartheid South Africa. Davis-Floyd, Lim, Penwell, and Ivry describe a low-tech, flexible, and mobile model of midwifery care that has been sustainably applied in multiple disaster settings, such as the 2004 tsunami in Aceh, Indonesia, the 2017–2018 volcanic eruptions in Bali, Hurricane Yolanda in the Philippines, and after the Great Sendai earthquake and tsunami in northeast Japan on March 11, 2011.

In our conclusion, we coeditors (Gutschow, Davis-Floyd, and Daviss) discuss how low-tech, high touch, and flexible models of midwifery care offer woman-centered and humanized care that mothers and newborns need in these disruptive times of climate crisis and pandemics. We return to the themes of sustainability and disruption while extending the lessons learned in our chapters about sustainable birth models that can improve outcomes and experiences for mothers, newborns, and providers.

Acknowledgments Gutschow thanks the mothers, providers, newborns, and ordinary folks she has engaged in India and the United States who have discussed and endured her endless questions about birth, midwifery care, obstetric care, neonatal care, and other topics that contributed to this chapter. Gutschow thanks Robin Sears for helping create the charts in this chapter and deeply appreciates her children for sustaining her with love and humor through the editing and writing process over the past years.

Appendix: The 7 Foundational Principles and 12 Steps of the *International Childbirth Initiative* (ICI): Promoting MotherBaby-Family Maternity Care

Our volume builds upon a recent focus on woman-centered and family-centered care based on women's rights that is epitomized in the *International Childbirth Initiative* (ICI): *12 Steps to Safe and Respectful MotherBaby-Family Maternity Care*. In this Appendix, we briefly present these 12 Steps as well as the foundational principles that they are based on. The ICI was created by two global organizations—the International Federation of Gynecology and Obstetrics (FIGO) and the International MotherBaby Childbirth Organization (IMBCO)—and was formally launched in October 2018 at the FIGO World Congress in Brazil (Lalonde et al. 2019). The ICI, whose wording Davis-Floyd and others helped craft, has been endorsed and adopted internationally by multiple international organizations and maternity care practices, including several described in this volume. Its proposed MotherBaby-Family Maternity Care Model embodies the following seven foundational principles:

1. *Advocate rights and access to care.* This principle recognizes women's and children's rights as human rights and attempts to ensure that all women, regardless of background, education, citizenship, age, or health status, have equal access to high-quality, affordable, or free maternity care. The principle uses the word "background" to index race, income, and ethnicity—three key variables that structure access to maternity care and produce significant health inequities within and between populations (Graham and Hussein 2006; Marmot et al. 2012).
2. *Ensuring respectful maternity care.* This principle insists on respect and compassion for all women as the foundation of maternity care and aims to protect women from abusive or disrespectful care, which remains prevalent and often unrecognized across the globe, in both high-income countries (HIC) and low- and middle-incomes countries (LMIC).
3. *Protecting the MotherBaby-Family triad.* This principle aims to treat the mother, baby, and family as a unified triad, even as it privileges the MotherBaby dyad as an essential unit. While the principle states that the woman should be the ultimate decision-maker and that shared decision-making is an *aspiration*, this principle could have more strongly worded guidance for when mothers and their families or communities disagree or where some women lack agency and informed choice in relation to reproductive rights, such as in extremely pronatalist societies or regimes (Goldberg 2009; Bongaarts and Guilmoto 2015).
4. *Promoting wellness, preventing illness and complications, and ensuring timely emergency referral and care.* This principle acknowledges that most labors and deliveries are normal physiologic events that most often require only supportive care for mother and newborn and that most pregnancy-related and newborn complications can be treated or prevented with timely emergency care.
5. *Supporting women's autonomy and choices to facilitate a positive birthing experience.* This principle aims to assure laboring women continuity of supportive care, access to evidence-based information, and the ability to make informed choices, including about place of birth. The principle explicitly states that women with low-risk pregnancies can safely birth at home, birth centers, or clinics— which is where 65% of the world's births still take place. Notably, this principle affirms low-risk women's right to out-of-hospital (OOH) or community birth, their right to continuous labor support and information about evidence-based care, while trying to "reduce the risk of psychological trauma" (Lalonde et al. 2019: 67). The mention of psychological trauma hints at pervasive patterns of obstetric violence and abusive care, which are routine in many hospitals across the world today and which our volume addresses.
6. *Providing a healthy and positive birthing environment: The responsibilities of caregivers and health systems.* This principle affirms that the birthing environment and caregivers' attitudes and practices influence a woman's confidence and ability for a healthy birth and a healthy newborn, with potential lifelong conse-

quences for both. It expressly notes that a caring and supportive atmosphere can be enhanced or diminished by every caregiver she encounters, encouraging listening to the mother and her family and women's self-expression. This principle also states that the needs of MotherBaby must take precedence over the needs of providers, even as it acknowledges that providers themselves require supportive maternity care systems within which to function. This principle reaffirms the importance of the relationships between mother and provider, between provider and family, as well as among the providers within a healthcare system. It recognizes that providers can vary—some can be respectful while others are not—and that the structural factors influencing quality of maternity care can be wideranging, including whether there are providers who have the skills, essential supplies, and support to care for the MotherBaby dyad.

7. *Using an evidence-based approach to maternal health services based on the MotherBaby-Family Maternity Care Model.* This principle insists that mother and newborn be given only evidence-based care and explicitly be "protected from unnecessary and potentially harmful interventions, practices, and procedures, and from both overuse and underuse of medical technology" (Lalonde et al. 2019: 67–68). It affirms a broader theme raised by Miller et al. (2016), who warn against care that is "too much too soon" (TMTS) and causes iatrogenic harm or "too little too late" (TLTL) and fails to offer timely benefit when it should have. This principle affirms the value of physiologic labor against the overuse of technology in an effort to save costs and optimize health outcomes for mother and baby. It also notes that the MotherBaby-Family care model *can be used in all settings by all providers*, even during obstetric or neonatal complications. As such, it affirms that compassionate, evidence-based care should always be the priority, regardless of birth setting or provider, and that even obstetricians can provide midwifery model care.

The ICI 12 Steps to Safe and Respectful MotherBaby-Family Maternity Care

(abridged, see www.internationalchildbirth.com for full text):

1. Provide respect, dignity, and informed choice in care to every woman and her family.
2. Provide free or affordable care with cost transparency for prepartum, intrapartum, and postpartum care.
3. Routinely provide MotherBaby-Family maternity care to all clients so as to optimize the biopsychosocial processes of childbirth, with multidisciplinary collaboration with other providers during obstetric or neonatal complications.
4. Offer continuous support in labor and delivery with doulas, partners, and/or TBAs so as to optimize safe vaginal delivery with fewer analgesics and better Apgar scores.

5. Provide drug-free pain relief measures such as breathing, touch, massage, relaxation, and water immersion if possible. If pharmacological pain relief options are available or requested, explain their benefits and risks.
6. Provide evidence-based practices including but not limited to:

    • Allowing labor to unfold at its own pace
    • Providing mothers access to food/drink as needed during labor
    • Ensuring that women have access to care and well-being in early labor but refrain from admitting women until they are in active labor
    • Supporting labor by allowing women to walk and move about freely and choose the birthing position of their choice as well as tools supportive of upright positions
    • Providing mothers with privacy during labor and delivery
    • Training staff to safely deliver breech babies vaginally or turning them to cephalic lie if possible
    • Facilitating immediate and sustained skin-to-skin contact between mother and newborn for warmth, stimulation, and breastfeeding
    • Delaying cord clamping to facilitate nutrient transfer from mother to newborn
    • Carrying out all elements of essential newborn care including allowing mothers to have skin-to-skin contact and breastfeed preterm babies where possible.

7. Avoid harmful practices such as:

    • Episiotomies
    • Enemas
    • Routine sweeping or artificial rupture of membranes
    • Frequent vaginal exams
    • Supine or lithotomy position
    • Keeping mother in bed or immobilized
    • Caregiver-directed pushing
    • Fundal pressure
    • Immediate cord clamping
    • Separation of mother/baby
    • Withholding of food/water from mother

8. Enhance wellness and prevent illness by providing access to:

    • Clean water, clean toilets, and WASH (water, sanitation, hygiene) measures
    • Education on and treatment or prevention of HIV, malaria, tetanus, syphilis, hepatitis B, and toxoplasmosis
    • Family planning services and reproductive rights
    • Culturally sensitive and competent prenatal education
    • Adequate education around postnatal and neonatal care before discharge

9. Provide emergency care and transport to skilled emergency care for life-threatening complications, including referral and consultation with tertiary centers as needed.

10. Have a supportive human resource policy that ensures a respectful and positive workplace to aid in retention of skilled staff.
11. Provide a continuum of care for mother and newborn during pregnancy, labor, and delivery that links mothers to all providers including traditional birth attendants and educators within a multidisciplinary care system.
12. Promote breastfeeding and skin-to-skin contact between mothers and newborns according to the 10 Steps of the Baby-Friendly Hospital Initiative.

References

Amnesty International (2010) Deadly delivery: the maternal health care crisis in the USA. Amnesty International Publications, London

Berry NS (2010) Unsafe motherhood: Mayan mortality and subjectivity in post-war Guatemala. Berghahn Press, New York

Bhutta Z et al (2014) Can available interventions end preventable deaths in mothers, newborn babies, and stillbirths, and at what cost? Lancet 384:347–370

Blencowe H, Cousens S, Oestergaard M, Chou D, Moller AB et al (2012) National, regional, and worldwide estimates of preterm birth rates in the year 2010 with time trends for selected countries since 1990: a systematic analysis. Lancet 379:2162–2172

Bohren MA, Vogel J, Hunter EC et al (2015) The mistreatment of women during childbirth in health facilities globally: a mixed-methods systematic review. PLoS Med 12(6):1–32. https://doi.org/10.1371/journal.pmed.1001847

Bongaarts P, Guilmoto C (2015) How many more missing women? Excess female morality and prenatal sex selection, 1970-2050. Popul Dev Rev 41(2):241–269

Byass P, Graham W (2011) Grappling with uncertainties along the MDG trail. Lancet 378:1119–1120

Campbell O et al (2016) The scale, scope, coverage, and capability of childbirth care. Lancet 388:2193–2208

Conrad P, Mackie T, Mehrotra A (2010) Estimating the costs of medicalization. Soc Sci Med 70:1943–1947

Darmstadt G, Shiffman J, Lawn JE (2015) Advancing the newborn and stillbirth global agenda: priorities for the next decade. Arch Dis Child 100(suppl 1):s13–s18. https://doi.org/10.1136/archdischild-2013-305557

Davis-Floyd R (2003) Birth as an American rite of passage. University of California Press, Berkeley

Davis-Floyd R (2018) Ways of knowing about birth: mothers, midwives, medicine, and birth activism. Waveland Press, Long Grove

Davis-Floyd, Cheney (eds) (2019) Birth in eight cultures. Waveland Press, Long Grove

Davis-Floyd R, Sargent C (1997) Childbirth and authoritative knowledge: cross-cultural perspectives. University of California Press, Berkeley

Davis-Floyd R, Barclay L, Daviss B-A et al (2009) Birth models that work. University of California Press, Berkeley

Davis-Floyd R, Gutschow K, Schwartz D (2020) Pregnancy, birth, and the COVID-19 pandemic in the United States. Med Anthropol. https://doi.org/10.1080/01459740.2020.1761804

Declerqc E, Shah N (2018) Maternal deaths represent the canary in the coal mine of women's health. Statnews. https://www.statnews.com/2018/08/22/maternal-deaths-women-health/

Freedman L (2016) Implementation and aspiration gaps: whose view counts? Lancet 388:P2068–P2069. https://doi.org/10.1016/S0140-6736(16)31530-6

Freedman LP, Ramsey K, Abuya T et al (2014) Defining disrespect and abuse of women in child-birth: a research, policy and rights agenda. Bull World Health Organ 92(12):915–917. https://doi.org/10.2471/BLT.14.137869

Goldberg M (2009) The means of reproduction: sex, power, and the future of the world. Penguin, New York

Graham W, Hussein J (2006) Universal reporting of maternal mortality: an achievable goal? Int J Gynecol Obstet 94:234–242

Graham W, Woodd S, Byass P et al (2016) Diversity and divergence: the dynamic burden of poor maternal health. Lancet 388:2164–2175. https://doi.org/10.1016/S0140-6736(16)31533-1

Greene M (2006) Obstetricians still await a Deus ex Machina. N Engl J Med 355(21):2247–2248

Gutschow K (2006) The politics of being Buddhist in Zangskar: partition and today. India Rev 5(3–4):470–498

Gutschow K (2011) From Home to Hospital: The Extension of Obstetrics in Ladakh. In: Adams V, Schrempf M, Craig S (eds) Medicine between science and religion: explorations on Tibetan grounds. Berghahn Press, London, pp 185–214

Gutschow K (2016a) Going beyond the numbers: maternal death reviews in India. Med Anthropol 35(4):322–337. https://www.tandfonline.com/doi/full/10.1080/01459740.2015.1101460

Gutschow K (2016b) On counting and miscounting maternal mortality: metrics and what matters in global health. In: Tamcke M (ed) Armut & gesundheit [poverty & health]. Göttingen, Üniversitätsverlag Göttingen, pp 131–146

Gutschow K, Dolma P (2012) In: Kappas M, Gross W, Kelleher D (eds) Global policies and local implementation: maternal mortality in rural India. Göttingen University Press, Göttingen, pp 153–166Global Health – A Challenge for Interdisciplinary Research

Hall KS, Samari G, Garbers S et al (2020) Centring sexual and reproductive health and justice in the global COVID-19 response. Lancet 395:1175–1178

Homer CSE (2014) The projected effect of scaling up midwifery. Lancet 384:1146–1157

Hoope-Bender t, de Bernis L, Campbell J et al (2014) Improvement of maternal and newborn health through midwifery. Lancet 384:1226–1235

Human Rights Watch (2009) No tally of the anguish: accountability in maternal health care in India. Human Rights Watch Publications, New York

Koblinsky M, Moyer C, Calvert C et al (2016) Quality maternity care for every woman, everywhere: a call to action. Lancet 388(10057):2307–2320. https://doi.org/10.1016/S0140-6736(16)31333-2

Lalonde A, Herschderfer K, Pascali Bonaro D et al (2019) The international childbirth initiative: 12 steps to safe and respectful motherbaby-family maternity care. Int J Gynecol Obstet 146:65–73

Lawn JE et al (2014) Progress, priorities, and potential beyond survival. Lancet 384:301–346. https://doi.org/10.1016/S0140-6736(14)60479-7

Leberghe V et al (2014) Country experience with strengthening health systems and deployment of midwives in countries with high maternal mortality. Lancet 384:1215–1225

Marmot M, Allen J, Bell R, Goldblatt P (2012) Building of the global movement for health equity: from Santiago to Rio and beyond. Lancet 379:181–188

Miller SE, Abalos E, Chamillard M et al (2016) Beyond too little, too late and too much, too soon: a pathway towards evidence-based, respectful maternity care worldwide. Lancet 388:2176–2192. https://doi.org/10.1016/S0140-6736(16)31472-6

Renfrew MJ, McFadden A, Bastos MH et al (2014) Midwifery and quality care: findings from a new evidence-informed framework for maternal and newborn care. Lancet 384:1129–1145

Sadler M, Santos M, Ruiz-Berdún MD et al (2016) Moving beyond disrespect and abuse: addressing the structural dimensions of obstetric violence. Reprod Health Matters 24(47):47–55

Shaw et al (2016) Drivers of maternity care in high-income countries: can health systems support women-centered care? Lancet 388:2285–2295

Simmons LE, Rubens CE, Darmstadt G et al (2010) Preventing preterm birth and neonatal mortality: exploring the epidemiology, causes, and interventions. Semin Perinatol 34(6):408–415. https://doi.org/10.1053/j.semperi.2010.09.005

Singh P, Hashmi G, Swain PK (2018) High prevalence of cesarean section birth in private sector health facilities- analysis of district level household survey-4 (DHLS-4) of India. BMC Public Health 18:613–623

St. Clair N, Batra M, Kuzminski J et al (2014) Global challenges, efforts, and controversies in neonatal care. Clin Perinatol 41:749–772

Strong A, Schwartz D (2016) Sociocultural aspects of risk to pregnant women during the 2013–2015 multinational Ebola virus outbreak in West Africa. Heathcare Women Int 37(8):922–942

Strong A, Schwartz D (2019) Effects of the West Africa Ebola epidemic on health care of pregnant women: stigmatization with and without infection. In: Schwartz DA (ed) Pregnant in the time of Ebola. Springer Nature, New York

Tuncalp O et al (2015) Quality of care for pregnant women and newborns – the WHO vision. Br J Obstet Gynecol. https://doi.org/10.1111/147-0528.13451

UNICEF (2019) Levels and trends in child mortality, report 2019: estimates by the United Nations inter-agency group for child mortality estimates. UNICEF Publications, New York

UNICEF (2020) Global delivery care coverage and trends: percentage of births assisted by a skilled birth attendant, by country, 2014–2019. Accessed at https://data.unicef.org/topic/maternal-health/delivery-care/

Wendland C (2010) A heart for the work: journeys through an African medical school. University of Chicago Press, Chicago

WHO (2006) Quality of care: a process for making strategic choices in health systems. WHO Publications, Geneva

WHO et al (2012) Born too soon: the global action report on preterm birth. WHO Publications, Geneva. Available via: https://www.who.int/maternal_child_adolescent/documents/born_too_soon/en/

WHO et al (2015) Trends in maternal mortality 1990–2015: estimates developed by WHO, UNICEF, UNFPA, The World Bank, and the United Nations Population Division. WHO Publications, Geneva. Available via: https://www.who.int/reproductivehealth/publications/monitoring/maternal-mortality-2015/en/

WHO et al (2019) Trends in maternal mortality 2000–2017: estimates developed by WHO, UNICEF, UNFPA, The World Bank, and the United Nations Population Division. WHO Publications, Geneva. Available via: https://apps.who.int/iris/handle/10665/327596

Part I
Sustainable Maternity Solutions in High-Income Countries

Chapter 2
Sustainable Midwifery

Elizabeth Davis

2.1 Three Models of Care: Holistic, Humanistic, and Technocratic

What is sustainable midwifery? It is that which has characterized midwifery practice for millennia, plus new skills and approaches that have proven useful since midwifery's resurgence in the last century. For much of human evolution, midwifery has been present, while obstetrics, having developed in Europe during the 1600s, is but a tiny dot on our timeline.

In the contemporary high-resource countries of Europe, Japan, New Zealand, and others, midwife-assisted birth is still the norm. In fact, the countries with the lowest perinatal mortality rates in the world all make generous use of midwives, who attend approximately 70% of all births in those nations. In the United States, where midwives assist only 9.1% of births (Martin et al. 2018) due to opposition from obstetricians and legislators, perinatal and maternal mortality rates are alarmingly high (Davis-Floyd 2018b). Out of 121 countries analyzed by the WHO, the United States ranked 43rd in lifetime risk of maternal mortality (WHO 2015). In short, pregnant women have a greater chance of dying in the United States than in any Western European nation, Puerto Rico, Libya, Serbia, Slovenia, and Belarus (WHO 2015).

So why is midwifery not the standard of care for *all* healthy birthing persons? In Europe, midwifery's oppression dates back to the "Burning Times" of the Inquisition. During this period, midwives became targets because they healed by way of nature and in alignment with the wisdom of the body, rather than relying on God (who was considered by the church to be the only real healer). As the *Malleus Maleficarum*, handbook of the Inquisitor and originally published in 1486, declared: "No one does

E. Davis (✉)
National Midwifery Institute, Inc., Middlebury, VT, USA
e-mail: elizabeth@elizabethdavis.com

© Springer Nature Switzerland AG 2021
K. Gutschow et al. (eds.), *Sustainable Birth in Disruptive Times*, Global
Maternal and Child Health, https://doi.org/10.1007/978-3-030-54775-2_2

more harm to the Catholic faith than do midwives" (cited from Henrich and Sprenger 1972). I ask my midwifery students to imagine living in this era and bearing witness to their peers or family members being tortured or killed for providing healthcare to mothers and children, and to consider the fear that this instilled regarding female power in general. Obstetrics evolved by feeding on this fear as well as that engendered by the well known biblical passage suggesting that God chose to greatly multiply woman's pain in childbirth.

To this day, midwifery continues to be subjugated to obstetric guidelines and political machinations, which have worked against the professional autonomy of midwives as well as their legal defense and the legislation needed to protect their practices. Institutional biomedicine has repeatedly demonstrated its greed for the power and revenues that accrue from assisting childbirth. During the last decade in the Netherlands, under the guise of "consumer choice," the obstetric lobby managed to undermine the long-standing tradition that all pregnant persons start care with a midwife, and the midwives, having grown complacent with time, are scrambling for a solution (Davis-Floyd et al. 2013; Cheney et al. 2019). In Germany, midwives are threatened by the skyrocketing premiums of mandated malpractice insurance, and although their outcomes are consistently superior to those of obstetricians, their practice is dwindling, and many smaller towns no longer have midwives who attend home births. It has never been more imperative that midwives articulate their unique approach to caregiving and lay claim to the body of midwifery skills that have proven themselves over the course of time and human evolution (Trevathan 1987; Davis 2010, 2017a, 2019; Cheyney and Davis-Floyd in press).

First and foremost, midwifery's resilience has been based on its adaptability to the needs of mothers and families. Skills for detecting complications have evolved over time, but the intention has always been to promote the health of mothers and babies and to preserve birth as a normal process. Here we will briefly explore the skills that have endured while evaluating new innovations in practice that have allowed midwives to improve maternal and neonatal outcomes despite political interference from institutional medical paradigms (Davis 2010, 2016, 2019).

In order to achieve its full potential, midwifery must align itself with the holistic model of care. Whether by shift work in hospital or by continuity of care in birth centers or at home, midwifery's survival depends on this model of care as the only one that truly addresses the needs of both client and provider.

What is holistic care? Robbie Davis-Floyd (2001, 2018b) has articulated three models of perinatal care, of which holism is the most evolved:

- The *technocratic model* is based on beliefs that the body is a machine, that disease comes from outside the body, that standardized care is superior because it minimizes the risk of the unexpected, and that the provider knows best. *This model is based on separation and control.*
- The *humanistic model* modifies the tenets of the technocratic model by treating the body as an organism and striving to support the normal physiology of birth by making practices more sensitive and humane. It has two facets: superficial and deep humanism. *Superficial humanism* may involve pretty labor rooms and

compassionate practitioners who still perform all sorts of technological interventions, while *deep humanism* involves facilitating the "deep physiology" of birth with minimal intervention. *This model is based on kindness and good intentions.*

- The *holistic model* is a radical departure from humanism in that it redefines the body as an energy system that can be affected by the energy of others, for better or for worse. It codes a pregnant person not as a patient but as a client and decision-maker in her perinatal experience, with the authority to make healthcare decisions in the best interests of her emotional, psychological, and physical well-being. *This model is based on relationship, integration, and empowerment.*

Although superficial humanism focuses on concern for the client's feelings and needs, in practice it may be little more than a kinder, gentler technocratic approach, whereby the provider gives care rather than empowering the client to care for herself. Even in deep humanism, the provider is still in charge. The holistic model redefines the provider/client relationship as one of equals—which has both benefits and pitfalls, especially for birth providers schooled in technocracy or humanism.

Care providers trained in the technocratic model soon learn to set their emotions and instincts aside for the sake of clinical detachment. Detachment is a prime value of this paradigm, based as it is on control, and the separation of patients from providers, mothers from babies, women from their bodies/relational selves, and providers from their emotions. Technocratic training is quite militaristic; students are expected to obey their superiors, and so they expect the same from their patients. Abnormally long work hours and high patient loads result in sleep deprivation and malnourishment—hardly optimal conditions for facing tough challenges in childbirth with minimal experience. Even if we have little personal experience with technocratic care, we may know it from TV shows like *Grey's Anatomy* or *Chicago Med*, which highlight the trials and tribulations of its practitioners.

Above all else, the technocratic model of care makes little allowance for providers to feel fear, which is seen as a disabling weakness. Yet as an ideology that codes all births as risky, the technocratic model of care is indeed fear based. Its birth management protocols seek to avoid risk by intervening too soon or too often, thereby causing adverse effects that stem from disrupting the normal physiology of birth. Cheyney and Davis-Floyd (2019: 7) have termed this phenomenon the "obstetric paradox": intervene in birth to avoid risk, thereby generating risk and causing iatrogenic damage. The overuse of interventions in perinatal care is called TMTS (too much, too soon), while the underuse of interventions is known as TLTL (too little, too late); both occur across the globe, due to the rapid spread of obstetric models without sufficient training or provider/institutional capacity (Miller et al. 2016). Cheyney and Davis-Floyd (2019: 235) recommend replacing TMTS and TLTL with "RART" or the "right amount at the right time," and Betty-Anne Davis (2020) suggests JOT care ("just enough on time"). Both RART and JOT are consistent with core tenets of midwifery practice.

Note that with regard to fear, in the humanistic model of care, only the client is allowed to express it, while the holistic model encourages both provider and client to express fear fully and legitimately.

2.2 Midwifery Education and the Three Models of Care: Technocratic, Humanistic, and Holistic

Now let us consider the content of technocratic medical education. Diagnostic methods and surgical remedies are strongly emphasized. But in terms of childbirth, which is not a disease but a normal, physiologic event, these have a very limited function. And regarding the role of emotions in health status, imagine asking a technocratic practitioner if grief, guilt, or fear might be affecting an illness; the likely answer would be "no." Yet we see, time and again, how these emotions can very much affect the course of labor. Along these lines, it continues to amaze me that most medical instruction does not include wellness aspects of nutrition, exercise, or stress reduction—they may be mentioned as possible factors in certain conditions, but courses to fully enlighten students on these subjects are notably absent from most techno-medical curricula. As another example, at a typical annual gynecological visit, most women are never asked to bring a 3-day diet record nor are they questioned about sexual satisfaction, family relationships, or stress/sleep patterns that could affect health status (all of which are standard in holistic care) (Davis 2017b, 2019).

Humanistic education, on the other hand, can be confounding for a student by virtue of its confused values: partly technocratic, partly holistic. Consequently, it generates a model of care based more on good intentions than on practice realities, so that providers in this model focus on giving everything they have to their client's care, but frequently more than is needed or appropriate. Codependence is a real pitfall, as the client is not a full partner in the exchange, and so the provider may feel inadequate for not "doing enough" or, conversely, may feel resentful at having little personal space, time, or respect from the client. The same is often true of students being schooled in this model. Humanism is the bridge between technocracy and holism, but at times, that bridge can feel shaky, without solid footing at either end.

Holistic education is a radical departure from both of the above methods because the hierarchy between teacher and student is dissolved. No matter their personal circumstances, the two are on a level playing field, with the understanding that they are both adults with their own life experiences and expertise. In practical terms, holistic education does not just "value" student input; it requires it (Davis 2010, 2017a). The interaction between teacher and student is a two-way street, with healthy function based on honesty, integrity, and transparency. Nobody gets to pull rank, because there is no rank.

In practical terms, teaching or practicing holistically may appear as threatening to privacy and personal space as humanism, but the critical difference lies in truthful communication. I make it a regular practice to check in with my students at the beginning of each class session: we go around the circle and are honest about the energy—physical, emotional, or mental—we are bringing to the day's work. As Davis-Floyd notes, energy is at the heart of holism because the body is viewed as an energy system in constant interaction with the other energy fields around it (Davis-Floyd 2018a: 28–31). In the holistic classroom, this is primary and essential. The first time we do this check-in, I let students know that it is critical to speak from the heart, not the head, as the latter can lead to lengthy and tedious processing. I once considered check-in to be extraneous to the day's work, but I have learned that without it, students will track each other emotionally and become distracted by what they discern that has not been named. Bringing the truth into the open each time we meet has more than proven itself in the way students are able to fully focus on their studies and get things done (Davis 2017a).

One of my favorite examples to help differentiate humanistic from holistic care is with the challenge of nutritional counseling. A humanistic practitioner may be full of ideas on what the client should eat, perhaps with handouts or other resources offered regardless of the client's interest or participation. In contrast, the holistic practitioner deliberately avoids giving advice, instead asking the client what she likes to eat, how she feels eating as she does, if there are any foods she is craving or denying herself, and, if so, what obstacles stand in the way. Holistic practitioners do not deny their expertise; for example, they may note a protein deficiency in a diet, but rather than make recommendations will ask the client about their favorite protein foods and which ones they would most like to increase. The psychological impact of this kind of care is subtle but significant: the client is put in charge of defining and improving their own health status, and the practitioner is freed of emotional and mental entanglements that could result from a client's dependence. This is particularly important for midwives, who must be ready for their next birth while leaving their last client on firm footing (Davis 2016, 2019).

For another, more personal example: imagine that you, as a holistic practitioner, are about to see a client just after a horrible argument with your partner or a very difficult birth with an upsetting outcome. Working in transparency, you expect your client to notice changes in your mood or affect, and, bottom line, you *want* her to notice, as that is your commitment to each other. In humanism, you might try to hide how you are feeling because you believe that you should put yourself aside, but in holism, it is unethical to do so. You certainly shouldn't "dump" on your client, but a simple acknowledgment of your situation, without processing, will do the trick and put your visit on the right track, as long as you reassure her that you are glad to see her and are looking forward to your time together.

In my experience, a great many midwives at this time are walking the line between humanism and holism; those caught up in humanism are far more likely to burn out or cop out on their professional values and personal care, whereas those stepping into holism are discovering rewards of increased energy and resilience, greater self-determination, and healthier relationships in general. Holistic practitioners understand that they must take care of themselves first in order to be able to fully care for their clients. In short, these are the midwives who can advocate for autonomous midwifery practice, promote their clients' agency, and ultimately seed sustainability for their work within society (Davis 2017b).

2.3 Practicing Holistic Midwifery Care

There are three ways to practice midwifery holistically, each with advantages and disadvantages:

(1) One-on-one midwifery, in which a client hires a midwife who promises to be there for her 24/7. Sometimes that midwife has a partner who will also get to know the client and may also come to the birth. This model ensures total continuity of care and care provider but can be hard on the midwives who practice it, as they are almost always on call and often miss important family events like birthday parties and graduations. A partial solution to this dilemma has been found in larger collective practices. For example, the San Francisco Bay Area Homebirth Collective, comprised of anywhere from 10 to 20 private practices at any given time, not only provides a pool of midwives to choose from for reasonably priced and highly skilled assistance at every birth, but also emergency backup should the chosen midwife have a critical personal engagement, family crisis, or serious illness. Most one-on-one midwives are community midwives attending births outside of hospitals.

(2) Caseload midwifery, in which a group of midwives form a practice, and each of them gets to know every client, promising that at least one member of the group will be there for the birth. This model provides continuity of care but not of care provider, so there is not as much intimacy in relationship, and the midwife who attends the birth may not be the one with whom the client is most deeply bonded. Caseload midwives may work inside or outside of hospitals, and they take turns being on call.

(3) Shift midwifery, in which midwives are hospital or birth center employees who work on shift for a certain number of hours and then are replaced by another midwife when their shift ends. This model provides no continuity of care provider for the woman, who may be in the middle of pushing when her midwife suddenly leaves because her shift is over. When a new, unknown midwife enters the room, this immediately changes the atmosphere and energy field—termed the *psychosphere* by holistic OB Ricardo Jones (2009). However, shift midwifery enables midwives to establish a known schedule, which can be helpful if they are raising small children or must deal with a personal crisis or emergency.

Independent midwives working out of hospital with private clients often find holistic practice quite attainable. Continuity of care makes holistic practice so much easier to realize. Midwives working on a caseload basis in hospitals can still find creative ways to incorporate components of holistic care, although hospital protocols may present obstacles. Midwives working on shift rather than caseload are at a decided disadvantage because a lack of communication during shift exchanges can make a holistic overview of their client's health status difficult if not impossible to provide. Even if a shift midwife is practicing holistic care, she cannot guarantee that the midwife replacing her will practice in this model, leaving the client potentially exposed to technocratic or fragmented care.

It bears mentioning that where midwifery has long been mainstreamed—for example, in the Netherlands—midwives find it difficult to limit the number of clients they take on, resulting in caseloads of two to three times what home birth midwives in the United States will accept and making the possibility of finding the time or energy to work with clients holistically very challenging. To earn their full salaries, Dutch midwives are expected to attend around 90–100 births per year, not to mention all the prenatal and postpartum home checks they must perform (Cheney et al. 2019). This figure averages out to around eight births per month, but because births may cluster, a Dutch midwife might find herself attending far more than that in any given month. On the other hand, most US community midwives consider 2–5 births a month to be quite sufficient and would be horrified at the thought of attending 8 or more births a month, precisely because they intend to provide the most holistic care possible.

And although every woman has access to a midwife in Germany and Norway, she will have different ones for her prenatal care and birth attendance. This fragmentation of the midwife's traditional scope of practice—care "from womb to tomb"—reflects the wider repression of female healers in which doctors have usurped midwives as primary care providers for both pregnant and nonpregnant clients, including those in menopause. Again, this situation points to midwives' need to strategize regarding ways to reclaim full scope practice, at least with regard to childbirth: a practice that reflects midwifery standards and core skills as addressed below.

Practical details of giving holistic care are numerous, but the core values of transparency, honesty, and integrity set the stage. Perhaps one of the most effective techniques for realizing holism in almost any practice situation is what I call "The Scale of 1 to 10." For example, when your client comes for a prenatal visit and you ask how she is doing, she reports feeling stressed. Rather than offer advice on relaxation, diet, or adequate sleep, you ask her to rate her stress on a scale from one to ten, with ten being the highest stress level. When she replies, "8," you ask, "What would it take to bring it down to 1 or 2?" She might respond, "A week on the beach in Hawaii, but that's impossible." Go further on this, and ask her, "Is there anything else that gives you that beach-in-Hawaii feeling?" She might respond that she could use a massage, or that she wants a long private bath, or that she needs a day off from the kids: the important thing is that *she is articulating her own health status and doing her own problem-solving*, which is key to her autonomy and self-realization. This also keeps her from becoming overly dependent on you, allowing you to care for your next client without lingering emotional entanglement (Davis 2017b, 2019).

Besides stress levels, other indicators of well-being can be ranked on a scale of 1 to 10, with 10 being the most desirable:

- Vitality
- Security
- Happiness
- Sexual satisfaction
- Nourishment
- Personal fulfillment

Note that when utilizing this process, it is critical to trust the first number that pops up and not overthink it. Not only can clients use this process but providers can too, as a means of self-assessment when they feel troubled or unwell and as a means of assessing what they observe in a client. Yet another benefit is that it can be used in situations outside continuity of care; for example, when meeting a client for the first time during her labor and she reports being afraid, tired, or stressed, she can do the rating and problem-solving on the spot. This tool works best when the provider is truly open to listening. Early in their instruction, I have my students practice listening to each other, first using just their mental faculties and then, while engaging all their senses, listening with an open heart. What a difference this makes in their ability to receive information!

Still, providing holistic care is not without its pitfalls. Here are some of the risks and challenges:

- Lack of privacy, "nowhere to hide"
- Increased need for self-nurture by aligning lifestyle with practice reality and maintaining optimal health on an ongoing basis
- Burnout from lack of nourishment, support, resources (for which self-care can be both antidote and treatment)

2.4   Holistic Care: Oxytocin, Theta, and Trauma

At the time of birth, physiology renders opportunities that are unacknowledged in technocratic care. Oxytocin, also known as the "love hormone" because it is released with sexual activity, orgasm, and arousal apart from physical contact, reaches levels many times higher during labor than at any other time in the female life cycle. Oxytocin is responsible for uterine contractions, and it peaks at the moment of birth—nature's design for separating the placenta efficiently with minimal blood loss. Both the mother's and the baby's oxytocin levels are high at this moment, so that both are emotionally and physically primed for bonding and falling in love.

However, there is a downside to this physiology. Increasing oxytocin levels during labor correlate to changes in brain activity, which, in addition to promoting deep relaxation and bonding, may also trigger any history of trauma. This is particularly true for mothers experiencing uninterrupted birth with no artificial hormone augmentation or pain relief: their brain waves will reach the theta frequency—a mental state correlated to forming or reliving strong positive or negative associations neurologically (Davis E, Pascali-Bonaro D 2010, Davis 2019). To better

Four Categories of Brain Wave Patterns	
beta (14–100 Hz)	Concentration, arousal, alertness, cognition Higher levels associated with anxiety, dis-ease, feelings of separation, fight or flight
alpha (8–13.9 Hz)	Relaxation, superlearning, relaxed focus, light trance Increased serontonin production Pre-sleep or pre-waking drowsiness Mediation, beginning of access to unconscious mind
theta (4–7.9 Hz)	Dreaming sleep (REM sleep) Increased production of catecholamines (vital for learning and memory), increased creativity Integrative, emotional experiences, potential change in behavior, increased retention of learned material Hypnagogic imagery, trance, deep mediation, access to unconscious mind
delta (.1–3.9 Hz)	Dreamless sleep Human growth hormone released Deep, trance-like, non-physical state, loss of body awareness

Fig. 2.1 Four categories of brain wave patterns. (Open source)

understand how/why brain wave changes correlated to labor may cause memories of trauma to arise, please see Fig. 2.1.

To better understand the link between trauma and theta, consider the fight/flight/ freeze response. A person in mortal danger will first release huge amounts of adrenaline and cortisol (correlated to the beta frequency) to help them either flee or fight back, but if they feel they can't save themselves, they freeze or collapse via a dorsal dive response that is correlated to the theta frequency (Van der Kolk 2014). In short, we neurologically encode trauma in the theta frequency but may have no conscious recollection of it until we reach that frequency again. This is why rape survivors sometimes experience flashbacks of their trauma during labor (Halvorsen et al. 2013). The implications of this deep neurological encoding point the way to effective trauma therapy, as it is increasingly understood that to get at the roots of trauma, we need to replicate the brain wave state wherein it is lodged, using body-based therapies such as EMDR, hypnotherapy, and so forth (Davis E, Pascali-Bonaro D 2010;

Van der Kolk 2014). Talk therapy, which occurs primarily in beta frequency, doesn't go deep enough to facilitate release and healing.

This explains why upholding the tenets of holism can be particularly challenging when assisting at births. In this model of care, clinical detachment is an illusion, as the energy fields of the client and the care provider are merged. For both the birthing person and the care provider, the choice may not be simple, but it is clear: to participate with the energy of oxytocin (love) or with the energy of adrenaline (fear). There is no in-between, because oxytocin and adrenaline *oppose* one another. Anything that causes adrenaline's release—the disruption of privacy, the feeling of being observed, bright lights, or extraneous conversation—leads to decreased oxytocin levels and impaired progress in labor. And herein lies the pitfall for the provider who engages with a laboring person's hormonal lead: their own traumatic memories may be activated by the mother's theta frequency. It is no wonder technocratic practitioners hold so tightly to the clinical detachment model.

However, technocratic providers determined to stay "objective" may find detachment impossible to maintain, which can lead to unconscious acting out or irresponsible and disconnected practice. In other words, when complications of labor or birth arise requiring full attention and participation, technocratic providers may fall short. I recall a hospital birth with a shoulder dystocia, one of the most challenging, life-threatening complications for a baby that demands an immediate and effective response (Davis 2019). My colleague, a physician I knew well and respected as highly skilled, lost control and began to do things that no medical textbook would advise, and I literally had to push his hands away to complete the birth safely. Later, he was humble enough to admit that he had acted irresponsibly. Sadly, this is not an isolated instance; I have seen similar occurrences in a number of hospital births. The point here is not to place blame but rather to illustrate the deficiencies of the technocratic model of care in disallowing the connection and presence whereby instinct and intelligence unite.

It is also critical to realize that spontaneous birth rarely progresses at a steady pace in the way that institutional models of birth would suggest (Davis E, Pascali-Bonaro D 2010, Davis 2019). Instead, there are major turning points during labor when birthing persons tend to plateau—typically at 4 cm, 8 cm, and the crowning phase—that present new emotional and physical challenges. Distinct from the pathological arrests of obstructed labor, these thresholds enable women to process fears and previous traumas either consciously or unconsciously, with great long-term psychological benefits. Holistic midwifery really shines at these junctures, because the midwife and client have established a depth of communication and trust that can facilitate free expression of whatever the client is feeling. When a midwife is able to be present to the mother's theta state, the mother can heal her own traumas. In other words, sex-positive and body-positive midwifery can heal all manner of previous traumatic events (Davis E, Pascali-Bonaro D 2010, Davis 2018).

Robbie Davis-Floyd recounts that during her second labor, she was terrified of repeating the unnecessary cesarean she experienced with her first birth, when she was diagnosed with "failure to progress" after 26 h of labor. This was a misdiagnosis, as she never got past 4 cm and was still in the latent phase, which can last for hours or days—in other words, she was not in active labor. The resultant cesarean was deeply traumatic, but she was able to heal during her second labor. At exactly 26 h, and still at 4 cm, she and her attendants made a circle with candles, and everyone present voiced their fears and symbolically threw them into the candle flames. Robbie's contractions then stopped for some hours, during which she slept. Soon after she woke, active labor began, and before long, trauma-free, Robbie joyfully birthed a healthy 10 lb. baby boy.

Even if trauma is not an issue for client or midwife, note that if both are in theta frequency, the midwife will bond with the client and vice versa. Midwives owe it to their clients to disclose how this bonding may impact the client's ability to be critical of their care. Time and again, I have asked groups of midwives at conferences how many had midwifery care for their own births, and most of the audience responds affirmatively. Then, I ask how many in the audience were in some way dissatisfied or disempowered by their care—and, surprisingly, many raise their hands again. But when I enquire further as to how many have shared this information with their midwife, only a few hands go up. To me, this shows failure in our mission: no more walking wounded mothers who have not had timely opportunity to process their births! Midwives need to explain the physiology of birth to every client: the oxytocin-induced bonding, the emergence of unprocessed trauma, and the potential for healing that these moments of labor afford. They also need to give clients ample and repeated opportunities postpartum—on day 1, day 3, day 10, and at the 6-week visit, all of which are turning points physiologically and socially for many mothers—to verbalize ways that they were dissatisfied with their care, so that these negative experiences are not embedded as traumas but may be released in fruitful dialogue and/or body-based healing techniques (Davis 2019).

Ideally, I think midwives should tell their clients about the physiology of labor and bonding *in late pregnancy,* as the afterglow of birth and challenges of early parenting can override, at least for a time, any dissatisfactions they may have regarding their care and so impede honest disclosure of less than positive feelings. I must emphasize again how critical this disclosure is, both to the client's ability to move forward to the next phase of life and to the midwife's continual improvement of her practice.

2.5 Holistic Midwifery: A Case Study

Finally, let us to return to the theme of autonomous midwifery practice and examine how our model of care is consistently unrepresented in perinatal standards of practice. To this end, I will share an account of a young woman, a member of my community I had known for several years, having her first baby. Intelligent, self-determined, and well informed, she chose to birth at home unassisted by any practitioner—often known as "freebirth." Not surprisingly, others in my community told me I must "do something" to change her mind. I refused to take that role, as I believed that trying to talk her out of it would only alienate her from any further communication we might have. Around 18 weeks by her calculations, she contacted me to ask if I could see her to make sure her dates were correct. She hoped they were, as then the date of conception would correlate to a particularly powerful love-making experience with her partner. Using one of the midwife's tricks of the trade, I planned to see her in two more weeks, knowing that at 20 weeks, the uterus, regardless of fetal size, is at the umbilicus and round, whereas uterine size at 16 or 24 weeks is markedly less or more (Davis 2017b, 2019). And indeed, she was exactly at 20 weeks.

I didn't hear from her again until around 32 weeks, when she asked if I would see her to determine if the baby was head down and growing normally. It was, and I showed her how to palpate the baby's head and how to track normal fetal activity, as well as gave her a few tips on nutrition and hydration. Weeks went by, as well as her due date, and she contacted me again at 42 weeks, asking if there was anything she should do to get labor going. We went over the options, the means of both natural and hospital induction, and she declared that she would wait. I asked her a few critical questions, improvised in the moment to be most essential to determining her baby's well-being and her readiness to labor:

1. *Is the baby moving as much as before?* (With her positive response, I reminded her how to count fetal movements for an hour each day right after a meal).
2. *Does your uterus feel squishy, like the baby has plenty of fluid to move around in, not tightly compacted?* (She said yes, and I reminded her to drink at least two quarts of water per day to maintain amniotic fluid volume).
3. *Are you and your partner feeling loving and being intimate together?* (Again yes, and I told her to keep it up).

What was my rationale for each of these questions? For the first, in routine post-dates screening, normal fetal movements (8–10 per hour after mother has a meal) are considered indicative of normal muscle tone and breathing movements and also indicate a normal fetal heart rate, which I would be checking for if she were my client. For the second question, I know that reduced amniotic fluid volume is the most significant indicator of fetal dysmaturity syndrome; if amniotic fluid decreases, the umbilical cord is likely to be compressed, which can lead to growth restriction, periods of hypoxia, or, in rare cases, fetal demise (Eden et al. 1987). I also know that research has proven adequate hydration to be critical to normal amniotic fluid volume (Borges et al. 2011). For the third question, labor is initiated by oxytocin, which is also released with sexual activity, and if the mother is partnered with a male, prostaglandins present in seminal fluid soften the cervix to prepare it for dilating (Davis 2019).

She went to 42.5 weeks, 43 weeks, and 44 weeks and at 44.5 weeks successfully gave birth at home assisted only by her partner. I couldn't wait to see a picture of the baby—would this be the wizened, growth-restricted dysmature baby I had seen in obstetrical textbooks? But no—here was a pink, plump, just-term baby! And then she confided, "Well, my mom had me at 43 weeks, my aunties gave birth late, so I figured this was normal for my family."

It is not my argument that this woman would not have benefited from midwifery care—and in fact, I did my best to offer core elements of holistic care to help her determine what was best for her and her baby. But in California and other states, midwives are forbidden to assist clients past 42 weeks, mandated to refer them for induction. Induction is correlated to increased cesarean rates (Oxorn and Foote 1986), and cesarean birth carries its share of long-term complications such as placenta accreta due to uterine scarring, correlated to severe postpartum hemorrhage and possible hysterectomy (Gaskin 2003; Childbirth Connection 2006; Davis 2019). The rationale for routine postdates induction is based on insubstantial and flawed studies claiming to show an increased rate of stillbirth for postdates pregnancies, yet the problem is that methods of evaluation and diagnosis in the technocratic model of care are inadequate to determine normal amniotic fluid volume and continued fetal growth. Technocratic practitioners rely on ultrasound, which is notoriously inaccurate at evaluating amniotic fluid levels or gestational age. Consequently, there has been an alarming rise in prematurity rates correlated to induction for what are assumed to be postdates pregnancies but in fact are not (McGuire 2012).

I share this birth account to illustrate the difference between the orientation, assessment skills, and health status evaluations of holistic midwifery care and those of the technocratic model. Perhaps my premise in the opening paragraph—that midwifery must formally articulate not only its model of care but also its unique practice guidelines—may now be better understood. Our Hippocratic mandate as care providers is to "do no harm," and in holistic midwifery care, we take this mandate as seriously as we would expect it to be taken by our own caregivers. *But we can only practice holistically if we practice autonomously, no longer servants to technocratic practitioners or their model of care.*

Achieving professional autonomy will require political action, public education, and deep resolve, yet it is crucial to realizing a midwifery model of able to protect normal, healthy birth, which in turn supports the growth of healthy families. As I often remind my students, the practice of midwifery is not just about being at births or catching babies, it's about reshaping the priorities of society so that families come first. This has always been midwifery's mission, and as our societies shift to establish global priorities, never has our mission been more timely.

References

Borges V, Rososchansky J, al AF (2011) Effect of maternal hydration on increase of amniotic fluid index. Braz J Med Biol Res 44(3):263–266

Cheney M et al (2019) Giving birth in the United States and the Netherlands: midwifery care as integrated option or contested privilege? In: Davis-Floyd R, Cheyney M (eds) Birth in eight cultures. Waveland, Long Grove, pp 165–202

Cheyney M, Davis-Floyd R (in press) Birth and the big bad wolf: the biocultural evolution of human childbirth, parts 1 and 2. Int J Child

Childbirth Connection (2006) What every pregnant woman should know about cesarean section, 2nd ed. Childbirth Connection, New York. http://childbirthconnection.org

Davis E (2010) Midwifery education: trauma or transformation? Midwifery Today 96:40–41

Davis E (2016) The enduring qualities in midwifery. Midwifery Today 117:41–42

Davis E (2017a) Midwifery education for autonomous practice: the time is now! Midwifery Today 123:8–10

Davis E (2017b) Prenatal care: what really matters! Midwifery Today 124:8–10

Davis E (2018) Plateaus in labor and our sexual nature. Midwifery Today 126:14–16

Davis E (2019) Heart & hands: a midwife's guide to pregnancy & birth, 5th edn. Ten Speed Press, Berkeley

Davis E, Pascali-Bonaro B (2010) Orgasmic birth: your guide to a safe, satisfying, and pleasurable birth experience. Rodale Press, Pennsylvania

Davis-Floyd R (2001) The technocratic, humanistic, and holistic paradigms of childbirth. Int J Gynecol Obstet 75(Suppl 1):S5–S23

Davis-Floyd R (2018a) The technocratic, humanistic, and holistic paradigms of birth and health care. In: Davis-Floyd R, Colleagues (eds) Ways of knowing about birth: mothers, midwives, medicine, and birth activism. Waveland, Long Grove, pp 3–44

Davis-Floyd R (2018b) American midwifery: a brief anthropological overview. In: Davis-Floyd R, Colleagues (eds) Ways of knowing about birth: mothers, midwives, medicine, and birth activism. Waveland, Long Grove, pp 165–188

Davis-Floyd R, Faber M, DeVries R (2013) An update on the Netherlands. Midwifery Today 105:54–59

Eden RD, Seifert LS, Winegar A et al (1987) Perinatal characteristics of uncomplicated postdates pregnancies. Obstet Gynecol 69:296

Gaskin IM (2003) Ina May's guide to childbirth. Bantam Dell, New York

Halvorsen L et al (2013) Giving birth with rape in one's past: a qualitative study. Birth 40(3):182–191

Henrich K, Sprenger J (1972) Excerpts from the Malleus Malificarum, part 1, question XI. In: Kors AC, Peters E (eds) Witchcraft in Europe, 1100–1700: a documentary history. University of Pennsylvania Press, Philadelphia

Jones R (2009) Teamwork: an obstetrician, a midwife, and a doula in Brazil. In: Davis-Floyd R, Barclay L, Daviss B-A et al (eds) Birth models that work. University of California Press, Berkeley, pp 271–304

Martin JA, Hamilton BE, Osterman MJ et al (2018) Births: final data for 2018. Natl Vital Stat Rep 28(13) https://www.cdc.gov/nchs/data/nvsr/nvsr68/nvsr68_13-508.pdf

McGuire M (2012) September is national infant mortality awareness month. Michael McGuire's Blog, August 31

Oxorn H, Foote WR (1986) Human labor & birth, 5th edn. Appleton & Lange, Norwalk

Trevathan W (1987) Human birth: an evolutionary perspective. Aldine de Gruyter, New York

Van der Kolk B (2014) The body keeps the score: brain, mind, and body in the healing of trauma. Penguin Books, New York

WHO (2015) Trends in maternal mortality: estimates by the WHO, UNICEF, UNFPA, World Bank Group, and the United Nations Population Division. WHO Publications, Geneva

Chapter 3
Bringing Back Breech by Reframing the Language of Risk

Betty-Anne Daviss, Anita Hedditch, Vijaya Krishnan, and Helen Dresner Barnes

3.1 Introduction: The Language of Risk vs. the Language of Rights[1]

The language of risk has historic and modern commonalities in arenas as disparate as seafaring and childbirth. Alaszewski and Burgess (2007: 349) explain that risk perceptions in challenging areas of decision-making like these have collectively taken an unintentional turn in society:

> The initial conceptualization of risk…was based on the use of knowledge from past events to provide the context for choices which minimize harm in the future. … In the late twentieth century a more precautionary approach has emerged, in which the fear of future [harm] is given precedence over evidence or lack of evidence of past harm. The precautionary

---

[1] Daviss wrote Sects. 3.1, 3.2, 3.3 and described the birth models at hospitals in Ottawa, Atlanta, Aabenraa, and Frankfurt. Hedditch, Krishnan, and Dresner Barnes described the birth models in the UK and India as noted in the text and contributed and agreed to the interpretations and analysis expressed in the rest of the chapter.

B.-A. Daviss
The Pauline Jewett Institute of Women's and Gender Studies, Carleton University, Ottawa, ON, Canada
e-mail: bettyannedaviss@gmail.com

A. Hedditch
Oxford Radcliffe Hospitals NHS Foundation Trust, Oxford, UK
e-mail: Anita.hedditch@ouh.nhs.uk

V. Krishnan
Director Healthy Mother Wellness & Care, The Sanctum, Natural Birth Center, Hyderabad, India
e-mail: hm@healthy-mother.com

H. Dresner Barnes (✉)
University of Bradford, West Yorkshire, UK
e-mail: H.Dresner-Barnes@bradford.ac.uk

© Springer Nature Switzerland AG 2021
K. Gutschow et al. (eds.), *Sustainable Birth in Disruptive Times*, Global Maternal and Child Health, https://doi.org/10.1007/978-3-030-54775-2_3

approach is future oriented and casts the future principally in negative, potentially catastrophic terms.

Heyman (2010: 24) concurs and argues that, in healthcare, the language of risk is
shortsighted because it provides only one approach to look at "future alternatives,"
predominantly worst-case scenarios, and "once their presence has been recognized
by a social group, contingencies generate substantive responses." The presence of
risk with breech birth has been recognized and amplified by obstetricians, a social
group that generates substantial control over birth in individual nations so that their
chosen response to risk often becomes the standard of care.

True to Alaszewski and Burgess' timeline, prior to 2000, although obstetricians
were still doing breech births in Western medical hospitals, their comfort was wan-
ing (Daviss et al. 2010; Daviss and Bisits 2021). Although our legislated scope of
practice as midwives across all provinces in Canada except Quebec included vaginal breech deliveries, few hospitals actually permitted midwives to do them. I was
only able to persuade the obstetricians in my hospital in the 1990s that I could manage breeches because of my experience gained internationally. The obstetricians on
call usually wanted to be in the room; it appeared they tolerated me, some less enthu-
siasm than others.

The Term Breech Trial (Hannah et al. 2000) was pivotal in diminishing that tol-
eration in most centers around the world, for obstetricians and midwives alike, especially if the teams were involved in the study (Hogle et al. 2003). Its initial (later
adjusted) findings suggested that the neonate presenting breech was at considerable
increased risk if the mother had a vaginal birth instead of a cesarean. As a result,
obstetricians at most hospitals in the West stopped offering vaginal breeches,
although some pockets in Europe doing their own research on innovative protocols
continued to perform them (Daviss et al. 2010).

Then the follow-up to the Term Breech Trial (TBT) demonstrated that cesarean
birth for breech "is *not* associated with a reduction in risk of death or neurodevelopmental delay in children at two years of age" (Whyte et al. 2004, emphasis
mine). This qualification was important because vaginal breech babies tend to have
low APGARs and other negative sequela at birth, yet the follow-up showed that
those effects are not long-lasting. Subsequently national guidelines in Britain,
Canada, and the USA began to support vaginal breech birth again, based on maternal choice and careful selection (Tsakiridis et al. 2019).

Subsequent research also supported the view that vaginal breech birth is not only
safe but better practice than cesarean section (CS), especially given the risks of CS
to the mother (Goffinet et al. 2006; Deneux-Tharaux et al. 2006; Verhoeven et al.
2005). Yet the focus on the potential catastrophic event remains difficult to break. In
2006, with the support of the Vice Executive President of the Society of Obstetricians
and Gynaecologists of Canada (SOGC), Andre Lalonde, I carried out a survey to see
how the Canadian hospitals with 3000 or more deliveries were affected by the Term
Breech Trial and compared the results with the period after the more reassuring
follow-up was published. These results speak to the reticence to return to a practice
once it is classified as "high risk":

When the findings from the Term Breech Trial suggested that a policy of Caesarean section for breech delivery decreased the risk for the neonate, Canadian institutions were almost five times more likely to adopt such a policy than they were to reintroduce the option of vaginal breech delivery when the difference between the two modes of delivery was *rendered insignificant* by the same group of investigators. (Daviss et al. 2010; italics mine)

In short, with a focus on neonatal risk, some obstetric providers in Canada followed research when it *increases* intervention but ignored the research that recommends *decreasing* intervention. Even when governing obstetric societies review the literature and acknowledge that a positive outcome is most likely with a vaginal breech delivery by a skilled provider, some providers practicing on the ground focus on the level of neonatal risk and, because they feel lack of support from peers or governing and disciplinary bodies, become unwilling to perform vaginal deliveries, regardless of their skill (Leeman 2020). Rather than some providers being encouraged by all the positive findings in new research, the language of risk has increased. It was not until 2012 that I first heard graphic language like the following, stated to a mother in the middle of labor with a planned vaginal breech birth:

Your baby's head can get stuck, the baby could develop cerebral palsy, and we might have to decapitate.[2]

I thought this was an isolated event but soon found out from our breech clients, who are required to have an obstetric consultation, that this line was being used to obtain informed consent at two of the hospitals in my hometown. The consumer groups and midwives have been working hard to request more balanced language and a more balanced approach. Analyzing the breech situation in sociological terms, applying Heyman's concept of "future alternatives" (2010: 14), we could see that some providers were using unprecedented language to influence how women may regard their imagined personal futures. It demonstrates in these times of risk aversion in obstetrics (Ballantyne et al. 2016), how the management of breech delivery has become a litmus test around which providers and hospital administrators make decisions based on a medical perception of risk rather than evidence-based analysis of outcomes or childbearers' rights.

Most hospitals in North America have not returned to offering vaginal breech delivery, and only a paucity of European and UK teams do (Daviss et al. 2010; Leeman 2020). Hospitals that do offer vaginal breech deliveries rely on a provider comfortable with breech being on call, and that may only be a rare possibility in many hospitals. This creates a highly emotional situation for a childbearer, who may not know until they go into labor whether or not they will be permitted to have a vaginal birth or will be asked to endure a major operation. Even when advised to offer vaginal breech by their obstetric societies (i.e., RCOG or SOGC), staff may

---

[2] I have never seen in the medical literature over the last century a report of a practitioner intentionally doing this. I know it has happened as a rare, *accidental* process, but only in preterm breech babies born at 33 weeks or less, usually after PROM (premature rupture of the membranes), when the mothers were not necessarily fully dilated and delivered the baby in the lithotomy position. If under duress, physicians have generally pushed the baby back up rather than decapitate.

promote a deadline for scheduling a cesarean, which is not done routinely with a cephalic presentation. In my experience, women have been made to feel uncooperative and noncompliant if they hesitate or refuse, when the day of their scheduled cesarean at 39 or 40 weeks arrives.

This chapter provides a comprehensive list of the elements that are needed in sites where successful, sustainable models of breech birth have been developed. We also present some examples of sites where providers have managed to collaborate to take a broader view not focused on catastrophic risk by deploying some or all of these elements.

3.2 Regenerating Focus on the Normal in Breech Birth

In 1997, I proposed that practitioners take a departure from the language of medical/clinical "risk" and explore instead start to understand the language of the different types of "logic" that childbearers use for their decision-making. I developed an analytical framework that laid out eight types of logic competing for attention among both practitioners and clients in any community: clinical, scientific, personal, intuitive, political, legal, and economic logic (Daviss 1997: 443).

Using this alternative language, and working with midwives in Quebec and Ontario while we obtained midwifery recognition and legislation, I could not sit back and watch our clients continue to be denied vaginal breech when the literature emerged showing the safety of vaginal breech delivery. I traveled to Paris, Dublin, Bergen, and Frankfurt to study protocols and observe breech deliveries, with the express intention of bringing best practices back to Canada (Daviss and Bisits 2021). Although I had never needed forceps for a breech, I approached my college about getting privileges and training to use forceps so that I could be permitted hospital privileges to deliver breeches.

When I made it to Frankfurt, I learned that forceps were not needed for breech. I could relate better to the Frankfurt model than any other I saw across Europe because Frank Louwen was doing births the way I had first learned from traditional midwives in Guatemala and Mexico back in the 1970s—in an upright position or on all fours. Knowing that obstetricians in my city would never heed a traditional midwifery method, I persuaded Andre Lalonde, then president of the Society of Obstetricians and Gynaecologists of Canada (SOGC), to bring Frank Louwen from Frankfurt to speak in Canada at the meeting where the new SOGC protocols on permitting vaginal breech birth were going to be launched. You could hear a pin drop in the room when Frank showed his videos to over 400 obstetricians in Halifax in June 2009. Yet there was no change in practice in Canada, except in Ottawa later that year.

Breech birth, like all birth, is governed by risk perception, societal norms, and patient and provider preferences. To change birth, one needs plausibility, acceptability, desirability, and comfortability (Daviss et al. 2010) in any given jurisdiction. The other important ingredient: a strong group of demanding women. The latter is required because otherwise by default, it is usually provider preference that governs whether a change is made, and our experience as midwives is that the status quo is not challenged unless it is forced by consumer demand. It was the women who had unnecessary cesareans for breech who largely planned and organized the conferences on breech, and those two conferences marked a new direction.[3] Focus on the risk of vaginal versus cesarean breech birth was replaced by rethinking the physiology of vaginal breech birth and teaching it in another way: in upright, all fours positions, squatting, sitting on a birth stool, kneeling, or even standing—as opposed to the way it has been done for centuries by obstetrics, on the back. Since these first two conferences, the positions of crouching rather than being supine (Reitter et al. 2014) and squatting compared to standing (Hemmerich et al. 2019) have been demonstrated to provide a wider pelvic opening that facilitates breech delivery.[4]

Since the consumer-driven North American conferences, international conferences on breech have concentrated exclusively on the development of this "new" physiology and positioning of breech birth in Sydney (2012), Sheffield (2014 and 2017), Amsterdam (2016), and Denmark (2018 and 2019). Breech research has also taken a regenerative turn from contrasting vaginal with cesarean modes of management toward the intricacies of how to provide vaginal birth with these new modes of delivery (Borbolla Foster et al. 2014; Bogner et al. 2015; Louwen et al. 2017). As popular as the new research[5] and conferences have been, trying to find sustainable models for breech has still proven difficult because there has been a repetitive pattern since the upright breech conferences started:

- An obstetric provider or midwife, or group, goes to an exciting conference on breech in upright positions.
- The providers return to their communities and continue to provide care for breech if they were already doing it, with some new ideas. Or, for the first time, they become brave enough to change the paradigm and offer upright breech.
- Conservative elements that don't think vaginal breech birth should be offered at all, let alone on all fours, raise their eyebrows. One obstetrician calls this group "the misery brigade."
- A few low APGARs occur, typical of breeches, but shown not to have long-term consequences (Whyte et al. 2004). The babies need resuscitation, and pediatrics starts to complain.
- A serious morbidity occurs—forceps damage, lengthy stay in the NICU, or even a baby death.

---

[3] I acted primarily as the scientific coordinator, choosing and bringing in the speakers.

[4] In our article about the Frankfurt data, to adhere to word length, we suggested that "upright" would include hands and knees, although we know it is not exactly upright, as when you are squatting.

[5] Our article on the Frankfurt data (Louwen et al. 2017) was the most accessed article in the *International Journal of Obstetrics and Gynecology* in 2017 and in the top 5% of all research outputs ever tracked by Altmetric.

• When an event occurs that produces conflict, regardless of whether or not there is a bad outcome, the participating hospital has two choices: (1) deal with the conflicts among the staff, investigate, and then continue on a better path with honesty and better communication or (2) close down the breech program.

Closing down a vaginal breech program is the easier choice for hospitals that follow risk averse paths, but it is not the solution. With the support of the SOGC, I invited Drs. Louwen and Anke Reitter from Frankfurt, Dr. Marek Glezerman from Israel, homebirth obstetrician Stuart Fischbein from California, Andrew Bisits from Australia, Savas Menticoglou (coauthor of the SOGC guidelines) from Winnipeg, Jane Evans from Britian, and Andre Lalonde to the breech conference in 2009 in Ottawa. Although obstetricians across Ottawa seemed to be boycotting our conference, I brought several of the same speakers to rounds at our French l'Hôpital Montfort. This became the catalyst for a model of breech delivery where midwives lead, which falls into the first category that we present in 3.4 below.

3.3 Three Themes, Three Proven Elements, and Three Categories of Sustainable Breech Birth Models

In all the places I have worked in the past 45 years—the 14 hospitals in my own area, other North American hospitals where I have attended breech births, high- and low-resource countries where I have worked and/or taught—I find that the sites that work best for childbearers focus are principled around three themes: *honesty, instinct, and diplomacy.* The focus on honesty requires providers to be honest about their skills or lack thereof and to sacrifice their image or comfort to protect childbearers and newborns. The instinct to protect normal birth and childbearers may need to trump the wish to be compliant with obstetric norms that are not keeping up with new findings. Finally, providers require infinite diplomacy in withstanding and mitigating inevitable conflicts among staff or with disciplinary bodies when difficult situations arise. In the process of applying these three themes and the three elements of sustainable models described below, a formula for success developed that increasingly resonated with the authors as they described their own experience in the chapter. They have edited and dubbed this formula "the Daviss model."

3.3.1 Three Proven Elements of Sustainable Breech Delivery Models

• First, final decisions are made by those who will be most affected by them—*the childbearers.*
• Second, providers who attend breeches cultivate:

- Honesty about their level of experience and those of their colleagues with patients/clients and each other
- Mastery over the best techniques
- An instinct to protect the childbearer, the baby, and normal birth
- An understanding that the client needs autonomy in spite of hospital rules
- An awareness of the limitations of protocols and the need for flexibility
- An ability to live with uncertainty understanding the research conflicts and limitations
- An ability to express confidence to clients and persuade colleagues
- A capacity to withstand marginalization, bullying, and harassment
- An ability to mitigate fear: fear of colleagues, fear of being sued, fear of birth
- Permissions to explore new ideas, let go of prejudices, and change
- Desire to learn and share skills with international colleagues

- Third, administrators (including lead or heads of departments) are:

  - Engaged in processing conflict resolution and in limiting jealousies and competition both inter- and intra-professionally so that a progressive infrastructure and program can facilitate change
  - Able to recognize and accommodate the breech experience of midwives
  - Willing to enforce communication (such as debriefs after every breech birth), recognizing that breech is an emotional issue
  - Able to give up on prediction and control while facing unfolding realities
  - Willing to act democratically even within Western medical hospital hierarchies
  - Willing to afford both practitioners and childbearers autonomy in their decision-making, allowing them to both take responsibility for their own actions and also work with the team
  - Willing to be public about problems and solutions so that other units can learn from past mistakes

3.3.2   The Three Categories of Vaginal Breech Delivery in Facilities

Because midwives have been a large part of bringing back breech, with most physicians more anxious to keep the prevailing system in place, almost all models that have been successful in bringing back breech since the Term Breech Trial use midwives in some capacity. Below we present three categories of vaginal breech delivery in facilities and provide several concrete examples for each category:

- Breeches managed by the midwife as the lead, without obstetricians required in the room
- Breeches managed by the midwife, with an obstetrician required to be in the room
- Breeches managed by the obstetricians, with midwives and/or doulas as support

To be clear, there are various versions of these seemingly distinct models: models that supposedly exclude physicians (except for CS) do not always do so, and in the ones where an obstetrician is the lead, sometimes the midwives take over or vice versa. As one physician said of a recent experience that was considered "golden":

> The obstetrician was not a requirement at delivery in our model, but I'm not sure the MW [midwife] was always the lead in the delivery room either. We worked together, collaboratively and saw each other very much as bringing different skills to the service...[the midwife] taught me her midwifery skills and I taught her obstetric skills—it was very much a two-way process.

In one hospital discussed below, the midwives were permitted to attend breeches for four and a half years without an obstetrician in the room. During this time period, the medical staff were usually welcomed in because the midwives and clients wanted them to learn the new upright techniques. When there was a change in administration, however, an external review was launched that was poised to stop the midwives being the lead. Instead, the review confirmed the model was reasonable *with the midwife exclusively managing the birth unless a cesarean was needed*. When the new administration then decided to make it a recommendation that an obstetrician be in the room anyway, the laboring women simply refused because they felt that the situation would be out of their control and therefore an imposition.

3.4 Category A: Breeches Managed by the Midwife, Without Obstetricians Required in the Room

3.4.1 The Breech Clinic in the Oxford Radcliffe Hospital, NHS Foundation Trust, Oxford, England, Described by Anita Hedditch

We meet families in our breech clinic where ECV (external cephalic version) is offered as the primary option. If this fails or is declined, cesarean section (CS) and vaginal breech birth (VBB) are discussed. Families are counseled in risks and benefits in VBB and strict inclusion criteria followed. If families choose a VBB, continuity of care and carer (UK requisites) are offered in a weekly breech clinic, and when labor starts, the wish to pursue VBB is again confirmed.

Breech birth is supported by a small group of midwives who work within the delivery environment of the obstetric unit, and we all commit to covering a rota (shift) to ensure 24/7 service provision. Our midwives have the support of our lead obstetrician as well as other breech-experienced obstetricians for VBB care. Care provision now includes two VBB-experienced midwives, who are present to facilitate a birth. If there is maternal consent, an obstetric observer attends. An experienced obstetrician is always in the department and available for support if needed. Each breech birth includes multidisciplinary planning about when a transfer to obstetric management might be considered. In practice, however, this now rarely happens.

As a team, we conduct rigorous training in normal physiology of breech labor and birth, using videos and mannequins. In my first breech birth, I was watched by two senior obstetricians; I followed Jane Evans' teaching like a mantra, and everything she said would happen did. After numerous conferences and training sessions, I developed local guidelines based on theory and practical experience. At each birth, the midwives gain video consent, take notes, and debrief with any obstetric observer who attends. Obstetricians train alongside midwives in both upright care provision and "emergency" lithotomy breech delivery, as this has emerged to be their preferred method.

The service has gradually evolved as an ongoing learning process that requires humility, honesty, dedication, and a certain amount of emotional strength. We look back and see that we conducted cesareans for deliveries that we could now conduct vaginally.

Breech birth within the UK is challenging as for so many years it has been an obstetric domain. However, because as midwives, we are experts in labor care and normal birth, we have applied this to breech delivery, while obstetricians and midwives continue to have defined roles. At times it feels like a fragile service because breech birth evokes strong beliefs and feelings among the wider multidisciplinary team. We have learnt that the successful births have been from labors that progress well and that is largely what we now expect and prefer. There is some robust support, but there are some less certain.

As a multidisciplinary group that has now delivered 101 births, we have weathered three births that proved more difficult; these babies were all discharged home well with their parents, and vaginal breech care continued to be provided. For sociopolitical reasons we still only serve the local population. Future collaborative learning and support with other UK breech centers would be fruitful.

3.4.2   The Breech Clinic in l'Hôpital Montfort, Ottawa, Canada, Described by Betty-Anne Daviss

After the Ottawa conference in 2009 described above, I was permitted to teach the Montfort staff, including the obstetricians, about upright and all fours breech. Finally, because of my research and experience, in 2013 I was given privileges to attend breeches without a physician present. The story of how we managed to override the prejudice against midwives managing vaginal breech deliveries, which no other midwives in Canada have yet been permitted to do (except undiagnosed in the far North), in a hospital where not all of the physicians are on board with attending vaginal breeches, is told in Daviss and Bisits (2021).

At a larger hospital in Ottawa, where two midwives who have more breech experience than many of the obstetricians but have not been permitted breech privileges, one of the chiefs suggested that l'Hôpital Montfort was able to make the changes because it is smaller, with less bureaucracy. We and the midwifery clients suggest that, regardless of size, midwives' full scope should be respected. We believe that the elements of francophone culture—the less conservative nature, the willingness to engage in social debates, and the admission that this is an emotional issue—have all weighed in on the breech innovations taking place at l'Hôpital Montfort.[6] We have been through many hurdles, but our midwives have stood with me to preserve vaginal breech delivery. Risk management, nurse management, and most recently, a new chief of staff have been willing to work out protocols and mitigate conflict among staff.

At the Montfort, we now have another midwife who has attended 20 breeches and is following in my footsteps; she should soon be able to provide backup care when I am away. And finally, the first anglophone hospital to grant midwives privileges in Canada has opened its doors to midwives with experience in breech to practice there—the Michael Garron Hospital in Toronto, although they have not yet found an experienced practitioner. The British Columbia midwives have also recently been making steps toward opening the issue in their province.

Fig. 3.1 In 2015 l'Hôpital Montfort of Ottawa won the Hospital Integration Award for Ontario, largely because they recognized midwives full scope of practice, including management of breech delivery. From left to right, Laurence Tsorba, incoming head midwife at the time, Teresa Bandrowska, outgoing head midwife, and Betty-Anne. Published with kind permission of © Ken Johnson. All Rights Reserved

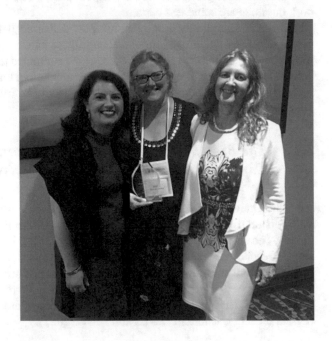

⁶ For a comparison of francophone and anglophone personalities, see Gibson et al. 2008.

3.4.3 The Sanctum Natural Birth Center in Hyderabad, India, Described by Vijaya Krishnan

The Sanctum Birth Center, which I founded, is a freestanding birth center, not attached to any hospital yet with emergency infrastructure built into it. After 8 years of having provided collaborative backup partnership, our main obstetrician, Dr. Jayanthi Reddy, became a full-time partner. In 2016, we moved to a larger facility— a 10,000 square-foot freestanding birth center, with an inbuilt operating theater where cesareans can be performed, a Level 1 NICU, pharmacy and lab facilities, and an ambulance. Since there is no recognition of "birth centers" in India, we are registered as a Level 3 hospital for legal and regulatory purposes. We also offer gynecology and pediatric services under our roof, thereby extending continuity of care and collaborative care to beyond just maternity care. Our natural birth rate (including complex pregnancies, VBACs, twins, and breeches) currently stands at 92.7%.

It is important to understand that what we are doing is a large step in India. With breech presentations, mothers and families rarely use a "rights and responsibilities" paradigm, but accept the physician's authority which usually directs them to plan for a caesarean for a breech. Many are not being afforded the right to wait to go past 37 weeks so we end up with preterm caesarean babies. What makes the Sanctum different from the freestanding birth centers one might see in middle- or high-resource countries is that we are not restricted to taking on low-risk clients because we have the skills, facilities, and backup required to manage clients with complex needs or complications. This includes women with twins, gestational diabetes, gestational hypertension, breech babies, etc. because we have the full support of backup obstetricians, pediatricians, and other physicians. If their help is required, all are available to come in if not already on site. We have enjoyed teaching upright breech, which comes naturally to us anyway as midwives. Since 2016, we have facilitated nine vaginal breeches and nine sets of twins born vaginally. There is good synergy between the obstetricians and midwives in the city, as the Chair of the Fernandez Foundation, Evita Fernandez, has made it a priority to develop a midwifery program. At Fernandez Hospital, midwives perform the normal births without complex needs including vaginal breeches that do not require intervention/surgery. The physicians also attend (though not required to do so) as they are also anxious to bring vaginal breech back (Fig. 3.2).

3.4.4 A Hospital in the North of England, Described by Helen Dresner Barnes

Our service began as a midwife-led format and became a multi-professional service between 2012 and 2019 with a midwife and obstetric team working together, with a dedicated clinic for planned breeches. Restructuring within the unit in 2019 resulted

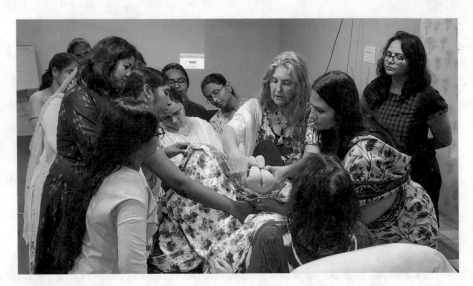

Fig. 3.2 Breech workshop organized by Dr. Vijaya Krishnan at The Sanctum Natural Birth Center in Hyderabad. Betty-Anne, holding the doll, provided a full-day breech training for midwives and obstetricians. Dr. Vijaya is to her immediate left (and at the right in the photo) in the colorful sari. February 2020. Published with kind permission of © Ken Johnson. All Rights Reserved

in the cancellation of this ideal model away from the dedicated clinic, and while vaginal breeches are still accommodated, they are now attended *either* by a midwife *or* an obstetrician. I would not have chosen to do breeches on my own as that's a lonely place to be, because a midwife who dares to do something that not all midwives are doing can be marginalized or reported to a disciplinary body by her peers.

I learnt my skills for managing breech births from Jane Evans, another independent midwife, and have attended one at home with her. Jane in turn learnt her skills from Mary Cronk, and together they had developed the "Day at The Breech" teaching workshop. I also worked with Dotty Watkins, an enlightened, women-centered head of midwifery in the UK National Health Service, who supported me to do another one at home.

In 2011, a women-centered obstetrician arrived at our unit, and we quickly established a shared interest in providing choice for women, for vaginal breech deliveries as well as VBACs (even after two cesareans) viewed with some suspicion by some peers. After attending the breech conference in Washington DC in 2012, we returned to the UK with the goal of establishing a sustainable breech service. We sought to learn from experienced breech practitioners, attended conferences together, and traveled to Dr. Frank Louwen's clinic in Frankfurt to observe his practices and techniques for a week.

Over time, we developed a multi-professional service where women with a suspected breech presentation were referred to us. Those who were confirmed breech were interviewed about their birth plans, counseled about breech birth and cesarean delivery, and then asked to make an informed choice. We were always honest about our skills level, and we did not claim specialist knowledge but offered structured support. Those women who chose vaginal breech birth were screened for suitability with ultrasound and offered external cephalic version (ECV). Initially the obstetrician conducted most of the accepted ECVs, but we were at our most successful when I began to perform ECV. This may be because midwives have a holistic perspective and take time, while the obstetricians tend to squeeze ECVs between other labor ward duties.

We offered a 24/7 on call service for women who elected for vaginal breech birth. When labor started women would call me or one of my two caseload colleagues, if I was on leave, and we would attend them at the hospital. If labor occurred during the day, the obstetrician would attend the first stage of labor, if duties permitted, and they would always attend as the mother approached the need to push. Hence the majority of our women were attended by an experienced midwife and an obstetrician with whom they had established a relationship.

Several key elements of the Daviss model we propose above were present: mothers were respected, providers met the needs of childbearers in consistent and continuous 24/7 manner, providers engaged in supportive, interactive management while staying in the background, every breech birth was debriefed, and we had regular meetings regarding the service. This collaborative effort resulted in national recognition from the UK Royal College of Midwives (RCM) in 2016, when we won an RCM Award for Excellence in Maternity Care for our breech birth service.

With the backing of our management, we organized two UK Breech Conferences in 2014 and 2017, where the Frankfurt data, the Frank Nudge (Louwen et al. 2017), and Jane's mechanisms were presented (Evans 2012). On the morning of the second day of our 2014 conference, the head of the UK Royal College of Obstetricians and Gynaecologists took the role of chair and opened the day thus:

> One of the things I reflected on last night was that I've spent 25 years doing something wrong…not everything wrong, but I think one of the things I have been doing wrong, clearly is how I've been supervising the management of breech birth. Hopefully today, we are going to be addressing the inevitable problems that arise and these problems will come, whatever we do, however clear we are, however normal things are, things are always occasionally going to go wrong. I hope to see this afternoon what we should be doing when things go wrong in the delivery room and at home.

Our experience confirms the validity of the Daviss model of sustainable models of vaginal breech delivery proposed above and draws attention to the necessary role of administrators, who are vital to provide support for practitioners and parents when poor outcomes occur. The strength of our service lay in the commitment to exchange skills internationally, while the main limitation of our 2012–2019 service was its reliance on a small group of practitioners.

3.5 Category B: Breeches Managed by the Midwife, with an Obstetrician Required to Be in the Room

3.5.1 SeeBaby Midwifery, Atlanta, Georgia, Described by Betty-Anne Daviss

This practice meets all the elements of a sustainable model for *all births*, with breeches being just one of many birth situations. They provide care for twins, triplets, and VBACs and encourage women to have births without epidurals and without augmentation if possible. They are honest about who has skills and therefore allow a midwife to perform vaginal breech births if she has experience, although the physician, Dr. Bootstaylor, is in the room for the second stage of labor. Ellen Adamo, the CNM who works closely with Dr. Bootstaylor, said that he "just always did breeches. He never stopped." As their website states, Dr. Bootstaylor "is in alignment with a less invasive and more holistic approach to prenatal care and birth…Top Doctor allowing our Midwives to actually practice Midwifery." (http://seebaby) The team welcomes homebirth midwife transfers and recognizes the value of certified professional midwives (CPMs). For 5 consecutive years, Dr. Bootstaylor has earned the title of "Top Doctor" in *Atlanta Magazine*, and he recently published a book *Shared Decision-Making, Bring Back Birth Into the Hands of Mothers* (Bootstaylor and Gaskin 2020), that outlines the importance of allowing the mother to choose her own options for delivery.

In the USA, where some members of the obstetric community are unsympathetic to both VBAC and breech, this model has been able to mitigate fears and provide supportive care from across the region. Clients are coming from far beyond Atlanta, Georgia, including Tampa, Florida, because similar choices for vaginal breech delivery may not be available near them. Because the unit offers harmony among providers and choice for women, and experience in many kinds of deliveries, this unit should be sustainable, as long as the current providers find successors who will continue the care after they are gone.

3.5.2 Hospital of Southern Denmark in Aabenraa, Denmark, Described by Betty-Anne Daviss

Dr. Nielsen has engaged her entire country in the vaginal breech issue by bringing in foreign practitioners who are managing breech in their own countries to teach. She was inspired while working in New Zealand when she attended a breech seminar with Maggie Banks, an Australian midwife. At the conference in Aabenraa in 2019, Dr. Nielsen presented impressive data on their overall cesarean rate, which was 11.8%. They deliver 34% of all breeches vaginally, whereas the Danish average is 14%. As in Frankfurt, their criteria for vaginal breech births include premature babies, gestational age greater than 34 weeks, flexed hips, and a weight range of 2500–4000 grams.

This hospital meets the parameters of our sustainable model, in particular with regard to honesty about their experience level from the first day that they started up, listening to mothers, debriefing of the staff, and a truly supportive female Head of Obstetrics, Katrin Löser, and Head of Department, Bo Sultan. Most mothers allow videos to be taken of their births so that the collaborative team of midwives and physicians can learn in their requisite debrief after each birth. The couples get the video afterward.

Breech birth in Aabenraa is managed by the team on call, who will have a briefing beforehand about division of roles. The midwife will support the normal birth. If maneuvers are necessary, they are done by the midwife coordinator or the doctor present. If a doctor is not yet thoroughly trained, an expert doctor will be present as well.

I had an opportunity to debrief from the conference on a 4-h ride back to Copenhagen with an obstetrician who had been a confessed sceptic before attending the conference. He told me he was encouraged to hear from the practitioners who were using these new techniques in their own hospitals. Two things he thought particularly groundbreaking: the upright position and the "crowning touch"—a forceps replacement maneuver I had invented and presented in which you grasp with one hand the entire the top of the baby's head and rotate and flex to retrieve the aftercoming head (Daviss 2017; Daviss and Bisits 2021). As in Northern England and Ottawa, the cross-pollination of ideas that have proliferated in Denmark and desire to learn from and share skills with international colleagues has become contagious.

3.6 Category C: Breeches Managed by Obstetricians, with Midwives and/or Doulas as Support

3.6.1 Goethe Klinikum in Frankfurt, Germany, Described by Betty-Anne Daviss

In Germany, by law every birth requires a midwife in attendance. At birth centers they can be primary care providers. Yet in hospitals, midwives rarely take the lead. Louwen is a dynamic negotiator and an energetic and disarming speaker, whose vision of vaginal breech birth began when he took the position of Head of Obstetrics at the hospital in 2002; in this position, he became determined to try to keep interventions to a minimum. One of Louwen's first actions as the new head was to study episiotomies. He was shocked to find that they were being done routinely by the midwives and obstetricians alike. Yet breech ultimately became his fascination.

When I first met him in person in 2008, he described to me how he was absent-mindedly looking at a book opened to a page on Bracht, the German obstetrician who created a maneuver to simulate how chimpanzees deliver on all fours. When

Dr. Louwen realized that the book was upside down, he decided to do what Bracht should have done: suggest that women get upright for their breech births (Daviss 2017). I first sought Dr. Louwen out in 2006 when I realized that he was doing births with the mother kneeling over the back of the hospital bed, on all fours or sometimes squatting—the way I had learnt from traditional midwives in Latin America. He told me that he honestly did not pretend to know how to do breeches in upright or all fours positions when he started; he reasoned it out and was equally honest with his patients.

Dr. Louwen's lead has had a great effect on us here in Ottawa. With senior epidemiologist Ken Johnson, I wrote up the analysis for Dr. Louwen's obstetric department at the Johann Goethe Klinikum Institute, which demonstrated that upright vaginal breech delivery was associated with reductions in duration of the second stage of labor, maneuvers required, maternal/neonatal injuries, and cesarean rate when compared with vaginal delivery in the dorsal position (Louwen et al. 2017).

In October 2014, Dr. Anke Reitter, who had been working side by side with Frank, became the Lead Consultant Obstetrician and Maternal-Fetal Medicine Specialist at the nearby hospital, Krankenhaus Sachsenhausen. She is one of several obstetricians now who have left the Johann Goethe Klinikum with knowledge and skills of upright and all fours vaginal breech birth and taken it to other settings.

3.7   Conclusion: Changing the Focus on Risk

Concepts of risk have been adulterated by healthcare systems in the twenty-first century that continue to increase intervention. We have included here the good models that we have encountered or in which we have been involved, which have managed to change this risk-based approach. This does not of course include all of the hospitals that have managed to continue or regroup to offer breech services since the notorious Term Breech Trial almost completely ended vaginal breech deliveries in hospitals around the world and the follow-up results were not heeded. However, because there still appear to be few practices that have had the courage to return to offering women the choice, we have presented some here in order for others to be encouraged and to glean from their experience.

We are hopeful and excited about the future of vaginal breech because of the models presented herein, which have been able to sustain ongoing or new services. As we move forward, the *honesty, instinct, and diplomacy* of our units will continue to be needed. Being honest about our skills and knowledge of the research, about best practice to normalize breech, and about the politics and how they affect our practice will keep us vigilant. For instance, several of the breech practitioners contacted in the UK and India suggested that there is some concern about the use of the term "breech specialist," as it does not have clear qualifications and could generate fraudulent representations of inexperienced midwives.

Meanwhile, as we move toward development of the new breech practices of upright and all fours delivery, we need to be cautious about each new message that comes out in the research. Here, we heed the concerns expressed by Armstrong (1995) about the invasion of surveillance into normal populations because it tends, like the focus on risk, to pathologize the normal. Strident micromanaged measurements in surveillance, Armstrong argues, have led to "blurring the lines of normalcy." With researchers lining up to "be the first" to study the new approach to breech, micromanagement of the normal becomes tempting but worrisome. A case in point is a new algorithm that was proposed by Reitter et al. (2020). In an approach comparable to Friedman's in the 1950s, this algorithm appears to introduce and impose unnecessary and nonproven time limits on the descent of the breech, in particular in primiparas. As it took us decades to undo the Friedman curve, which set unnecessary and misleading time limits on normal labor, we suggest that this approach is neither based on good evidence nor desirable (Daviss and Johnson in press).

The UN has declared resolutions to protect human rights (1948), Indigenous rights (2007), and maternal rights not to die in childbirth (2009). Yet in all of the legal and political protections internationally, there have been no overtures to create an international declaration that protects *normal birth, the practitioners who provide it,* and *the parents who seek it.* Access to vaginal breech birth has been so decimated over the last two decades that the issue provides worthy fodder for the suggestion by Daviss (Daviss 2021) to debate whether or not the time has come to provide political and legal means to require systems to institutionalize such protection. The models in this chapter offer sustainable alternatives to the focus on risk and surveillance of the normal, to promote systems that bring honesty, instinct, and diplomacy into facilitation of breech birth.

References

Alaszewski J, Burgess A (2007) Risk, time and reason. Health Risk Soc 9(4):349–358

Armstrong D (1995) The rise of surveillance medicine. Sociol Health Illn 17(3):393–404

Ballantyne A, Gavaghan C, McMillan J, Pullon S (2016) Pregnancy and the culture of extreme risk aversion. Am J Bioeth 16(2):21–23

Bogner G, Strobl M, al SC (2015) Breech delivery in the all fours position: a prospective observational comparative study with classic assistance. J Perinat Med 43(6):707–713

Bootstaylor B, Gaskin IM (2020) Shared decision making: bring birth back into the hands of mothers, vol 1. Serebal 360 Publishing

Borbolla Foster A, Bagust A, al BA (2014) Lessons to be learnt in managing the breech presentation at term: an 11-year single-centre retrospective study. Aust N Z J Obstet Gynaecol 54:333–339

Daviss BA (1997) Heeding warnings from the canary, the whale, and the Inuit. In: Davis-Floyd R, Sargent C (eds) Childbirth and authoritative knowledge: cross-cultural perspectives. University of California Press, Berkeley, pp 44–473. http://understandingbirthbetter.com/files/uploads/Heeding-Warnings-Betty-anne-Daviss-Childbirth-and-Authoritative-Knowledge.pdf

Daviss BA (2017/2020) Rethinking the physiology of vaginal breech birth. Informed Descent Publishers, Ottawa. Available at http://understandingbirthbetter.com/section.php?ID=25&Lang=En&Nav=Section

Daviss BA (2021) Introduction. In: Daviss BA, Davis-Floyd R (eds) Birthing models on the human rights frontier: speaking truth to power. Routledge, Abingdon

Daviss BA, Bisits A (2021) Bringing back breech: dismantling hierarchies and re-skilling practitioners. In: Daviss BA, Davis-Floyd R (eds) Birthing models on the human rights frontier: speaking truth to power. Routledge, Abingdon

Daviss BA, Johnson KC (in press) Upright breech birth: does new research risk reviving Friedman's curse?

Daviss BA, Johnson KC, Lalonde AB (2010) Evolving evidence since the term breech trial: Canadian response, European dissent, and potential solutions. J Obstet Gynaecol Can 32(3):217–224

Deneux-Tharaux C, Carmona E, al B-CMH (2006) Postpartum maternal mortality and cesarean delivery. Obstet Gynecol 108(3Pt1):541–548

Evans J (2012) The final piece of the breech birth jigsaw? Essentially MIDIRS 3(3):46–49

Gibson KL, Mckelvie S, de Man AF (2008) Personality and culture: a comparison of francophones and anglophones in Quebec. J Soc Psychol 148(2):133–165. https://doi.org/10.3200/SOCP.148.2.133-166

Goffinet F, Carayol M, Foidart JM et al (2006) Is planned vaginal delivery for breech presentation at term still an option? Results of an observational prospective survey in France and Belgium. Am J Obstet Gynecol 194:1002–1011

Hannah ME, Hannah WJ, Hewson SA et al (2000) Planned caesarean section versus planned vaginal birth for breech presentation at term: a randomised multicentre trial. Lancet 356(9239):1375–1383

Hemmerich A, Bandrowska T, Dumas GA (2019) The effects of squatting while pregnant on pelvic dimensions: a computational simulation to understand childbirth. J Biomech 87:64–74

Heyman B (2010) Values and health risks. In: Heyman B, Shaw M, Alaszewski A et al (eds) Risk, safety and clinical practice. Health care through the lens of risk. Oxford University Press, Oxford

Hogle KL, Kilburn L, Hewson S et al (2003) Impact of the international term breech trial on clinical practice and concerns: a survey of centre collaborators. J Obstet Gynaecol Can 25:14–16

Leeman L (2020) State of the breech in 2020: guidelines support maternal choice, but skills are lost. Birth 47:165–168

Louwen F, Daviss B, Johnson KC, Reitter A (2017) Does breech delivery in an upright position instead of on the back improve outcomes and avoid cesareans? Int J Gynaecol Obstet 136(2):151–161

Reitter A, Daviss BA, Bisits A et al (2014) Does pregnancy and/or shifting positions create more room in a woman's pelvis? Am J Obstet Gynecol 211:662.e1–662.e9

Reitter A, Halliday A, Walker S (2020) Practical insight into upright breech birth from birth videos: A structured analysis. Birth 00:1–9

Tsakiridis I, Mamopoulos A, Athanasiadis A et al (2019) Management of breech presentation: a comparison of four national evidence-based guidelines. Am J Perinatol 37(11):1102–1109

Verhoeven AT, de Leeuw JP, Bruinse HW (2005) Breech presentation at term: elective caesarean section is the wrong choice as a standard treatment because of too high risks for the mother and her future children [article in Dutch]. Ned Tijdschr Geneeskd 149:2207–2210

Whyte H, Hannah ME, Saigal S et al (2004) Outcomes of children at 2 years after planned cesarean birth vs. planned vaginal birth for breech presentation at term: the international randomized term breech trial. Am J Obstet Gynecol 191:864–871

Chapter 4
From Home to Hospital: Sustainable Transfers of Care in the United States

Bria Dunham and Sara Hall

4.1 Introduction

Rapport matters in patient[1]–provider relationships, and continuity of care improves outcomes for both mothers[2] and neonates (McLachlan et al. 2012). Over the course of many visits, a client may become more willing to disclose concerns and more trusting of the provider's clinical judgment. Yet for spontaneous vaginal deliveries within US hospitals, a patient may have little choice about who attends her birth. Indeed, this disconnect prompts a familiar refrain, "Oh, I hope I get *my* doctor when it's time for the baby to be born."

A shift in the practitioner attending a birth may be relatively common, but a shift in the site of delivery is not. A transfer of care from home to hospital—and potentially involving a different care team—brings a host of new concerns and costs, financially, logistically, and emotionally. This disruption can be buffered by the use of a coordinated and sustainable model for peripartum transfers, as developed by the Home Birth Summit (HBS 2014) in their Best Practice Guidelines for transfers of planned homebirths to hospital settings. This approach smooths inefficiencies,

---

[1] We alternate between the terms "patient" and "client" to describe the individual receiving maternity care, recognizing that "patient" more closely represents a role within the obstetric model of care and "client" more closely represents a role in the midwifery model of care.

[2] We default to the term "mother" and she/her pronouns in describing people who receive maternity care. We note that not all pregnant persons identify as women or as mothers, and not all mothers gestate or give birth to their children. We discuss pregnant transgender and nonbinary individuals and gestational surrogates in the Further Considerations section.

B. Dunham (✉)
Department of Health Sciences, Boston University, Boston, MA, USA
e-mail: dunhamb@bu.edu

S. Hall
Massachusetts General Hospital, Institute of Health Professions, Boston, MA, USA

© Springer Nature Switzerland AG 2021
K. Gutschow et al. (eds.), *Sustainable Birth in Disruptive Times*, Global Maternal and Child Health, https://doi.org/10.1007/978-3-030-54775-2_4

promotes optimal maternal and newborn outcomes, and best supports the needs and wishes of the mother, all while forging a sustainable system that conserves resources and recognizes the contributions of the transferring provider.

4.2   Transfers of Maternity Care: Who, When, Why, and to What End?

With a few exceptions, in the United States, the planned settings for birth include home, birth center (hospital-based or freestanding), or a hospital obstetric unit. Transfer of care may occur at any point during pregnancy, labor, or the immediate postpartum period; generally, this reflects a shift from a lower to a higher level of anticipated obstetric interventions. The protocols supporting these transfers and attitudes of providers involved deeply impact how smoothly the transfer proceeds for all parties.

Hospital transfers occur in approximately 9–13% of planned homebirths in the United States (Vedam et al. 2014). Transfers are more common for primiparas (23.4–45.4%; Blix et al. 2014), for subsequent births after cesarean (Cox et al. 2015), and for clients with preexisting conditions (Snowden et al. 2015). The most common indication for transfer is "failure to progress" (Blix et al. 2016; Cheyney et al. 2014a; Cox et al. 2015; Johnson and Daviss 2005), and only few transfers (0–5.4%) are due to obstetric emergencies (Blix et al. 2016). Even among women who plan a homebirth after cesarean (HBAC), the primary indication for transfer remains "failure to progress" (Rowe et al. 2015).

While a peripartum transfer does not preclude spontaneous vaginal birth, transfer can lead to instrumental or operative delivery. Rates of cesarean birth following transfer from homebirth settings in the United States ranged from 10.6% in primiparous women to 12.8% in women who attempted HBAC (Cox et al. 2015). Given the desire of those who plan out-of-hospital birth to avoid most obstetric interventions, the likelihood of instrumental or operative delivery may complicate or delay the decision to transfer for both providers and clients.

In addition to having an increased likelihood of obstetric interventions, transfers can be emotionally challenging. How might it be possible to better support the transferring client's psychosocial and clinical needs, especially if "failure to progress" or desire for pharmacological pain management suggests the non-emergent nature of most peripartum transfers?

4.3   A Sustainable and Humanized Approach to Transfers of Care

We build upon Robbie Davis-Floyd's (2018b) theoretical model for describing transfers of care in terms of disarticulation, fractured articulation, smooth articulation, and seamless articulation between homebirth midwives and hospital-based providers. Smooth articulation between providers is critical to mothers and mid-wives, and it can also influence decisions about transfers of care, as providers on both ends make future decisions based on past experiences (Johnson and Davis-Floyd 2006; Davis-Floyd 2018b; Cheyney et al. 2014b). Where can we find this smooth articulation and where do we not?

In the Netherlands, low-risk women routinely receive care from midwives and are transferred to secondary care directed by obstetricians if complications arise. Secondary care may also include care provided by clinical midwives, which is asso-ciated with decreased instrumental delivery (Wiegers and Hukkelhoven 2010, Bommarito, 2020). In determining whether a transfer should occur, the Dutch Obstetrical Indications List distinguishes between "physiological" and "pathologi-cal" birth—rather than between "low-risk" and "high-risk" as in the United States—and provides a framework for interprofessional collaboration (DeVries et al. 2009).

The United States has historically lacked a similarly cohesive and broadly accepted framework for transfers of care, although the Best Practice Guidelines (HBS 2014) seek to change that. The guidelines were based on the Smooth Transitions program, stemming from the work of the Midwives Alliance of Washington State (MAWS) to produce an evidence-based document that outlines the different indications for discussion, consultation, and transfer of care (MAWS 2016). In 2009, Smooth Transitions began reaching out to hospitals and asking them to voluntarily participate in the program, focusing on birthing sites where tensions between local community midwives and hospital staff appeared greatest. As part of the Smooth Transitions program, pairs of midwives and obstetricians visited hospi-tals and gathered information about liability, risk management, and the perspectives of the health care team, to better understand what went well and what went poorly during transfers. Smooth Transitions also educated healthcare professionals in the hospital setting, finding that staff often didn't know that midwives were licensed in Washington, what training they had, or what equipment and medication they car-ried. Smooth Transitions recommended that hospitals set up a planning committee with licensed midwives that would address what would make transfers go most smoothly. Due to this initiative in Washington State, non-emergent transfers of care have become relatively smooth, while emergent transfers of care, particularly neo-natal emergency transfers, could still use more support (Audrey Levine, personal communication).

The Best Practice Guidelines were developed by 11 delegates to the Home Birth Summits held in 2011 and 2013, including homebirth midwives, hospital providers and administrators, academic researchers, and advocates. The Best Practice Guidelines (HBS 2014) include 22 specified guidelines in three distinct categories: model practices for homebirth providers, model practices for hospital providers and staff, and quality improvement and policy development. The document emphasizes the importance of good communication between providers, a consideration of the transferring woman's psychosocial needs, opportunities for continued involvement of the transferring provider and interprofessional collaboration, and ongoing oppor-tunities to strengthen quality improvement and the development of policies and pro-tocols. Thus far the guidelines have had a scattered reception, with a possible greater integration in the Northwest and less integration in the Northeast (Audrey Levine,

Judy Norsigian, and Kristen Leonard, personal communication).[3] Part of this dynamic may be attributable to state-by-state differences in licensure, such that hospitals in states that do not formally recognize or license certified professional midwives (CPMs) would be unlikely to adopt the guidelines for reasons of liability (Judy Norsigian, personal communication).

We argue that the Best Practice Guidelines (HBS 2014), in conjunction with the related guidelines for interprofessional collaboration across the span of maternity care and the newborn period (HBS 2020), represent a *sustainable* framework for prenatal and peripartum transfers that may be particularly salient during times of disruption, such as during public health emergencies like the coronavirus pandemic. This approach is explicitly sustainable in that it embodies humanized birth, conserves resources, and provides a context for interprofessional collaboration and coordination of care. Humanized childbirth places the laboring woman at the center of her care and emphasizes that her experience and agency matter (McKay 1991; Wagner 2001, 2006, Davis-Floyd 2018a). A humanized approach to childbirth is sustainable, given its holistic focus on the pregnant individual's physical, social, and emotional needs as well as its reliance on evidence-based care. Indeed, we argue that a paradigm for birth that does not work for the person giving birth—by failing to fully recognize her humanity or causing her distress or poor outcomes—will itself not be sustainable over time. The principles of transfers of care are sustainable if they lower the incidence of costly interventions while remaining flexible and adaptable to the needs of mothers and babies so that their outcomes and experiences are improved. Where healthcare systems face increased stress or resource scarcity, ways to integrate community-based providers, reduce distress, and avoid unnecessary delays may be all the more vital.

The need for clear communication between out-of-hospital providers and receiving clinicians neither begins with nor ends when care is transferred. The Best Practice Guidelines (HBS 2014) recognize this through advocating for "[o]pportunities for education regarding home birth practice, shared continuing medical education, and relationship building." Midwives have voiced an unfulfilled need for post-transfer debriefing with hospital providers (Kuliukas et al. 2015) that might be further addressed via interprofessional working groups (Cheyney 2011; Bommarito 2020) and interprofessional education (Avery et al. 2012). Meeting this need would help acknowledge the important role played by community midwives and could positively impact decision-making about future potential transfers. This communication could further facilitate seamless articulation in peripartum transfers, wherein the transferring midwife remains with the client throughout her birth, working cooperatively with hospital providers.

Such coordination would further strengthen collaboration during transfers of care earlier in pregnancy (e.g., MAWS 2016). Many conditions considered to be higher risk can be safely monitored and managed by a homebirth midwife when

---

[3] Given limited published information about the implementation of the Best Practice Guidelines, we reached out to a small number of homebirth midwives and/or birth advocates, including several authors of the guidelines. Their insights are cited as personal communication.

there is collaboration with other providers, and having a multidirectional preexisting framework facilitates these prenatal transfers of care.

4.3.1 Maintain the Pregnant Client's Support Personnel

The indication and timing of prenatal and peripartum transfers impact both clinical and psychosocial outcomes. In a transfer prior to the onset of labor, a pregnancy complication may necessitate an urgent labor induction, without the time to develop a new patient–provider relationship. Alternately, some prenatal transfers may allow more time to establish a new patient–provider relationship that can take the patient's desires around birth into greater consideration.

When care is transferred after spontaneous onset of labor, whether due to "failure to progress" or obstetric complications, less time is available to develop a new patient–provider relationship. Hospital transfers may result in negative feelings about the birth experience (Geerts et al. 2014; Lindgren et al. 2011), which can increase the risk of postpartum depression (Bielinski-Blattmann et al. 2016). Such disarticulations in transfers can also leave midwives feeling invisible when their knowledge of the client is disregarded by the obstetric team (Davis-Floyd 2018b; Kuliukas et al. 2015). Maintaining continuity of the laboring woman's support personnel not only improves maternal and newborn outcomes (Shaw et al. 2016) but also improves maternal comfort, which may result in fewer interventions. This is recognized throughout the Best Practice Guidelines (HBS 2014), including recommendations (1) that transferring providers may continue to serve as the primary birth attendant if doing so is within their scope of practice and if they have admitting privileges; (2) that hospital staff support the presence of the transferring providers in addition to the patient's primary support person; and (3) that transferring and receiving providers coordinate in planning follow-up care, which may revert care for the postpartum woman to the transferring provider.

4.3.2 Avoid Unnecessary Replication of Tests and Procedures

Hospital births are generally more costly than out-of-hospital births (MacDorman et al. 2012; Boucher et al. 2009; Anderson et al. 2021), although out-of-pocket expenses may vary depending upon insurance coverage, local rates, interventions used, and the length of the hospital stay. While a peripartum transfer nearly always increases costs, the additional expense could be partially mediated by avoiding the unnecessary replication of tests and procedures already performed. Having accurate diagnostic information is important in clinically managing complications and ensuring that the receiving care team has access to all relevant information can reduce costs and increase efficiency. This is supported through the Best Practice Guidelines (HBS 2014) recommendations that the transferring midwife provide both a verbal report to the receiving provider and a copy of the relevant prenatal and labor charts. This may be especially relevant in prenatal transfers, where diagnostics should focus upon addressing any complication that precipitated the transfer and routine procedures for the remainder of the pregnancy, rather than repeating tests that had already been administered by the transferring provider.

4.3.3 Limit Obstetric Interventions to Those Medically Indicated and Desired by the Pregnant Client

Clinical outcomes are qualitatively different when care is transferred, including increased rates of interventions and adverse outcomes (Laws et al. 2014). This disparity is inherently related to the indications for the transfer but may also be impacted by the transfer itself, including coordination of care or lack thereof. The Best Practice Guidelines recommend following "[a] defined process to regularly review transfers that includes all stakeholders with a shared goal of quality improvement and safety" (HBS 2014), which could further illuminate both areas where needed interventions are refused as well as ones where unnecessary interventions were made. Elective obstetric interventions increase the resources—instrumental, pharmacological, and financial—used for birth, without necessarily improving outcomes. While the use of medically necessary obstetric interventions may save lives or preserve function, their usage when not indicated increases costs and may result in poorer outcomes for mothers or neonates.

4.3.4 Eliminate the Fragmentation of Care Between Sites and Providers During Transfers of Care

Collaborative relationships between community-based and hospital-based providers could eliminate the fractured articulations or fragmentation of care that can lead to poorer outcomes (HBS 2020). The National Institute for Health and Care Excellence (NICE) recommends that collaboration between homebirth and hospital-based providers in the United Kingdom be initiated during prenatal care and provided in all low-risk pregnancies (Shaw ct al. 2016). Within the United States, Declercq (2012) advocates for developing coordinated policies governing transfers and routes of communication between homebirth midwives and hospital staff, guided by professional organizations. This sentiment is echoed in the Best Practice Guidelines (HBS 2014), which include coordinated follow-up care for both the mother and neonate, as well as the potential for the homebirth provider to resume primary responsibility for care after discharge, as well as in the guidelines for interprofessional collaboration between community midwives and specialist providers (HBS 2020).

Preregistration of planned homebirths by the potential receiving hospital would result in swifter transfers while reducing last-minute replication of data entry or diagnostic tests (Blix et al. 2016). While registering and tracking the majority of planned homebirths that do occur at home would initially expend additional hospital resources, in the long term it could *save* hospital resources by reducing the hesitation that a provider or client would feel toward transfer, thus resulting in earlier transfers where indicated and potentially fewer operative deliveries. Significantly, the expanded dataset could be useful for research comparing home and hospital birth and thus could inform evidence-based childbirth practices, along with setting the framework for a regular review of transfers by all stakeholders specified in the Best Practice Guidelines (HBS 2014). Preregistration could further contribute to an easing of tensions between homebirth midwives and hospital-based providers, who often believe that homebirth is unsafe or are reluctant to assume responsibility for a homebirth transfer (Vedam et al. 2014; Davis-Floyd 2018b; Cheyney et al. 2014b; Declercq 2012).

Alternately, interprofessional collaboration can focus on future providers rather than existing practitioners, such as by incorporating interprofessional practice into academic programs in medicine, nursing, and midwifery (Vedam et al. 2014). This approach should emphasize system issues and support relationship-building between students and practitioners from different domains (HBS 2014). Exposure to a different knowledge base will give students a better understanding of one another's scope of practice and will prepare medical students to collaborate with midwives and other healthcare professionals, potentially altering attitudes toward out-of-hospital births and resulting in more harmonious, smooth, or seamless future transfers.

As this chapter is heading to press, the global community is grappling with the COVID-19 pandemic that has upended daily life and imposed restrictions, including limitations on support persons and visitors for individuals planning hospital births (Davis-Floyd et al. 2020). Fears of giving birth in overwhelmed hospitals have led to surging interest in homebirth among currently pregnant individuals (Gammon 2020), even as midwives struggle to secure adequate personal protective equipment and face their own risks of infection (Candib et al. 2020). In this time of disruption, Candib et al. (2020) have called for Massachusetts homebirth providers to be included in emergency planning for maternity care during the COVID-19 crisis and licensed to provide services. This call is consonant with a recent recommendation on COVID-19 by the American College of Obstetricians and Gynecologists (2020) advocating innovative collaboration between hospitals and community-based providers. As transfer presents additional risks of infection and engagement with strained hospital systems, implementation of the Best Practice Guidelines (HBS 2020) to support greater involvement of homebirth midwives during this time of disruption would help increase safety while preparing to support the needs of the community into the future (Candib et al. 2020; Davis-Floyd et al. 2020).

4.4 Further Considerations

While enhancing sustainability in transfers of care is important for all patients, some populations face increased vulnerability. These populations may include, but are not limited to, survivors of abuse, immigrants, transgender or nonbinary individuals, or gestational surrogates. As such, we have addressed how promotion of a sustainable, humanized approach to transfers of care can support these populations.

Birth may be particularly triggering for survivors of sexual abuse, who face a 13-fold increase in risk of cesarean and tenfold increase of risk of instrumental delivery (Nerum et al. 2010). Transfer to an unfamiliar provider may exacerbate prior trauma, especially when a survivor of abuse may have no choice but to receive care from a provider of a different gender than anticipated. Because the receiving provider may be unaware of the patient's history of sexual trauma, all providers should follow universal precautions (e.g., Coles and Jones 2009) by providing care that is trauma-informed and relevant to all patients, such as keeping the room temperature warm, asking before touching any body part, smiling and maintaining eye contact, or offering a same-sex provider (Gesink and Nattel 2015). Haen's (2017) emphasis on supporting the agency of the survivor to make decisions about her own care, ideally with the continuous support of a doula, is fully compatible with sustainable transfers.

Immigrant women, who already face additional challenges in childbirth relative to their nonimmigrant peers (Barclay and Kent 1998; Van Roosmalen et al. 2003; Bakken et al. 2015), represent another vulnerable population in peripartum transfers. There may be difficulties in both linguistic and cultural translation, wherein the client may bring expectations that vary from the care that she receives, where she may be unable to articulate her wishes to a new care team and where she may not receive fully informed consent prior to the administration of obstetric procedures. Within the United States, undocumented immigrant women, who can be underinformed about options for out-of-hospital birth (Cadena 2013), may fear legal repercussions if a planned out-of-hospital or community birth is transferred to a hospital setting. Given the anti-immigrant tenor of the Trump administration (Lancet 2016) and ongoing efforts to deport undocumented persons, a humanized approach to peripartum transfers must protect against exposure of the patient or any family members to Immigration and Customs Enforcement. Further, a sustainable approach should mobilize existing hospital resources for linguistic translation en route and enable opportunities for cross-cultural communication about expectations for birth.

Relatively little has been written about the maternity care experiences of pregnant transgender men, who choose out-of-hospital birth at a much higher rate (22%; Light et al. 2014) than does the US population as a whole (1.36%; MacDorman et al. 2014). Transgender men who have given birth after socially and/or medically transitioning report that they desired more effective support resources and that care providers were unfamiliar with their needs (Light et al. 2014). Existing challenges faced by transgender and nonbinary gestational parents include being misgendered by hospital staff and being reported to Child Protection Services (Light et al. 2014); these challenges may be exacerbated when care is transferred to new providers. A sustainable approach to transfers of care that creates pathways for seamless articulation between sending and receiving providers can help to minimize additional risks for pregnant transgender men and nonbinary individuals.

Unlike the other populations we have addressed, gestational surrogates may have limited choice in their own care due to the terms of the surrogacy contract or wishes of the commissioning parents, although the International Federation of Gynecology and Obstetrics (FIGO) emphasizes that the gestational surrogate maintains individual autonomy and that her wishes around childbirth should prevail (FIGO 2008; Söderström-Anttila et al. 2016). We do not know of any studies about homebirth among gestational surrogates, yet a humanized, sustainable approach to peripartum transfers in surrogate pregnancies necessitates an awareness of and sensitivity to the concerns of the gestational surrogate.

While increasing sustainability in transfers of care is an overarching goal, implementation must protect the most vulnerable populations. Additional resources—including staff who can devote time and sensitivity to addressing the needs of patients with diverse backgrounds and concerns—should be provided to fully meet the clinical and emotional needs of patients. This chapter has focused on transfers between sites of delivery rather than transfers within the hospital setting, but a recent retrospective cohort study in Ohio found that Black women were statistically more likely to transfer from midwifery to obstetric care both during prenatal care and peripartum (Weisband et al. 2018). Continued efforts to address enhancing sustainability in transfers of peripartum care must consider the role that race plays in maternity care and childbirth outcomes.

4.5   Conclusion

In improving the sustainability of peripartum transfers, our ability to make projections is only as strong as the available data and is thus hindered by systemic gaps in medical records. For instance, Lindgren et al. (2011) found that 15% of charts of homebirth transfers contained no information about the transferring provider. More effectively coordinated transfer of care, and better communication between providers working with different models of care—such as the obstetric versus midwifery models of care (Rothman 1982) or technocratic versus humanistic models of care (Davis-Floyd 1993, 2018a, c)—could lead to better data on transfers and ultimately improve transfers of care in the United States.

In the majority of cases, transfers of care involve an increase in obstetric interventions or technologies. However, these transfers can be made more seamless and sustainable by developing and implementing protocols and processes designed to support best practices (e.g., HBS 2014, 2020) and that make better use of available resources and supports, including the existing relationship between the transferring client and midwife. Simultaneously emphasizing sustainable and humanized transfers of care will support the patients' psychosocial and clinical needs while improving provider satisfaction. Furthermore, a coordinated system for review of these transfers can allow for continued quality improvement and opportunities for interprofessional collaboration and education (HBS 2014). While these changes will likely require adjustments to the operations of the receiving facility and within the belief systems of personnel involved in the transfer, they can ultimately pave the way to better outcomes for mothers and neonates.

References

American College of Obstetricians and Gynecologists (ACOG) (2020) COVID-19 FAQs for obstetrician-gynecologists, obstetrics. https://www.acog.org/clinical-information/physician-faqs/covid-19-faqs-for-ob-gyns-obstetrics. Accessed 12 Apr 2020

Anderson D, Daviss BA, Johnson KC (2021) What if another 10% of deliveries in the United States occurred at home or in a birth center? Safety, economics and politics. In: Daviss BA, Davis-Floyd R (eds) Birthing models on the human rights frontier: speaking truth to power. Routledge, New York. (in press)

Avery MD, Montgomery O, Brandl-Salutz E (2012) Essential components of successful collaborative maternity care models: the ACOG-ACNM project. Obstet Gynecol Clin N Am 39(3):423–434

Bakken KS, Skjeldal OH, Stray-Pedersen B (2015) Higher risk for adverse obstetric outcomes among immigrants of African and Asian descent: a comparison study at a low-risk maternity hospital in Norway. Birth 42(2):132–140

Barclay L, Kent D (1998) Recent immigration and the misery of motherhood: a discussion of pertinent issues. Midwifery 14(1):4–9

Bielinski-Blattmann D, Gürber S, Lavallee K et al (2016) Labour experience and postpartum stress and depression: a quantitative and qualitative examination. J Reprod Infant Psychol 34(2):162–174

Blix E, Kumle M, Kjaergaard H, Oian P, Lindgren HE (2014) Transfer to hospital in planned home births: a systematic review. BMC Pregnancy Childbirth J 14:179. https://doi.org/10.1186/1471-2393-14-179

Blix E, Kumle M, Ingversen K, Huitfeldt AS et al (2016) Transfers to hospital in planned home birth in four countries: a prospective cohort study. Acta Obstet Gynecol Scand 95:420–428

Bommarito R (2020) Structures for collaboration between midwives and obstetricians in the Netherlands: the obstetrics and midwifery manual and perinatal care partnerships. In Gutschow K, Davis-Floyd R, Daviss BA (eds) Sustainable Birth in Disruptive Times. Springer, New York

Boucher D, Bennett C, McFarlin B et al (2009) Staying home to give birth: why women in the United States choose home birth. J Midwifery Womens Health 54(2):119–126

Cadena M (2013) Delivering access: home birth for women and families of color in New Mexico. Master's Thesis, University of New Mexico

Candib LM, Norsigian J, Richardson M (2020) Home birth and the coronavirus crisis. Boston Globe 18 Apr

Cheyney M (2011) Born at home: the biological, cultural, and political dimensions of maternity care in the United States. Belmont, Wadsworth

Cheyney M, Bovbjerg M, Everson C et al (2014a) Outcomes of care for 16,924 planned home births in the United States: the midwives Alliance of North America statistics project, 2004–2009. J Midwifery Womens Health 59(1):17–27

Cheyney M, Everson C, Burcher P (2014b) Home birth transfers in the United States: narratives of risk, fear, and mutual accommodation. Qual Health Res 24(4):254–267

Coles J, Jones K (2009) 'Universal precautions': perinatal touch and examination after childhood sexual abuse. Birth 36(3):230–236

Cox KJ, Bovbjerg ML, Cheyney M et al (2015) Planned home VBAC in the United States 2004–2009: outcomes, maternity care practices, and implications for shared decision making. Birth 42(4):299–308

Davis-Floyd R (1993) The technocratic model of birth. In: Hollis ST, Pershing L, Young MJ (eds) Feminist theory in the study of folklore. University of Illinois Press, Champaign, pp 297–326

Davis-Floyd R (2018a) The technocratic, humanistic, and holistic models of birth and health care. In: Davis-Floyd R and Colleagues (eds) Ways of knowing about birth: mothers, midwives, medicine, and birth activism. Waveland, Long Grove, pp 3–44

Davis-Floyd R (2018b) Homebirth emergencies in the US and Mexico: the trouble with transport. In: Davis-Floyd R and Colleagues (eds) Ways of knowing about birth: mothers, midwives, medicine, and birth activism. Waveland, Long Grove, pp 283–322

Davis-Floyd R (2018c) The midwifery model of care: anthropological perspectives. In: Davis-Floyd R and Colleagues (eds) Ways of knowing about birth: mothers, midwives, medicine, and birth activism. Waveland, Long Grove, pp 323–338

Davis-Floyd R, Gutschow K, Schwartz D (2020) Pregnancy, birth, and the COVID-19 pandemic in the United States. Med Anthropol 39:413–427. https://doi.org/10.1080/01459740.2020.1761804

DeVries R, Wiegers T, Smulders B et al (2009) The Dutch obstetrical system: vanguard of the future in maternity care. In: Davis-Floyd R, Barclay L, Daviss B-A et al (eds) Birth models that work. University of California Press, Berkeley, pp 31–53

Declercq E (2012) The politics of home birth in the United States. Birth 39(4):281–285

Gammon K (2020) Should you have a home birth because of coronavirus? New York Times 30 Mar 2020

Geerts CC, Klomp T, Lagro-Janssen ALM et al (2014) Birth setting, transfer and maternal sense of control: results from the DELIVER study. BMC Pregnancy Childbirth 14:27. https://doi.org/10.1186/1471-2393-14-27

Gesink D, Nattel L (2015) A qualitative cancer screening study with childhood sexual abuse survivors: experiences, perspectives and compassionate care. BMJ Open 5:1–10

Haen LS (2017) Labor doula care for survivors of sexual violence. Master's Thesis, University of Pittsburgh

Home Birth Summit (HBS) (2014) Best practice guidelines: transfer from planned home birth to hospital. https://www.birthplacelab.org/best-practice-guidelines-for-transfer-from-planned-home-birth-to-hospital/

Home Birth Summit (HBS) (2020) Best practice guidelines for interprofessional collaboration: community midwives and specialist providers. https://www.birthplacelab.org/best-practice-guidelines-for-interprofessional-collaboration/

International Federation of Gynaecology and Obstetrics (FIGO) (2008) Committee report: surrogacy. Int J Gynecol Obstet 102:312–313

Johnson CB, Davis-Floyd R (2006) Home to hospital transport: fractured articulations or magical mandorlas? In: Davis-Floyd R, Johnson CB (eds) Mainstreaming midwives: the politics of change. Routledge, New York, pp 469–506

Johnson KC, Daviss BA (2005) Outcomes of planned home births with certified professional midwives: large prospective study in North America. Br Med J 330(7505):1416. https://doi.org/10.1136/bmj.330.7505.1416

Kuliukas LJ, Lewis L, Hauck YL et al (2015) Midwives' experiences of transfer in labour from a Western Australian birth centre to a tertiary maternity hospital. Women Birth 29:18–23

Lancet Editorial Board (2016) President Trump. Lancet 388(10059):2449

Laws PJ, Zu F, Welsh A, Tracy SK, Sullivan EA (2014) Maternal morbidity of women receiving birth center care in New South Wales: a matched-pair analysis using linked health data. Birth 4(3):268–275

Light AD, Obedin-Maliver J, Sevelius JM, Kerns JL (2014) Transgender men who experienced pregnancy after female-to-male gender transitioning. Obstet Gynecol 124(6):1120–1127

Lindgren HD, Radestad IJ, Hildingsson IM (2011) Transfer in planned home births in Sweden: effects on the experience of birth: a nationwide population-based study. Sex Reprod Health 2(3):101–105

MacDorman MF, Matthews TJ, Declercq E (2012) Home births in the United States, 1990–2009. US Department of Health and Human Services, Centers for Disease Control and Prevention, National Center for Health Statistics, Hyattsville

MacDorman MF, Matthews TJ, Declercq E (2014) Trends in out-of-hospital births in the United States, 1990–2012, NCHS data brief, no. 144. National Center for Health Statistics, Hyattsville

McKay S (1991) Shared power: the essence of humanized childbirth. J Prenatal Perinatal Psychol Health 5(4):283–295

McLachlan HL, Forster DA, Davey MA et al (2012) Effects of continuity of care by a primary midwife (caseload midwifery) on caesarean section rates in women of low obstetric risk: the COSMOS randomised controlled trial. Br J Obstet Gynaecol 119:1483–1492

Midwives Association of Washington State (MAWS) (2016) Indications for discussion, consultation, and transfer of care in a home or birth center midwifery practice. https://www.washington-midwives.org/uploads/1/1/3/8/113879963/maws-indications-2016.pdf. Accessed 29 Jan 2020

Nerum H, Halvorsen L, Oian P, Sorlie T, Straume B, Blix E (2010) Birth outcomes in primiparous women who were raped as adults: a matched controlled study. Br J Obstet Gynaecol 117:288–294

Rothman BK (1982) In labor: women and power in the birthplace. WW Norton, New York

Rowe R, Li Y, Brocklehurst P, Hollowell J (2015) Maternal and perinatal outcomes in women planning vaginal birth after caesarean (VBAC) at home in England: secondary analysis of the birthplace national prospective cohort study. Br J Obstet Gynaecol 123(7):1123–1132

Shaw D, Guise JM, Shah N et al (2016) Drivers of maternity care in high-income countries: can health systems support woman-centered care? Lancet 388(10057):2282–2295

Snowden JM, Tilden EL, Snyder J et al (2015) Planned out-of-hospital birth and birth outcomes. N Engl J Med 373(27):2642–2653

Söderström-Anttila V, Wennerholm UB, Loft A et al (2016) Surrogacy: outcomes for surrogate mothers, children and the resulting families—a systematic review. Hum Reprod Update 22(2):260–276

Van Roosmalen J, Schuitemaker NWE, Brand R, Van Dongen PWJ, Bennebroek Gravenhorst J (2003) Substandard care in immigrant versus indigenous maternal deaths in the Netherlands. Br J Obstet Gynaecol 109(2):212–213

Vedam S, Leeman L, Cheyney M et al (2014) Transfer from planned home birth to hospital: improving interprofessional collaboration. J Midwifery Womens Health 59(6):624–634

Wagner M (2001) Fish can't see water: the need to humanize birth. Int J Gynaecol Obstet 75:S25–S27

Wagner M (2006) Born in the USA: how a broken maternity system must be fixed to put women and children first. University of California Press, Berkeley

Weisband YL, Gallo MF, Klebanoff MA, Shoben AB, Norris AH (2018) Progression of care among women who use a midwife for prenatal care: who remains in midwife care? Birth 45(1):28–36

Wiegers TA, Hukkelhoven CWPM (2010) The role of hospital midwives in the Netherlands. BMC Pregnancy Childbirth 10(1):80. https://doi.org/10.1186/1471-2393-10-80

Chapter 5
Structures for Sustainable Collaboration Between Midwives and Obstetricians in the Netherlands: The Obstetric and Midwifery Manual and Perinatal Care Partnerships

Rachael Kulick Bommarito

5.1 The Collaborative Dynamic Among Midwives and Obstetricians

In most high-resource countries, at least 95% of women give birth in hospitals. In the Netherlands, however, a long-standing tradition of home birth attended by community midwives is integrated into the mainstream maternity care system. While the home birth rate in the Netherlands has declined significantly over the last half century, from 69% in 1965 to 36% in 1978 to 13% in 2019, it is still the highest of any high-resource country (Wiegers et al. 1998; Perined 2019). The high home birth rate depends, in part, on robust cooperation between community midwives to attend the vast majority of home births and obstetricians who provide hospital-based care. My ethnographic research in two locations, a town of 40,000 in North Brabant province and a village of 10,000 in Friesland, illustrates the collaborative dynamics of midwife and obstetrician interactions. This chapter shows how these dynamics both produce and maintain a sustainable maternity care system despite the challenges and disagreements faced by midwives and obstetricians today.

I begin by illustrating the collaborative dynamics via an exchange I observed at a monthly meeting of maternity care providers. Near the meeting's end, an obstetrician stood up to say that while he was not on the agenda, he would like to make a statement. The midwife chairing the meeting joked, to muffled laughter, that the obstetrician always gets the last word. The obstetrician then announced that he would like primary care midwives to refer their clients with suspected fetal or genetic anomalies to him and his team of secondary care providers at the local hospital, where they could receive faster care closer to home, rather than refer them to

R. K. Bommarito (✉)
Accreditation Coordinator, Midwifery Education Accreditation Council (MEAC),
Ann Arbor, MI, USA
e-mail: rachael@umn.edu

© Springer Nature Switzerland AG 2021
K. Gutschow et al. (eds.), *Sustainable Birth in Disruptive Times*, Global
Maternal and Child Health, https://doi.org/10.1007/978-3-030-54775-2_5

the tertiary care center at the academic hospital 90 km away. He described a recent situation in which a midwifery practice referred a client directly to the academic hospital after a midpregnancy anatomy scan revealed a serious fetal anomaly.

A senior midwife in the community who was a researcher and university lecturer stood up in front of nearly 100 colleagues to respond to the obstetrician. She said that the case in question, which involved her practice, was special because by the time the anomaly had been confirmed, the woman only had 7 days before she reached the deadline for termination of pregnancy. Because Dutch law mandated a 5-day waiting period for termination, and the procedure likely had to take place at the academic hospital, the midwives in the practice determined it was in the client's best interest to skip the secondary care providers and go directly to tertiary care so that if the client decided to terminate the pregnancy, she would not miss the legal deadline to do so. The midwife agreed with the obstetrician that, in general, primary care providers should refer their clients to a local hospital rather than tertiary care; however, this situation was unusual. After some back-and-forth, the obstetrician amended his statement and suggested that in *most* cases midwives should refer clients with genetic or fetal anomalies to him.

Another midwife spoke up and lightened the mood. She said she would like to make a deal with the obstetrician. Midwives in the community would send him their clients with fetal anomalies, if he would send them his clients who became pregnant using in vitro fertilization (IVF). In the Netherlands, IVF falls within the scope of obstetricians. However, once a woman becomes pregnant, she may transfer from an obstetrician to a midwife so long as there are no medical indications for specialist care (e.g., multiple gestation or a preexisting health condition that poses increased risk for pregnancy or birth). Midwives have been concerned that obstetricians are keeping IVF clients when they should be referring them to primary care midwives after their pregnancies are confirmed to be physiologically normal.

Such exchanges, in which midwives and obstetricians speak directly to one another on equal footing, do not occur in most countries. In the Netherlands, cooperation across disciplinary divides is facilitated by two structures: (1) the *Obstetric and Midwifery Manual* (OMM), which establishes a division of labor between midwives and obstetricians (College voor Zorgverzekeringen 2003), and (2) Perinatal Care Partnerships (PCPs) that operate in every region of the country and are tasked with the implementation of OMM guidelines at the local level (Koninklijke Nederlandse Organisatie van Verloskundigen 2013). These two structures are crucial to the long-term sustainability of home birth and independent midwifery in the Netherlands because they acknowledge the necessary interdependence of midwives and obstetricians and help build and maintain mutual respect via regular face-to-face interactions oriented around shared goals.

In this chapter, I provide an overview of how the OMM is used in everyday midwifery practice in the Netherlands and examine the effects of regular communication between midwives and obstetricians in one PCP. Data include ethnographic field notes collected during participant observation at midwifery appointments and PCP meetings as well as textual analysis of the OMM and of protocols and procedures published by one PCP from 2008 to the present.

5.2 Organization of Maternity Care in the Netherlands

Dutch maternity care is provided in an echelon system that is organized into three lines (Koninklijke Nederlandse Organisatie van Verloskundigen 2015a). Healthy women with normally progressing pregnancies receive care in the first line and can choose whether to birth at home, in a birth center, or in an outpatient clinic within a hospital. In 2018, 89% of all women started pregnancy in the first line, 51% remained in the first line at the onset of labor, and 28% gave birth under the care of a first-line provider (Perined 2019). Of those who gave birth in the first line, 13% gave birth at home. Midwives provide almost all care in the first line, with general practitioners (GPs) only responsible for roughly 1000 births per year (or 0.006% of all births) (Van der Velden et al. 2012). Since 2002, maternity care has not been taught in the GP curriculum (Cheyney et al. 2019). A short specialization in midwifery was offered for GPs until 2016 when that was discontinued as well. Therefore, I will refer to first-line maternity care providers as midwives.

Some women with preexisting conditions that place them at higher risk for obstetric complications begin prenatal care in the second line. Yet most women who receive care in the second line are referred by their first-line care provider during pregnancy, labor, or the immediate postpartum period. In 2018, 11% of women started pregnancy in the second line, 49% were referred to the second line before the onset of labor, and 72% gave birth in the second line (Perined 2019). Second-line births take place in inpatient maternity wards in hospitals under the supervision of an obstetrician. While some hospital-based clinical midwives work in the second line, obstetricians provide the majority of second-line care.

The third line provides specialized maternal and perinatal care for complex conditions and critically ill women, fetuses, and newborns. This care is provided by obstetricians at academic medical centers or regional hospitals. Third-line facilities include high-risk obstetric and neonatal intensive care units.

5.3 The Dutch *Obstetric and Midwifery Manual*

The three-line maternity care system rests on three assumptions: (1) pregnancy and childbirth are, in most cases, normal physiologic processes; (2) it is possible to identify pathology or increased risk if it develops in pregnancy, labor, birth, or the postpartum period; and (3) first-line care providers can identify pathology and risk and consult with and make timely referrals to the second or third line, as necessary (Bais and Pel 2006). This process of ongoing evaluation, consultation, and referral is called "risk selection."

To aid in risk selection, maternity care providers have constructed lists of medical conditions that require specialized obstetric care. The first list, published in 1959, was known as the Kloosterman List after Dr. Gerrit-Jan Kloosterman, a famous Dutch obstetrician. The most recent version, a consensus document developed by the Royal Dutch Organization of Midwives, the National General

Practitioner Association, and the Dutch Association for Obstetrics and Gynecology, is called the *Obstetric Indications List* or *Verloskundige Indicatielijst* (VIL) and is part of the *Obstetric and Midwifery Manual* (OMM) (College voor Zorgverzekeringen 2003). The VIL plays an important role in establishing the boundaries of professional jurisdiction and in generating a degree of cooperation between midwives and obstetricians that is unusual outside of the Netherlands (De Vries et al. 2009, p. 41).

The VIL catalogs conditions that may lead to complications during pregnancy, labor, birth, or the postpartum period. It labels these conditions as A, B, C, or D. Categories A through C align with increasing levels of risk or concern, while category D is more ambiguous. Category A conditions (e.g., gestational diabetes controlled by diet) may be handled in the first line. The client may choose to birth at home, in a birth center, or in an outpatient clinic, and her first-line midwife may attend her in any of those locations. Category B conditions (e.g., suspected fetal growth restriction) are indications for consultation between a first-line midwife and a second-line obstetrician. Place of birth and attendant depend on the outcome of the consultation. Category C conditions (e.g., amniotic fluid loss prior to 37 weeks of pregnancy) are indications for transfer from the first line to the second line, where responsibility for the client's care is taken over by an obstetrician, and the birth takes place in the inpatient maternity ward of a hospital. Category D conditions (e.g., previous postpartum hemorrhage) may be handled in the first line but are contraindications for home birth, so the client usually stays with her midwife but is advised to give birth in an outpatient clinic at a hospital.

It is important to note that the VIL is only a guide and that care providers can make autonomous decisions (Koninklijke Nederlandse Organisatie van Verloskundigen 2015a). Recent research describes additional considerations that factor into the everyday clinical decision-making of midwives in the Netherlands (Daemers et al. 2017). These include an understanding of the pregnant woman as a whole person, as well as characteristics of the midwife—her experience, intuition, and personal circumstances, as well as her attitude toward physiology, woman-centeredness, shared decision-making, and collaboration. Because issues occasionally arise that are not explicitly addressed in the VIL, the list should not be considered definitive.

5.3.1   *The* Obstetric Indications List *in Everyday Midwifery Practice*

Nadine,[1] 41 weeks pregnant with her first child, has come with her husband to the midwife's office for a routine prenatal appointment. The midwife, Charlotte,[2] discovers that Nadine's diastolic blood pressure is high, at 103. According to the VIL, consultation with an obstetrician is indicated for diastolic blood pressure over 95

---

[1] All names and identifying details were changed to protect the identities of individuals.
[2] All names and identifying details were changed to protect the identities of individuals.

(College voor Zorgverzekeringen 2003, p. 113). Next, Nadine explains that she thinks her water may have broken overnight. Charlotte asks her to lie down on her back on the exam table but is unable to determine whether Nadine's membranes have ruptured. Rupture of membranes without contractions for 24 h is an indication for transfer to the second line (College voor Zorgverzekeringen 2003, p. 117). As 24 h have not passed and Charlotte is not able to confirm that Nadine's membranes have ruptured, there is not a clear indication for consultation or transfer. However, upon palpation of Nadine's abdomen, amniotic fluid levels feel low, and the baby feels large.

Based on physical examination in combination with the fact that Nadine is 1 week past her official due date, Charlotte decides to refer her to the second line for evaluation. She calls the hospital maternity ward to inform them that she is sending in a client. The exchange is collegial and respectful, a normal part of day-to-day midwifery practice in the Netherlands. Charlotte then inputs information from the morning's appointment into her computer, prints an updated prenatal record, and hands it to Nadine. Charlotte also prints a consultation letter that Nadine is to give to the obstetrician when she arrives at the hospital.

Charlotte instructs Nadine and her husband to go home, have lunch, pack a bag, and head to the hospital sometime that afternoon. The care providers at the hospital will listen to the baby, do an ultrasound, assess whether the membranes have ruptured, and then make a plan. Nadine asks Charlotte, "Will they keep me at the hospital or send me home?" Charlotte says they will probably keep her and likely induce. She explains, "They'll see whether your cervix is ripe. If not, they'll probably introduce a prostaglandin gel. If the cervix is ripe, or if it ripens with the aid of the gel, they will start intravenous oxytocin to induce labor." Charlotte will not accompany Nadine to the hospital. For now, Nadine is going in for a consultation, but it is likely that the obstetrician will recommend induction, a category C condition, which will make the birth the responsibility of the second-line care provider.

Nadine begins to cry. She thanks Charlotte for her care and says, "I am mourning the loss of my beautiful home birth with my husband and trusted midwife." Her husband squats by her side, and she turns to face him. They sit, forehead to forehead, eyes closed. He puts his hand on the back of her head and whispers to her.

Later that afternoon, Nadine and her husband go to the hospital. Her labor is induced, and she gives birth to a healthy baby without complications. Following the birth, mother and child return home and to the first line where Charlotte provides in-home postpartum care.

5.4 Perinatal Care Partnerships

In addition to the *Obstetric and Midwifery Manual*, Perinatal Care Partnerships (PCPs) provide a critical structure for communication, negotiation, and cooperation between midwives and obstetricians in the Netherlands. PCPs are organized around every hospital with an obstetrics department (Inspectie voor de Gezondheidszorg

2014). In the province of North Brabant, for example, there are six PCPs, each made up of obstetricians and second-line midwives from the central hospital and first-line midwifery practices located within the hospital's catchment area. Many PCPs also include other health professionals such as general practitioners, pediatricians, and pathologists. Some include emergency medicine or ambulance personnel, representatives from postpartum home care agencies, or members of the health insurance industry. PCPs bring stakeholders together to work across lines of care.

To conduct their work, PCPs follow certain norms of organizational structure. They have regularly scheduled board meetings with a chairperson, agenda, and minutes. They have established agreements about decision-making and handling disputes. They have mechanisms for disseminating information from the board to the broader membership and for bringing the concerns of the membership to the board. The following vignettes illustrate the type of work a PCP undertakes and how it operates.

5.4.1 Two Board Meetings of a Perinatal Care Partnership

The board meeting takes place in a conference room at the local hospital where the seating arrangement is nonhierarchical, and the feeling is one of a "brown bag" discussion or working lunch. The tone of the meeting is collegial. Present are first-line midwives, each representing a different geographic area, and three second-line care providers (a hospital-based midwife, an obstetrician, and a pediatrician). Committee members are called to order by the chairwoman, a second-line midwife, who reviews the agenda for the meeting and then solicits topics for the PCP to consider in the future. Examples of future discussion topics include "Should women taking antidepressant medications be cared for in the first or second line?" "What does the scientific literature say about how to care for women with a body mass index over 30?" "How should we advise our clients on pain medication?" "Is there interest in creating a shadowing program in which first- and second-line care providers follow each other for a day or a week to build respect and understanding?"

After the initial round of comments, the discussion moves to current agenda items. The first item on the agenda involves the establishment of a protocol for returning clients to the first line after a consultation with an obstetrician results in remediation or a finding of no pathology. Currently, there is no such protocol, and when a first-line care provider refers a client to the second line for consultation, the client does not always return to the first line after the issue is resolved. Instead, sometimes the obstetrician will offer the client a choice about where to continue her care. A first-line midwife describes a situation that has come up in her practice. She says that an obstetrician said to one of her clients, "There is nothing wrong. You can now choose if you want to stay here in the second line with me or go back to your midwifery practice in the first line." Another first-line midwife comments, "There should be no choice. The obstetrician should send the woman back to the first line. That is in the best interest of the client, the system, and the division of labor." A third midwife adds, "We also have to work for our bread." There is one obstetrician in the room. He does not respond to these comments. The issue is not resolved. Yet the conversation on this issue has started and will be taken up again at future meetings.

The conversation shifts to a local shortage of maternity care aides (MCAs). MCAs are health professionals who assist midwives during labor and birth as well as care for the woman and infant in the home during the first week postpartum (Cheyney et al. 2019). Under their insurance plans, most women are guaranteed 49 h of postpartum home care by an MCA. However, due to a shortage of MCAs, many women are receiving only minimal care (such as 24 h of medically oriented care). The question at hand is whether this shortage is increasing the workloads of local midwives. The first-line midwives in the room agree that it is, particularly in the realm of breastfeeding support. The amount of additional work they are doing has not been quantified, and they are not currently being compensated for this work.

The group moves to agenda item three. A company based in another part of the country wants to open a postpartum "hotel" in the community. This facility would offer 1 week of postpartum care for the mother and baby, as well as education on topics such as infant feeding, bathing, and safe sleep practices provided by professional maternity care aides. This care has historically been provided in women's homes following a home birth or discharge from the hospital. First-line midwives are frustrated because the company has not consulted with them regarding the development of the postpartum care facility, even though the facility would be providing first-line care. A second-line midwife asks of the first-line midwives, "Why are you opposed to this? What are you afraid of?" A first-line midwife responds, "Before we know it, they will be hiring midwives and doing births at the facility as well." An action step is agreed upon. The PCP will write a letter to the company that is seeking to build the facility. It is the duty of the PCP to make sure that the facility is, above all, in the best interest of women who give birth.

After 90 min, the board meeting concludes with a final round of questions and comments, allowing members to articulate lingering concerns that will be placed on future meeting agendas. A date and time for the next meeting are set before the current meeting is adjourned.

Two months later, the PCP meets again. Present are first-line midwives and four second-line care providers (two hospital-based midwives, an obstetrician, and a pediatrician). Guests include a hospital administrator and the chief executive officer of a local postpartum care company. On the agenda are two topics: the hospital's newly opened birth suites and a local company's plans to open a postpartum care facility. Unlike the facility discussed at the previous meeting, which was to be built by a company from another region, this facility would be built by a local company.

First, the board members discuss the birth suites, which were developed in consultation with community midwives and are intended to offer low-risk women an alternative to home birth. Women who use the new suites will not be admitted to the hospital, and barring any complications, they will return home a few hours after giving birth. As the hospital administrator says, there are no "white coats." Birth support is provided by first-line midwives and maternity care aides, and no hospital staff is involved. Prior to the development of the birth suites, only women who had been transferred to the second line gave birth at this particular hospital.

Now that the suites have been open for 2 months, a hospital administrator is meeting with PCP members to provide an update about changes that have been made based on feedback from first-line midwives who have used the rooms. When the suites first opened, midwives were required to bring all their own supplies, including oxygen tanks. Because it was cumbersome for midwives to carry their oxygen tanks from the parking lot, the hospital will now provide oxygen in the rooms, as well as some disposable medical supplies such as absorbent underpads and gloves. Regarding access to the rooms, midwives will check in and pick up a key at the information desk, and desk personnel will be provided with additional training to avoid confusion. After the birth, the midwife will stay for approximately an hour to monitor the client. The first-line maternity care aide will stay for about 2 h and will be responsible for cleaning the room and returning the key to the information desk. Hallway lights will be left on as a result of feedback that the halls were dimly lit and made the rooms feel uninviting. Finally, the hospital will be offering sandwiches in the vending machines for women who give birth outside of normal business hours when room service is not available. The midwives are generally satisfied that the hospital is listening to them and responding to their concerns.

Next on the agenda is the development of the postpartum care facility. The CEO of the local postpartum care company announces that his company is collaborating with the hospital to develop a birth center, a postpartum hotel, and a perinatal specialty center. Some of the first-line midwives in the room look upset, as their profession was built around providing childbirth and postpartum care in women's homes. With the opening of the hospital's birth suites and now the likely development of a birth center, extended-stay postpartum care facility, and perinatal specialty center, some feel like their business model is under attack. These sorts of facilities already exist in other parts of the country, especially in large urban centers, but they are new to this region.

The CEO reassures the first-line midwives that his core business is first-line maternity care, and his goal is to keep as many births as possible in the first line. He says that his organization is trying to preserve first-line work by rethinking the delivery of care. Further, when he heard that a company from another region was considering building a postpartum hotel in the community, he decided that his company needed to move fast to prevent an outsider from coming in. The proposed facilities would allow low-risk women to give birth in the birth center with their first-line midwife and then move to the postpartum hotel for a week to be cared for by first-line maternity care aides. The perinatal specialty center would provide second- and, potentially, third-line care for complex maternal-fetal conditions during pregnancy, birth, and postpartum.

The CEO goes on to say that he has some bad news. He and the other developers had planned to invite the first-line midwives in the region to a meeting to inform them about plans for the hotel. Only after this meeting took place did they intend to unveil the plan to the community. Unfortunately, the local newspaper got ahold of the story and would be running it the next day. The first-line midwives are not happy. Some have scowls on their faces or arms crossed across their chests. The pediatrician says, "You all have been hearing about this for years. It's not like it's new. Why are you always reactive and not proactive?" The midwives do not respond. After a brief back-and-forth, the board meeting ends in the customary way, with the chairwoman going around the room and offering attendees the opportunity to make a concluding statement. No one says anything. The next day, I look at the local newspaper. The story about the postpartum hotel is on the front page.

This PCP meeting illustrates two disparate approaches to dealing with changes in the organization and delivery of maternity care that are occurring across the country—one in which first-line midwives work in partnership with second-line care providers and institutions to develop innovative solutions and one in which midwives are left out of the process. Midwives are not happy with the latter approach and are worried about what the future may bring for their professional autonomy and status as well as the long-standing practice of interprofessional cooperation.

5.5 The Dutch *Obstetric and Midwifery Manual*

The *Obstetric and Midwifery Manual* (OMM) establishes not only a division of labor between midwives and obstetricians but also an interdependence. While the current OMM was published in 2003, a fully updated OMM has not been produced since then because professional organizations representing midwives and obstetricians have not been in agreement about how to proceed (Cheyney et al. 2019). Revisions to the *Obstetric Indications List* (VIL) were adopted in 2014 and 2016 (College Perinatale Zorg 2014; Koninklijke Nederlandse Organisatie van Verloskundigen 2015b). However, the most recent VIL revisions process was interrupted by work on a new document called the *Care Standard for Integrated Maternity Care* (College Perinatale Zorg 2016).

The *Care Standard* calls for multidisciplinary and "line-transcending" collaboration among maternity care providers. It refers to the OMM as one of a number of sources of guidelines for clinical decision-making. It raises questions about the primacy of the OMM, the division of labor between midwives and obstetricians, and the future of the echelon system of maternity care in the Netherlands.

The creation of the *Care Standard* began with representatives of all parties involved in perinatal care participating in the process. However, the various parties could not agree on a number of tenets, and, after 2 years, the process was taken over by the Dutch Health Care Institute. As such, the *Care Standard* is not a consensus document like the OMM. Nonetheless, it is included in the Register of the Health Care Institute, and, therefore, midwives and obstetricians have an obligation to implement it. Perinatal Care Partnerships have been tasked with determining how to implement it at the local level.

5.6   Perinatal Care Partnerships

Perinatal Care Partnerships (PCPs) bring midwives and obstetricians together for regular, face-to-face communication and negotiation. My initial reflection on the meetings I observed left me disappointed, as it seemed as though little got resolved and few action steps were taken. First- and second-line care providers appeared to be odds with one another, and PCP meetings seemed to highlight conflict more than collaboration. However, I have since come to understand the value of these meetings in two ways.

First, while progress on particular issues may be slow, meaningful progress is made over time. For instance, the beginning of this chapter describes a meeting in 2008 in which an obstetrician argued that midwives should refer their clients with suspected fetal anomalies to him and his team at the local hospital. In 2016, the PCP published a formal protocol regarding referrals for suspected fetal anomalies. In another example from 2008, concerns about antidepressants, obesity, and pain relief during childbirth were brought to the PCP by the membership. In 2009 and 2010, the PCP published guidelines on these subjects, which were further updated in 2015. In these and other cases, dialogue between midwives and obstetricians leads to new or revised protocols, including guidance for interprofessional collaboration in patient care.

Second, these meetings have a more subtle yet potentially more important function. According to the Royal Dutch Organization of Midwives, a core feature of a PCP is that a recurring, fixed day is established for its meetings (Koninklijke Nederlandse Organisatie van Verloskundigen 2013). As a result, regardless of conflicts that arise, first- and second-line care providers come together every month in PCPs across the country to sit face-to-face with one another to discuss their shared concerns and try, above all, to put the needs of birthing people in their communities first. These meetings are part of a long history of collaboration among midwives and obstetricians in the Netherlands that are essential to the sustainability of home birth and independent midwifery in the country.

5.7   Conclusion: Is the Dutch System of Home Birth and Autonomous Midwifery Sustainable?

Despite the large drop in its home birth rate over the last 50 years, the Netherlands still has the highest home birth rate among high-resource countries and the most autonomous midwifery profession in Europe. My research has examined two structures that help sustain these features of the Dutch maternity care system: (1) national-level collaboration agreements like the *Obstetric and Midwifery Manual* that delineate the roles and responsibilities of midwives and obstetricians and affirm both their autonomy and interdependence and (2) regularly occurring meetings of associations such as Perinatal Care Partnerships that bring together midwives and obstetricians to interpret the agreements developed by their professional organizations at the national level and implement them at the local level while building relationship, respect, and trust among colleagues.

In recent years, the professional organizations representing midwives and obstetricians have not been able to reach consensus about how to revise or develop a new national-level collaboration agreement. At the same time, the organization and delivery of maternity care are changing, leaving some analysts and practitioners to wonder about the sustainability of the Dutch model of care. The Dutch case is instrumental, especially in this time of conflict and change, because it suggests that formal structures for collaboration and communication support resilient and sustainable systems, and may provide the foundation for compromise between a range of providers and institutions.

References

Bais J, Pel M (2006) The basis of the Dutch obstetric system: risk selection. Eur Clin Obstet Gynaecol 2(4):209–212

Cheyney M, Goodzari B, Wiegers T et al (2019) Giving birth in the United States and the Netherlands: midwifery care as integrated option or contested privilege? In: Davis-Floyd R, Cheyney M (eds) Birth in eight cultures. Waveland Press, Long Grove, pp 165–202

College Perinatale Zorg (2014) Herziene Onderwerpen Verloskundige Indicatielijst 2014 [Revised topics obstetric indications list 2014]. College Perinatale Zorg, Utrecht

College Perinatale Zorg (2016) Zorgstandaard Integrale Geboortezorg [Care standard for integrated maternity care]. College Perinatale Zorg, Utrecht

College voor Zorgverzekeringen (2003) Verloskundig Vademecum: Eindrapport van de Commissie Verloskunde van het College voor Zorgverzerkeringen [Obstetric and midwifery manual: final report of the Obstetrics Commission of the College for Health Insurance]. College voor Zorgverzekeringen, Diemen

Daemers D, Van Limbeek E, Wijnen H et al (2017) Factors influencing the clinical decision-making of midwives: a qualitative study. BMC Pregnancy Childbirth 17:345

De Vries R, Wiegers T, Smulders B et al (2009) The Dutch obstetrical system: vanguard of the future in maternity care. In: Davis-Floyd R, Barclay L, Daviss B-A et al (eds) Birth models that work. University of California Press, Berkeley, pp 31–53

Inspectie voor de Gezondheidszorg (2014) Mogelijkheden voor verberting geboortezorg nog onvollegdig benut [Possibilities for the improvement of maternity care that have not been fully utilized]. Inspectie voor de Gezondheidszorg, Utrecht

Koninklijke Nederlandse Organisatie van Verloskundigen (2013) Verloskundig Samenwerkingsverbanden (VSV) [Perinatal Care Partnerships (PCPs)]. Resource document. Koninklijke Nederlandse Organisatie van Verloskundigen. https://www.knov.nl/samenwerken/tekstpagina/330-3/verloskundig-samenwerkingsverband-vsv/hoofdstuk/56/verloskundig-samenwerkingsverband-vsv/

Koninklijke Nederlandse Organisatie van Verloskundigen (2015a) Midwifery in the Netherlands. Koninklijke Nederlandse Organisatie van Verloskundigen, Utrecht

Koninklijke Nederlandse Organisatie van Verloskundigen (2015b) Verloskundige Indicatielijst [Obstetric Indications List]. Resource document. Koninklijke Nederlandse Organisatie van Verloskundigen. https://www.knov.nl/vakkennis-en-wetenschap/tekstpagina/524-2/verloskundige-indicatielijst/hoofdstuk/733/verloskundige-indicatielijst/

Perined (2019) Perinatale Zorg in Nederland anno 2018 [Perinatal care in the Netherlands in 2018]. Perined, Utrecht

Van der Velden L, Hingstman L, Wiegers T et al (2012) Verloskundig actieve huisarts bestaat nog steeds [Obstetrically-active general practitioners still exist]. Huisarts en wetenschap 55(3):131

Wiegers T, Van der Zee J, Keirse M (1998) Maternity care in the Netherlands: the changing home birth rate. Birth 25(3):190–197

Chapter 6
Re/Envisioning Birth Work: Community-Based Doula Training for Low-Income and Previously Incarcerated Women in the United States

Rebecca L. Bakal and Monica R. McLemore

6.1 Introduction

Women of color face disproportionately adverse birth outcomes, especially within the context of race, class, mass incarceration, and other forms of structural violence in the United States today. This chapter explores how doula work can link women of color seeking meaningful employment to vulnerable populations. Doula work is sustainable because it provides doulas with valuable work experience and their clients with improved birth outcomes and experiences. We examine how the East Bay Community Birth Support Project (EBCBSP), based in Alameda County, California, helped shape the lives of doulas as well as their clients through a transformative project of community-based care. We look closely at a set of interviews with the doulas from the EBCBSP to consider how doula training can build human capacity, help transform communities from within, and offer a model of empowerment for women of color and previously incarcerated women. The history and goals of the EBCBSP provide a critical window into the scale of change that is necessary to link low-income doula care to clients in an economically sustainable way. We conclude by recommending policies to support the sustainability of doula vocational training programs in the United States.

R. L. Bakal (✉)
Chicago, IL, USA

M. R. McLemore
School of Nursing, University of California San Francisco, San Francisco, CA, USA
e-mail: Monica.McLemore@ucsf.edu

© Springer Nature Switzerland AG 2021
K. Gutschow et al. (eds.), *Sustainable Birth in Disruptive Times*, Global
Maternal and Child Health, https://doi.org/10.1007/978-3-030-54775-2_6

6.2 Racial Disparities in Birth Outcomes

The US healthcare system produces higher maternal morbidity and mortality for Black women than White women: Black women die of pregnancy-related deaths three times as often as White and Hispanic women (Eichelberger et al. 2016). Additionally, infant mortality is 2.3 times as high for Black infants as White infants, according to 2017 government statistics. For over two decades, the medical and research communities in the United States have investigated why Black and other people of color are less safe in pregnancy and childbirth than White people. Accounting for differences in income or education does not eliminate these disparities, but societal, institutional, and provider racism together explain many of the racial disparities in maternal and infant outcomes (Bridges 2011; Davis 2019). Racism causes toxic levels of stress, which impact maternal health as well as fetal growth and development (Villarosa 2018). Despite all these advances in understanding, US healthcare systems continue to fail women of color.

With 2.3 million people behind bars in 2018, the United States locks up more people per capita than any other nation in the world (Stevenson 2015; Sawyer and Wagner 2019). Incarceration disproportionately affects people of color, while police surveillance is an everyday reality for urban communities of color (Goffman 2014; Sufrin 2014). In the United States, African Americans are six times as likely to be incarcerated as Whites, while for Latinx people the incarceration rate is two and a half times that of Whites. While incarceration rates for women are far lower than those for men, the effects of female incarceration upon children, families, and communities are extensive as women frequently are the primary caretakers in their communities (Greenfeld and Snell 2000). Over two-thirds of incarcerated women have children under the age of 18, and mothers face a unique set of issues upon release: they must gain employment while also reconstructing their relationships with their children and their children's caretakers. Individuals with criminal records face compounded barriers to employment and housing security, as well as implicit and explicit bias on the basis of race and previous incarceration (Bloom et al. 2003). Providing vocational training and employment opportunities has been shown to reduce recidivism and build self-esteem (Garcia and Ritter 2012).

6.2.1 Doulas and Better Birth Outcomes

A birth doula is a person, usually a woman, who provides emotional, physical, and social support during labor, delivery, and the postpartum period (Gilliland 2002). Peer-reviewed epidemiological studies have linked doula support to decreased risk of cesarean section (CS), less need for pain medication, shorter labors, higher likelihood of successful breastfeeding, and better mother-infant bonding (Campbell et al. 2006; Gordon et al. 1999; Hodnett and Osborn 1989; Hofmeyr et al. 1991; Kennell et al. 1991; Klaus et al. 1986; McGrath et al. 2004; Sosa et al. 1980).[1] A national survey of doula certification programs in 2003 found that 93.8% of doulas were White; most had some college education and a household income of over $40,000 a year, to which doula work contributed marginally (Lantz et al. 2005). Many community-based doula projects in the United States have worked to expand access to doula care among women of color and other marginalized women and tried to diversify doula care by training women of color and low-income women to be doulas (Beets 2014; HealthConnect One 2019). These projects have shown promising results, with doulas often providing critical support while building their own skills and confidence (Breedlove 2005; Gentry 2010).

6.3   The East Bay Community Birth Support Project

The East Bay Community Birth Support Project (EBCBSP) began in 2014 by training 16 women to become birth doulas, 8 of whom were low-income and 8 of whom were previously incarcerated (Stanley et al. 2015). A team led by women of color developed and implemented the training program by applying birth traditions practiced in African, Black, and Latinx communities. The project was explicitly designed to address the stigma of incarceration by including both women who had been incarcerated and those who had not, which afforded participant anonymity, mentor support, and long-lasting professional networks, as we will explore. Each trainee attended five births of low-income women of color who were referred by local agencies. Previously incarcerated participants were compensated for their time at these births, while other participants volunteered their time, as is typical in other doula training programs. The EBCBSP ran until 2016, later becoming the Roots of Labor Birth Collective.

6.4   The Experiences of Doula Trainees and the Impact of Doula Training

We conducted semi-structured interviews with 12 doulas in the EBCBSP training, as well as with the 2 organizers of the training. Of our 14 interlocutors, 7 identified as Black and 5 as Latina; of the doulas, 4 had been incarcerated and 8 had not.[2] While some of the trainees had been looking explicitly for a low-cost doula training oriented toward low-income or people of color, the previously incarcerated trainees

---

[1] Doula support can have a pronounced impact in low-income settings, or when a birth companion is not present. For instance, doulas in resource-poor settings have been shown to dramatically decrease labor length (Campbell et al. 2006; Klaus et al. 1986; Sosa et al. 1980).

[2] The race/ethnicity of two interlocutors remains unidentified in order to protect confidentiality.

first heard about doula work when approached to be part of the program itself. For these women, the welcoming approach of the trainers and the focus on building community and trust was critical to their buy-in.

The trainers designed the doula curriculum to reflect the needs of communities of color by building in diversity and sensitivity. Tanya[3] explained: "We added resources that were particular to persons of color and Latino and Latina people and Black people and [were] trying to make the training more well-rounded and more encompassing of everyone instead of [just] maybe a privileged person who can afford a doula." They also updated the resource binder to reflect resources for low-income and previously incarcerated persons and brought in guest teachers who were women of color with experience in birth work.

Trainees learned the basic physiology of childbirth, including some of the tools, terms, and regulations they would encounter when supporting clients in hospital-based birth. The trainees also learned to be attuned to the social and emotional needs of their clients, which they found often took precedence over actual birth coaching. Roxane said:

> For people who might be more privileged, their only worry right now is their birth. But for many of the women, especially the women that we serve through the Project, there are things related to housing. There's things related to domestic violence. There's things related to finances, trauma. I mean racism big time. Like these are all things—just the way that historically our society has shaped our experiences and our communities, there's much more than pregnancy that is impacting this person.

The EBCBSP training employed an intersectional lens to empower doulas to address multiple axes of oppression that shape birth—including race, class, gender, and carceral history. As a result, the new doulas found that the scope of their care extended far beyond birth and into many other realms of their clients' lives. Several of our interlocutors used the language of sacred or safe space to describe their training, which implies a linkage between social connection and personal empowerment. Patricia Hill Collins (2009, 111) discusses the importance of "safe space" for Black women, calling it "a necessary condition for Black women's resistance... By advancing Black women's empowerment through self-definition, these safe spaces help Black women resist the dominant ideology promulgated not only outside Black civil society but within African-American institutions."

6.5   Negotiating Birthing Spaces

Practicing what they learned in their training, the EBCBSP doulas employed an ability to "boundary cross" between the medical realms and their clients' communities. The doulas used their familiarity with their clients' life circumstances to help

---

[3] Names and identifying details of all interlocutors have been changed to protect confidentiality, unless otherwise specified.

their clients feel more comfortable in a room full of medical personnel with rather different backgrounds. Having gained literacy in the medical management of birth and familiarity with hospital-based birth, the doulas wielded the symbolic capital their clients lacked to create a bridge between their clients and the healthcare providers. Sometimes the doulas advocated for their clients, and if that did not appear feasible, they served as a reminder that their clients were not alone in their struggles.

As women of color providing care for other women of color, the doulas often engaged in "medical translating," either helping to explain clinical information to their clients or literally translating between their clients and clinical staff. Their intersectional work included helping their clients communicate with their care providers, even if the solutions they found were compromises in a constrained environment. In one case, Rose had a client who did not speak English and whose care providers did not speak Spanish. Rose explained a situation in which a nurse frantically yelled at her client:

> So [the nurse] starts yelling at her like, "Stop pushing. Stop pushing." And then [the client] is like, "What's she saying?" I'm like, "Oh, she's telling you to stop pushing." And she's like, "But I'm not pushing." And the nurse is like, "What did she say?" And I was like, "She's saying she's not pushing." And I could tell that this nurse is just not helping.

The doulas helped mitigate or deflect the explicit or implicit bias their clients might face around race, socioeconomic status, national origin, drug use, age, or other factors.

6.6 Reflecting on Changes in Network

Many of the EBCBSP doulas established deep bonds with their fellow trainees that led to fruitful personal and professional partnerships, helping them further their education and work as doulas or find other employment. The training offered a clear path for low-income women of color and previously incarcerated women to create new social and professional networks that shaped subsequent career choices. Carla said, "I feel really close to my cohort. We still hang out a lot, I see people a lot. We share resources, we teach each other how to make each others' websites and business cards and stuff like that." The community that these doulas created helped them gain confidence in marketing themselves, as well as finding jobs and childcare, which made their birth work both more fulfilling and more fun. Dana said, "Two of the births I did with another trainee from the program, and those were really awesome because she and I worked really well together." Doula training had provided an opportunity for these women to connect to each other in ways that their other work, at a kennel and providing in-home care, did not. To overcome the difficulty of finding childcare at such short notice, the doulas who were moms created a "childcare pool" to free each other to sign up for births. The doulas also used social media and email listservs to connect with their cohort and establish a wider network of professional birth workers in the Bay Area. Doulas from the EBCBSP training use an active Facebook group to ask each other for advice, request backup doulas, and post job opportunities, as well as help their clients in a variety of ways.

6.6.1 Empowerment

Several of the doulas we interviewed used the language of empowerment to indicate how doula work reaches far beyond reproductive healthcare. In fact, empowerment was one of the main benefits of doula work both for doulas and their clients. Empowerment is a central theme in Black feminist scholarship, defined as the result of "what happens when an individual Black woman's consciousness concerning how she understands her everyday life undergoes change" (Hill Collins 2009: xi). For Brea, doula training helped her to trust in her own goals, because she had often felt trapped between what she "should" be doing as a college graduate and what she really wanted to be doing. The doula training helped her bring her dreams and life into alignment: "Taking this step and completing the doula training, becoming a doula, has kind of empowered me to say, 'You know what? What you actually really want is important, and seizing it in the moment that your heart wants it, is also really important. This is your life. You get to determine what happens with it.'" Many other doulas shared similar sentiments about taking control of their lives and recognizing their own agency. These changes in self-determination reverberated outward to the doula's families, clients, and their clients' families, as they assisted their communities in taking ownership over their health. The concept of empowerment came up in many different interviews and contexts, usually in reference to helping doulas and their clients feel more agency and ownership over their experiences.

6.7 Challenges to Sustainability

The doulas struggled to fit their doula work into their other responsibilities, including raising children, holding down other jobs, and caring for families. Brea, who was juggling waitressing and raising her 2-year-old, said, "When your tank's not full to begin with, it's hard to support someone else." While she struggled with finding childcare during her birth work, other doulas had trouble juggling jobs with volunteer doula work. Maria recalled a time when she was supporting a birth and had to call in sick:

> My husband was like, "You can't keep just calling in sick." Because I don't have benefits right now [at my job], so it's like losing a whole day worth of paid work to [volunteer]. I mean, I, it was still fulfilling to me, but then when it came time to pay the bills, my husband was like, "Are you gonna keep doing that, because we can't compensate for your lost hours." He would joke around and be like, "Feeling fulfilled doesn't the pay the rent."

While Maria felt that doula work was meaningful, her husband reminded her that it was financially untenable for their family. It was challenging for Maria to reconcile a commitment to financially support her family with a desire to do doula work for low-income women. Mediating between financial and family responsibilities is not unique to doula work, but doulas face special difficulty balancing volunteer doula work with inflexible shift-based jobs, family stressors, and financial worries.

6.7.1 "This is Where My Heart Lies, but Realistically Speaking I Can't Do It": Money as Barrier

Like Maria, many of the doulas we interviewed expressed frustration that they couldn't do doula work full-time for low-income women. They felt torn between a desire to serve low-income women and the need to make money. Brea knew that every time she supported a birth, she was losing money because of the cost of transportation, cancelling shifts at work, and childcare. Yet she wanted to stay true to the mission of the EBCBSP by serving low-income women:

> The kind of doula work I want to do, I refuse to take clients who are able to pay me, like $1500, which is what it would cost for me to be able to take the time away from my family like that. That's not the demographic that I'm drawn to serve. This is a service for me, you know. I feel really compelled to give back to my community or at least a community that isn't able to access birth support financially.

Seeking out paid doula work did not feel true to her values, because it would mean serving middle-class women while many low-income women of color needed birth support but lacked access. While some of the EBCBSP doulas did try to seek out paid birth doula work, they struggled to market themselves. Some looked to one of their trainers, Linda Jones[4]—who is one of the most experienced Black doulas in the East Bay—as an example, figuring that if she could make a living as a doula, so could they. Yet Linda supports herself not only with birth work but also with postpartum doula work—which includes caring for newborns, birth mothers, and parents in the postpartum period—primarily for paying clients, so that she can attend to low-income women as well. Linda has an established pay structure based on client income. Many of the doulas struggled to develop a pay structure that could work for them. Maria described her thinking about doula work so far:

> Your value is based on the work that you do and how the person that you helped values you. And even so, some of the births that I attended, there would've been no way for me to expect them to pay anything [because they couldn't have afforded it]. And just knowing that I made a difference, right now, is good enough for me, but I can't live off of x, y, and z thinking I was awesome and that they couldn't have had their babies the way they did if I hadn't been there.

---

[4] Linda Jones's name and identifying information are used with permission.

Like Maria, many doulas feel torn between the satisfaction of doula work for clients who appreciate them and the need to make a living. The ambivalence of being stuck between the goal of caring for others and the need for income prevents other low-income women from becoming doulas.

6.7.2 "I'm Down for Birth": Making It Work

The EBCBSP doulas and trainees who were most financially successful had three ways of moving past this dilemma: (1) they took on some paying doula clients in order to subsidize their volunteer work with the demographic they preferred to serve; (2) they did other work for pay so that they could volunteer birth support; and (3) they moved into allied professions like midwifery and nursing, so that they could help birthing women as part of an established pay structure.

(1) *Taking on paying clients*: For the doulas who took on paying clients, it was often feasible to set aside money from clients who paid the full fee to cover the costs of supporting low-income clients. Carla said that she was in the process of working out the logistics of this kind of system. "I'm down for birth. I know that's a possibility where I can have someone pay me and then let them know that part of their payment is going to someone that can't and establish some kind of relationship like that between my clients so that I could do that work." In Carla's vision, her clients would know that their full payment includes part of the cost of another woman's birth. So, rather than Carla needing to sacrifice income, she enables a transfer of care from middle-class clients to lower-income clients. Tanya has a basic payment plan, but she talks through the costs of her care with all clients and explains that she is open to alternate payment options. This puts the onus on her clients to request to pay less and allows those clients who can pay the full fee to help subsidize those who cannot.

(2) *Doing other work for pay*: Several of the EBCBSP doulas do other work for pay, either to supplement their birth doula work long-term or just temporarily, until they can get their doula practice off the ground. Many of them do work that is related to birth, like placenta encapsulation, postpartum doula work, or childcare. Others work as medical assistants or at universities and public health nonprofits. Dana decided to go back to school to become a massage therapist. She sees it as a compromise that will allow her to continue doing doula work: "If I have to do work as a massage therapist to allow me to be able to do work with low-income doula clients, then that's what I'll do." Gabrielle said: "As a doula I'm doing pretty well, because I also do postpartum doula work, and that's where there's a lot of money because people that can afford a postpartum doula can usually fork out the full amount for it." She found that she could supplement her volunteer birth doula work with paid postpartum work.

(3) *Moving into allied professions*: For some, like Gabrielle, paid employment has helped them train to be a direct-entry midwife. At least 3 of the 16 EBCBSP

doulas had begun to pursue additional training as midwives or nurses in the year after their training. It is common for doula work to be a gateway to other medical careers (Morton and Clift 2014). Rose, who was considering midwifery training, said:

> I can't do volunteer work forever. I need to eat. I need to pay bills. And the women in my community who we assist, most of them cannot afford to pay for a doula. So, that's why I'm considering being a midwife, because when you're a midwife you can get more money paid or maybe a little bit more stability than being a doula.

Rose sees becoming a midwife as a way to keep serving women from her own community but without having to worry as much about finances. Maria had a similar logic: "Nurses make a lot. And in the hospitals, you know, a doula will only get paid as much as she sells herself by, but as a nurse you have a degree, and you have all this schooling behind you, so I'm not saying they're worth more, but you know, to people that hand out checks, you're worth more as a nurse than a doula." Rose and Maria felt that, if they wanted to work in the birthing field, doula work would not be a well-compensated option. Yet those who sought to become clinicians often recognized that leaving doula work was a missed opportunity for birth support in underserved communities. Martina, who is pursuing direct-entry midwife training, noted that one of her doula trainers said, "I hope you stay a doula."

Many of these strategies represent compromises that enable low-income women to provide birth support to other low-income women. Yet doula work is still undervalued—not recognized monetarily for its potential to improve birth. Brea captures this gap between the current landscape of doula care and what could exist:

> I don't think the space has been carved out yet for that person to exist, for someone who does view birth as something very political to have it generate the bulk of their income. It's not there because the two things just kind of clash. It's uber-capitalist for you to be like, "I'm gonna generate all this income." But you can't serve a certain community in that. I mean, I think that's the community that you really need to target if you think that this is political work or work for the social good. So I think that they'll exist one day, but we're doing the work right now to make that a possibility.

Brea claims that while it is difficult to provide doula support only for low-income women, this kind of doula work could be sustainable if it were properly subsidized and recognized as a social and public good.

6.7.3   "I Could Be Part of the Solution": Doulas Envisioning Their Role in Systemic Change

Doulas see their individual-level work as possibly leading to systems-level change. Some of the systemic changes they hoped to see were in policy, like Medicaid reimbursement for doulas. Other changes were more grassroots, like increasing the number of doulas of color and the accessibility of doula care for women of color. There is a growing trend of low-income women of color acting as advocates for healthcare in their communities as well as other transformative change (Mullings and Wali 2001). The EBCBSP doulas saw doula work as a way to envision a world of better healthcare for women in their communities. By helping women to aspire toward their ideal births, the doulas also began to create larger-scale visions for better maternity care and healthcare.

Through the training process, many of the doulas realized they might be able to help fix a broken maternity care system where lack of access and discrimination lead to poor outcomes for women of color. Tanya, who had helped organize the training, said, "I think it just made me confront the issues around health equity and health disparities. And I'm just feeling really action-oriented around it, and I'm feeling really ticked that doula services are not accessible for everyone." Like Tanya, Brea recalled her experience of becoming aware as to how she might move the needle toward community empowerment through doula work. The training led her to reflect on her own birth and how she had felt judged as a young Black woman trying to have a natural birth. She realized, "I could be part of the solution to my own problem. I didn't think it was quite fair that I was in a position where I couldn't pay almost two grand for someone to support me in my labor." By becoming a doula, Brea felt that she could meet the needs of other women of color during their births.

Additionally, many doulas believe diversification of the pool of doulas should improve access to maternity care among low-income women and women of color. Roxane said:

> My hope is that there are going to be more trainings like this offered and that it could be sustainable and actually where the woman can get paid and that Medi-Cal reimbursement will become something that's definitely available. Yeah, that's my hope, is that more women of color are able to serve as doulas in their communities, that women are able to serve the communities that they're from and receive care from the communities that they're from.

Roxane and Desiree specifically mentioned the importance of providing care to incarcerated women. Desiree said, "I really want to make sure that—that was my goal—that people that have been incarcerated or have had pasts at least have some support where the person doesn't care." In Desiree's view, a person who "doesn't care" is someone who doesn't judge: someone who accepts the birthing person and does not view her as lesser because of a history of incarceration or drug addiction. Carla connected doula support for communities of color to the more global well-being of those communities: "[If] we're really thinking about supporting communities of color to thrive, then we need to put people of color that are from those communities there to do that work."

Several of the other doulas we interviewed tied improving birth for women of color back to a larger goal of improving society and health. Brea considers providing emotionally supportive birthcare for women of color "a Step One in curing some of what ails society." Brea said that encouraging mothers and parents to take "ownership" over their birth experiences can lead to emotional reinvestment in their families and communities. The notion that birth can be a platform for societal change is common among doulas who believe that "birth is inextricable from people's lives as a whole, not reducible to a set of measurements or a single experiential moment" (Basile 2012: 98).

6.8   Conclusions: The "Roots of Labor Collective" and Policy Implications

In January 2017, the EBCBSP refocused their work and developed the Roots of Labor Birth Collective in order to make doula work more sustainable for members. The collective developed a website (http://www.rootsoflaborbc.com/) and social media pages and expanded their referral relationships. These changes allow for a central repository for doula referrals and collective capacity for backup doula support as well as structural support for mentoring new doulas who are most vulnerable in their early years of work. The collective has developed an application for not-for-profit status and obtained a fiscal sponsor to expand and diversify its funding. The doulas are working toward sustainability in an imperfect system.

The EBCBSP was an answer to two critical injustices: (1) low-income women of color, including those with a carceral history, need self-directed employment that draws on their skills and interests; and (2) low-income birthers of color would benefit from better support throughout the prenatal, birth, and postpartum periods. One of the greatest barriers to doula care is cost. Paying out of pocket for a doula is unaffordable for many low-income women, while serving as a volunteer doula can be unsustainable without supplemental income and support from the community and family. The ideal policy solution would use a third-party payment system to allow low-income birthers to access doulas and assist low-income doulas in generating income. The integration of doula services into the social safety net would resolve the barriers that doulas face in marketing themselves, while the improved birth outcomes would more than pay for the programs. In order to meet the demand that this system would create, it is critical to offer low-cost or free doula trainings.

6.8.1   Medicaid Coverage of Doula Care

Seeking third-party reimbursement is critical to creating sustainable access to doula care. This would enable low-income women on Medicaid to access doula care and would allow doulas to earn a living from serving women who can benefit from their care but could not otherwise afford it. Public funding for doula care could save money by reducing the use of costly medical interventions in birth and improve maternal and neonatal health (Strauss et al. 2016). Access to doula care could lead to a savings of $58.4 million each year for Medicaid in the Midwest alone—partly because doula care reduces the high risk and costs of preterm birth (Kozhimannil et al. 2016).

Medicaid reimbursement for doula care is not a cure-all. Minnesota implemented such reimbursement in 2013 and is currently navigating several challenges: low reimbursement rates that are a barrier for doulas, lack of available doula trainings that focus on trauma, poverty, or other challenges specific to low-income birthers, and lack of awareness about doula coverage among both Medicaid beneficiaries and providers (Kozhimannil et al. 2015). Even so, Medicaid coverage for doula care is a critical step to improving maternal health outcomes and experiences of low-income women, especially women of color.

Within the past few years, several additional states have begun to build pathways for Medicaid reimbursement for doula care, including Oregon, New York, New Jersey, Indiana, and Washington—and several more have introduced legislation to do so (HealthConnect One 2019). Doula care is an evidence-based way to reduce the incidence of cesarean sections, preterm birth, and other costly health outcomes. This is *especially* true for low-income women, who would benefit from Medicaid coverage of doula care (Campbell et al. 2006).

6.8.2 *"A Starter Kit to Your Baby": Doula Care as an Institutionalized Social Service*

Medicaid reimbursement will only increase access to doula care if it is coupled with programs to disseminate information about birth support coverage and with programs that match clients with doulas. Gabrielle told me that she thinks the United States should give everyone a "starter kit to your baby." She was not just referring to physical objects like diapers and baby clothes but to the state doing a better job of supporting women before, during, and after delivery. Integrating doula care into prenatal care would create an access point, while linking it to postpartum care improves both maternal and neonatal outcomes (see Chap. 14, which shows that neonatal mortality is a huge fraction of infant mortality). Until these programs exist, most low-income women may not know that doula care is an option, especially *for them*. While Medicaid coverage for doula care has become a rallying cry, nonprofit and government organizations will help ensure that Medicaid coverage is not underutilized.

6.8.3 *Vocational Training for Previously Incarcerated Women*

Folding doula care into the social safety net will lead to improved birth outcomes, increased demand for doula care, and better maternity care for Medicaid recipients. Many of the doulas we interviewed recognized that women from at-risk populations could meet these needs by giving back to their community and becoming more empowered through birth work. Doula work allowed women to develop skills that they could use to serve their communities, support themselves, and draw on interpersonal skills and experiences in a way that many other jobs do not. As reentry training programs become key to mitigating the impacts of mass incarceration, policymakers should consider vocational trainings that allow participants to use life experiences (e.g., having given birth) to inform their work. Funding for such trainings is paramount to the successful reintegration of formerly incarcerated women while being a gateway to other paid employment and personal fulfillment. We propose Medicaid coverage for doula care, the integration of doula services into other social programs, and vocational trainings to equip formerly incarcerated individuals to serve their own communities. Together, these could systemically address lack of employment opportunities for formerly incarcerated low-income women of color and meager social support in maternity care for at-risk families. In an ideal world, all women should be able to birth and work in meaningful ways that empower themselves and their communities.

References

Basile MR (2012) Reproductive justice and childbirth reform: doulas as agents of social change. PhD dissertation, University of Iowa

Beets VD (2014) The emergence of U.S. hospital-based doula programs. PhD dissertation, University of South Carolina

Bloom BE, Owen B, Covington SS (2003) Gender-responsive strategies: research, practices, and guiding principles for women offenders. US National Department of Justice

Breedlove G (2005) Perceptions of social support from pregnant and parenting teens using community-based doulas. J Perinat Educ 14(3):15–22

Bridges K (2011) Reproducing race: an ethnography of pregnancy as a site of racialization. University of California Press, Berkeley

Campbell D et al (2006) A randomized controlled trial of continuous support in labor by a lay doula. J Obstet Gynecol Neonatal Nurs 35(4):456–464

Collins PH (2009) Black feminist thought. Routledge, New York

Davis DA (2019) Reproductive injustice: racism, pregnancy, and premature birth. NYU Press, New York

Eichelberger KY et al (2016) Black lives matter: claiming a space for evidence-based outrage in obstetrics and gynecology. Am J Public Health 106(10):1771–1772

Garcia M, Ritter N (2012) Improving access to services for female offenders returning to the community. Natl Inst Justice J 269:18–23

Gentry QM (2010) 'Going beyond the call of doula': a grounded theory analysis of the diverse roles community based doulas play in the lives of pregnant and parenting adolescent mothers. J Perinat Educ 19(4):24–40

Gilliland AL (2002) Beyond holding hands: the modern role of the professional doula. J Obstet Gynecol Neonatal Nurs 31(6):762–769

Gordon NP et al (1999) Effects of providing hospital-based doulas in health maintenance organization hospitals. Obstet Gynecol 3:426–444

Goffman A (2014) On the run: fugitive life in an American city. University of Chicago Press, Chicago

Greenfeld LA, Snell TL (2000) Women offenders. Bureau of Justice Statistics. https://www.bjs.gov/index.cfm?ty=pbdetail&iid=568

HealthConnect One (2019) HealthConnect One issue brief: Creating policy for equitable doula access. https://www.healthconnectone.org/new-hc-one-issue-brief-creating-policy-for-equitable-doula-access/. Accessed 4 Apr 2020

Hodnett ED, Osborn RW (1989) Effects of continuous intrapartum professional support on childbirth outcomes. Res Nurs Health 12:289–297

Hofmeyr GJ et al (1991) Companionship to modify the clinical birth environment: effects on progress and perceptions of labour and breastfeeding. Br J Obstet Gynaecol 98:756–764

Kennell JH et al (1991) Continuous emotional support during labor in a US hospital: a randomized controlled trial. J Am Med Assoc 265:2197–2201

Klaus MH et al (1986) Effects of social support during parturition on maternal and infant morbidity. Br Med J 293:585–587

Kozhimannil KB, Voselgang CA, Hardeman RR (2015) Medicaid coverage of doula services in Minnesota: preliminary findings from the first year. Interim report to the Minnesota Department of Human Services July 2015

Kozhimannil KB et al (2016) Modeling the cost-effectiveness of doula care associated with reductions in preterm birth and cesarean delivery. Birth 43(1):20–27. https://doi.org/10.1111/birt.12218

Lantz P et al (2005) Doulas as childbirth paraprofessionals: results from a national survey. Womens Health Issues 15:109–116

McGrath S et al (2004) Doula support and breastfeeding success. J Dev Behav Pediatr 25:373–374

Morton CH, Clift E (2014) Birth ambassadors: doulas and the re-emergence of woman-supported birth in America. Praeclarus Press, Amarillo

Mullings L, Wali A (2001) Stress and resilience: the social context of reproduction in Central Harlem. Kluwer Academic/Plenum Publishers, New York

Sawyer W, Wagner P (2019) Mass incarceration: the whole pie https://www.prisonpolicy.org/reports/pie2019.html

Sosa R et al (1980) The effect of a supportive companion on perinatal problems, length of labor, and mother infant interaction. N Engl J Med 303:597–600

Stanley D et al (2015) The East Bay community birth support project, a community-based doula program to decrease recidivism in previously incarcerated women. J Obstet Gynecol Neonatal Nurs 44(6):743–750

Stevenson B (2015) Just mercy: a story of justice and redemption. Spiegel & Grau, New York

Strauss N, Sakala C, Corry MP (2016) Overdue: Medicaid and private insurance coverage of doula care to strengthen maternal and infant health. J Perinat Educ 25(3):145–149. https://doi.org/10.1891/1058-1243.25.3.145

Sufrin, CB (2014) Jailcare: the safety net of a U.S. women's jail. PhD dissertation, University of California, San Francisco

Villarosa L (2018) Why America's black mothers and babies are in a life-or-death crisis. New York Times, 11 Apr 2018

Chapter 7
Sustainable Metrics: Using Measurement-Based Quality Improvement to Improve Maternity Practice While Avoiding Frustration and Pitfalls

Kathleen H. Pine and Christine H. Morton

7.1 Introduction

Quality measures are powerful tools used by change agents to illuminate persistent problems within maternity care that can support the trend toward evidence-based clinical practice. Increasingly, systems of accountability and reimbursement are also using quality measures. Additionally, widespread availability of information and communication technologies (ICTs) and perceptions that data are more readily available have ushered in a new era of accountability in healthcare. Healthcare in general has seen a rapid digitization of work systems, including the mass adoption of electronic health record (EHR) systems. In the era of ICT-embedded accountability, performance measurements have proliferated and are accessible to hospitals more quickly than ever before. Quality measurements are used to highlight underperforming areas of clinical practice, evaluate the outputs of practice changes, and establish performance baselines for providers and healthcare staff, a process known as quality improvement (QI).

Change agents are working to ensure that organizational and individual practices develop capacities to calculate, report, and incorporate quality measures in order to significantly improve US maternity care and quality. In the context of obstetrics, such efforts are relatively recent, as there have been few external reporting requirements. Despite widespread adoption of data-driven accountability tools and practices, maternity care organizations and clinicians face a number of challenges to engaging in quality measurement.

K. H. Pine (✉)
College of Health Solutions, Arizona State University, Phoenix, AZ, USA
e-mail: khpine@asu.edu

C. H. Morton (✉)
Stanford University School of Medicine, Palo Alto, CA, USA
e-mail: cmorton@stanford.edu

© Springer Nature Switzerland AG 2021
K. Gutschow et al. (eds.), *Sustainable Birth in Disruptive Times*, Global Maternal and Child Health, https://doi.org/10.1007/978-3-030-54775-2_7

We provide a practical guide to the landscape of quality measurement in maternity care. We consider ways to utilize quality measurements in appropriate and beneficial ways while avoiding some of the pitfalls of the intensively quantitative regime of data-driven accountability and QI. Maternity care systems and clinicians are now required to report an array of external quality measures; we show how these quality measures can be integrated into and contribute to a sustainable maternity care system. Our insights are focused on the United States but may be relevant abroad as maternity care clinicians grapple with the promises and perils of quality measurement.

7.2 Maternal Care QI: A Recent Focus

Maternal quality measures have been advanced as one of the key mechanisms for improving maternal outcomes, including infant and maternal mortality and morbidity, through aligning obstetric practice with evidence-based standards (Janakiraman and Ecker 2010; Main and Bingham 2008). Yet until recently, maternity care was left out of the larger QI movement in medicine (Jolivet and Main 2010). A major reason for the omission of maternity care is that Medicare (the program that provides public insurance to senior citizens and people with disabilities) has dominated much of the development and utilization of quality measures. Medicare is administered through the federal government, while Medicaid, the public insurance program that pays for 43% of all US births, is administered at the state level (Martin et al. 2018). While the federal government has long tied performance criteria to Medicare payments, states began to explore tying Medicaid reimbursement rates to hospital performance on certain quality measures in the mid-2000s (Kuhmerker and Hartman 2007). The 2010 Patient Protection and Affordable Care Act (ACA) includes several provisions relevant to childbearing women, which are expected to escalate the use of maternity care quality measures over time. Section 2701, for example, provides a directive to develop a healthcare quality measurement program for adult beneficiaries of Medicaid; this program is viewed as an opportunity for newly adopted maternity care quality measures to be used for evaluation of Medicaid programs that include maternity benefits (Wier and Andrews 2011).

7.3 Key Organizations and Advances in Maternal Care Quality Measurement

7.3.1 National Organizations

The National Quality Forum (NQF) is an organization charged with considering, evaluating, and endorsing quality measures in the United States. A wide variety of organizations work to develop measures, including The Joint Commission (TJC),

Centers for Medicare & Medicaid Services (CMS), professional organizations, and hospital systems. These organizations draft and submit potential quality measures to NQF for endorsement consideration. NQF is the sole organization responsible for endorsing quality measures and plays a significant role in shaping US quality improvement. Once endorsed, measures can be adopted by organizations for quality improvement activities at the local and national levels by health departments, payers, purchasers, and perinatal quality collaboratives, to name a few.

In 2008, NQF endorsed 17 submitted maternity care quality measures (Morton et al. 2017). This action created a pool of vetted measures from which hospitals, regulatory agencies, and other stakeholders could select measures for QI efforts and reporting requirements. NQF published these measures as the *National Voluntary Consensus Standards for Perinatal Care 2008* (Table 7.1). The NQF updated these measures in 2011 and again in 2016 (NQF 2018).

TJC is a key player in assessing and publicly reporting maternity care quality. As of 2016, hospitals with 300 or more births per year were required to collect data and report a new perinatal care (PC) measure set (Table 7.2). Most hospitals that provide maternity services meet this requirement. The set of five measures was re-endorsed by TJC in 2016, with an additional PC measure added in 2019 on unexpected newborn complications, designed to be a balancing measure for PC-02 (Lyons 2018).

Table 7.1 NQF voluntary consensus standards for perinatal care 2008 (Data from (NQF 2009))

Measure title	Level of analysis
Elective delivery prior to 39 completed weeks gestation	Facility
Incidence of episiotomy	Facility
Cesarean rate for low-risk first birth	Facility, group, integrated system, or community
Prophylactic antibiotic in cesarean sections (CS)	Facility
Appropriate deep vein thrombosis prophylaxis in women undergoing CS	Facility
Birth trauma rate measures	Facility
Appropriate use of antenatal steroids	Facility
Infants under 1500 g delivered at appropriate site	Facility, integrated system, or community
Nosocomial bloodstream infection in neonates	Facility
Birth dose of hepatitis B vaccine and hepatitis immune globulin for newborns of mothers with chronic hepatitis B	Facility
Exclusive breastfeeding at hospital discharge	Facility, integrated system, or community
Paired measures	Facility
First temperature of newborn within 1 h of admission to NICU	
And	Facility
First NICU temperature < 36°C	
Retinopathy of prematurity screening	Facility
Timely surfactant administration to premature neonates	Facility
Neonatal immunization	Facility

Table 7.2 TJC perinatal core measure set (Data from (The Joint Commission 2009))

Measure description and developer	Explanation (summary)	Data elements	Type
PC-01. Percentage of patients with elective vaginal deliveries or elective cesarean sections at greater than or equal to 37 and less than 39 weeks of gestation completed	Elective inductions result in more CS deliveries, longer maternal length of stay	Documentation patient was in active labor	Process
	Repeat elective CS before 39 weeks results in higher rates of adverse outcomes for newborns	ICD-10-PCS principal procedure code	
		ICD-10-PCS other procedure codes	
		Documentation SROM	
PC-02. Percentage of nulliparous women with term, singleton baby in vertex position delivered by CS	CS rates have skyrocketed	ICD-10-PCS principal procedure code	Outcome
	No data that higher rates improve outcomes	ICD-10-PCS other procedure codes	
	Term labor CS in nulliparous women accounts for majority of the variable portion of the overall CS rate		
PC-03. Percentage of pregnant patients at risk of preterm delivery at 24–32 weeks' gestation receiving antenatal steroids prior to delivering preterm newborns	Full course of antenatal corticosteroids should be given to women <32 weeks to reduce risks of respiratory distress syndrome, prenatal mortality, and other morbidities	Antenatal steroid delivered (baby)	Process
PC-04. Healthcare-associated bloodstream infections in newborns	Healthcare-associated sepsis and bacteremia are a problem for hospitalized infants	ICD-10-CM other diagnosis codes (baby)	Outcome
	Centers with prevention protocols will likely have success in reducing rates		
PC-05. Percentage of newborns fed with breast milk only during newborn's entire hospitalization	Exclusive breast milk feeding for first 6 months is a goal of the World Health Organization, American Academy of Pediatrics, and others	Documentation of exclusive breast milk feeding (discharge summary, flow sheets, nursing notes, etc.)	Process
PC.06. The percentage of infants with unexpected newborn complications among full-term newborns with no preexisting conditions	Serves as a balancing measure for other maternal measures such as PC-01 and PC-02, to guard against unanticipated or unintended consequences of quality improvement activities for these measures	ICD-10-CM diagnosis codes	Outcome
		Birth certificate	
		Medical record	

In the above table, ICD stands for International Classification of Diseases.

Another organization influential in hospital quality assessment, Leapfrog, surveys hospitals on rates of early elective deliveries and NTSV (nulliparous, term, singleton, vertex) cesareans using the same measurement algorithms as TJC core measures PC-01 and PC-02. Leapfrog also surveys hospitals on additional maternity care measures including rate of episiotomy, performance on standard processes of care, and delivery outcomes for high-risk births.

7.3.2 The State Level

Quality measurement is playing out in important ways at the state level, particularly through perinatal quality collaboratives (PQCs)—single or multistate networks working on maternal-infant QI. Many states have active collaboratives, and others are in development. The Centers for Disease Control and Prevention (CDC) Division of Reproductive Health (DRH) provides support for several state-based PQCs, including California, Colorado, Delaware, Florida, Georgia, Illinois, Louisiana, Massachusetts, Minnesota, Mississippi, New Jersey, New York, Oregon, and Wisconsin (CDC 2018). PQC members identify healthcare processes in need of improvement and use the best available methods to make and record real-time changes. PQCs have contributed to important improvements in perinatal healthcare and outcomes, including (1) reduction in elective births before 39 weeks of pregnancy, (2) reduction in healthcare-associated bloodstream infections in newborns, and (3) reduction in severe pregnancy complications (CDC 2018).

California has been an outsized influence in the maternal quality measurement landscape. The California Maternal Quality Care Collaborative (CMQCC) at Stanford University, with funding from the California Department of Public Health, developed maternal safety and quality toolkits to address QI opportunities identified from a statewide review of maternal death (California Pregnancy-Associated Mortality Review). The work involved multidisciplinary clinicians and other experts representing partner organizations, developing toolkits, and coordinating implementation collaboratives among California hospitals focused on key contributors to maternal death. Additionally, CMQCC produced toolkits focused on quality measures around early elective deliveries and primary cesareans among low-risk women (Smith et al. 2016; Main et al. 2010). Tens of thousands of California's open source toolkits have been downloaded across the world and implemented widely throughout the United States. CMQCC also operates the Maternal Data Center (MDC), a resource for hospitals and clinicians in California, Oregon, and Washington, facilitating reporting of near real-time data and enabling hospitals to track their performance. The California Maternal Quality Care Collaborative (CMQCC) has developed and submitted three quality measures (PC-02, PC-05, PC-06) that are currently used by government and quality review agencies such as TJC and Leapfrog.

7.3.3 Advances in Maternal Care Quality Measurement

Maternal quality measures work by making an entity's processes and outcomes of care visible, comparable, and actionable. Well-designed measures minimize sources of variation in performance that are outside the control of those being evaluated for effective comparisons. For example, some providers serve high-risk patient populations, making CS (cesarean section) more likely. The NTSV CS algorithm modulates this variation by only measuring cesareans that are low risk, singleton, vertex, first-time births—a subset of all births that can be isolated at any level of care or size of clinic, regardless of the wider population served.

Quality measures provide a tool for public-facing accountability and are increasingly reported on websites such as qualitycheck.org, hospitalcompare.org, and leapfrog.org. In California, maternal quality measures for hospitals can be viewed on Yelp, a consumer rating application. Because of easy access to performance data and ability to compare a wide array of providers, quality measures are raising the stakes for hospitals and healthcare systems. As quality measures are collected at the group and individual clinician level, results could increasingly influence how payers and purchasers reimburse and how women choose their maternity hospitals and providers.

Well-constructed quality measures shift maternity care practices and are clearly tied to practices that can be altered to produce better results. For example, to reduce the rate of early elective deliveries (EEDs), hospitals and maternity care groups can adopt and enforce policies that prevent clinicians from scheduling inductions without indication or repeat cesareans before 39 weeks' gestation. To reduce NTSV cesareans, hospitals can implement policies to limit admission of women in early labor (i.e., up to 4–5 cm) and further limit other practices known to increase cesareans such as early inductions and continuous electronic fetal monitoring in low-risk births.

In one of the hospital field sites studied, the hospital set a "bold goal" to reduce NTSV cesarean rates. A multidisciplinary team including nursing and physician leaders championed and collaborated on the effort and identified multiple evidence-based practices that, if implemented, would lower the NTSV cesarean rate. One such practice was not admitting women in labor until they were at least 6 cm dilated. Another practice change was implementing a cesarean checklist that had to be signed off on by a physician and a nurse. The educator shared individual cesarean rates with physicians upon request. The hospital monitored and successfully lowered its NTSV cesarean rate.

Hospitals can tailor approaches using precision QI—if the data show that most NTSV cesareans are clustered among a group of providers, the QI actions will be different than if the driver for NTSV cesareans is labor dystocia (Smith et al. 2016). In that case, QI measures would focus on lowering the CS rate of that particular group. "Moving the dial" on EED and NTSV CS can be much more complex than simply taking these specific actions, but we offer these as examples of how stakeholders can utilize quality measures to create links between data and action, so providers receive feedback about how their actions directly impact their rates.

7.4 Design Considerations

7.4.1 Designing an Actionable Problem

Framing in our usage means the particular ways that people construct a phenomenon, such as "premature birth." Instead of thinking of problems as existing independently of those who seek to solve them, we argue that change agents inherently design problems as they measure them, regardless of whether this process is conscious or not. "Frames" have been described as a "definition of a situation" that becomes apparent as people negotiate meaning in their interactions, reflecting actors' organizing principles and structuring their perceptions of a situation (Goffman 1974). How a problem is "framed" can profoundly shape how it is understood and how institutions or actors seek solutions or ways to manage it.

Creating a maternal quality measure is an act of framing a maternity care problem. Selecting quality measures to collect and use presents a key decision point, because the way a problem is framed in turn delimits the potential pathways for acting on it. Measurements open up particular pathways to action and close off others (Pine and Liboiron 2015). For example, the TJC PC measure for EED is defined as number of births occurring after 36 and before 39 weeks completed gestation (normal pregnancy is 40–42 weeks). Since the EED measure defines an acceptable boundary line for elective deliveries, it creates a pathway for action where clinicians and hospitals may continue to perform elective deliveries that occur after 39 weeks. In this measure, the specific time period is the focus, not the act. If the quality measure were calculated as *rate of elective deliveries performed before labor began on its own*, the measure would create a different pathway to action, one where clinicians would need to wait for labor to begin spontaneously before labor augmentation or conducting an elective CS. When stakeholders design or set quality measures, it is crucial to consider how problems are being framed, how well the design of a measure fits the particular problem, and how the measure will influence action during implementation.

Another key concept related to the design of measures is "wicked problems" which are defined in relation to "tame problems." A wicked problem is characterized as having incomplete, changing, and unpredictable requirements, making solutions extremely difficult. These situations, summarized by Ferlie et al. (2011), are those in which (1) there is no obvious solution; (2) many individuals and organizations are necessarily involved; (3) there is disagreement among stakeholders; and (4) desired behavior changes are part of the solution. Since no single entity is responsible for wicked problems, success requires broad systemic response, collaborative policy-making, and implementation.

Several persistent issues in maternity care quality are wicked problems, including rates of maternal mortality, infant mortality, preterm birth, and cesarean delivery. In each case, many actions are possible, but no single solution exists. Maternity care quality measures tend to work best when there are specific actions that can be taken to move in the desired direction (up or down, toward the goal or benchmark).

We believe measurement-based QI initiatives may be more successful when they focus on a small piece of a wicked problem, essentially creating a tame problem with clear boundaries and goals.

The following anecdote is drawn from Morton et al. (2017). This mixed qualitative interview and archival study revealed that EED measure developers initially saw lowering EED rates as a way to impact three intersecting issues in maternity care: (1) pre-term birth, (2) infant mortality, and (3) overutilization of inductions and cesareans. However, developing measures to address these issues proved exceedingly complex. As one informant involved in measurement development and reporting for maternal care quality at the national level noted in an interview, a cesarean measure was originally slated to appear in a national survey, but the complexity of scenarios involving cesareans made the necessary data collection unfeasible: "One hospital system said they would have to collect something like … they'd have to review 10,000 charts or something. It just wasn't going to work. And we tried sampling but even then, it was not feasible. …the measure was not ready for primetime … so we had to pull the measure from the survey." Developing a quality measure for cesareans, a wicked problem, had proven too challenging, both politically and practically.

However, the EED measure found support and success where the cesarean measure did not. One informant, a physician who spearheaded a large-scale EED reduction initiative, noted that EED reduction was a compelling issue "because it was something that you could just put a finger on and say … well, you just actually go to the obstetricians and say, 'Hey, this is no good.' ACOG—the American College of OBGYN—has long ago stated that you shouldn't electively induce anybody." Further, interlocutors suggested that the EED initiative was easier to mobilize because it was easier to share information about both the initiative and the reasons behind it and the results. As one interlocutor, who was responsible for one of the first comprehensive EED incidence surveys, stated, "It was transparency and accountability and that can really have a galvanizing affect … all we did was make everyone that we knew in the world aware of it and really try to encourage action. That's what we did. We didn't act, though. We just encouraged the action and lots of really smart, committed people went out and acted." The limited scope of EED reduction strategies enabled both robust measurement-strategies and a coherent narrative for change.

Stakeholders assumed that implementing EED reduction efforts would lower preterm birth and infant mortality. This frame achieved buy-in from multiple stakeholders because it isolated a tame problem, with clear boundaries and a clear endpoint (a rate of zero or close to zero of EEDs indicates success) that all could agree was achievable and appropriate. Creating a clear tame problem amid the wicked problem of preterm birth worked because it was easy for stakeholders on the ground to tie the results of the measure to specific actions. Hospitals that established hard-stop policies against scheduling elective inductions or cesareans prior to 39 weeks could clearly see the positive effect, in both numbers and visible proof of fewer 37–38 week babies in the NICU, a harmful potential outcome of EEDs.

7.4.2 Additional Design Considerations for Quality Measures

AHRQ and NQF provide criteria for evaluating quality measures. These criteria group desirable attributes into three broad conceptual areas: measure importance, measure feasibility, and scientific soundness. These criteria provide an excellent starting point in designing or evaluating measures for potential use in improving clinical practice. Our research on the micro-practices of data collection and the contingencies of data work, and the social and organizational factors underlying successful uptake of quality measures, has uncovered additional design considerations that we suggest have large impacts on implementation and sustainable use of a measure over time.

7.4.3 Data Issues

Data elements and their sources are a crucial consideration in designing or selecting quality measures. "Data elements" are processable units of data. Each quality measure specifies both data elements and acceptable sources, and measure developers must carefully balance data economy and quality. Some elements may provide high-quality data yet be difficult to extract. In general, administrative data—particularly billing data such as ICD-10 diagnosis and procedure codes associated with patient records—are easier to extract and use than clinical data drawn directly from electronic or paper records. But administrative data offer less depth and accuracy, in part because medical coders are trained to code patient charts to maximize fiscal payouts for clinical activity, rather than to maximize or assess the degree to which a coded chart reflects clinical reality (Pine et al. 2016).

The precision with which data elements and their sources are specified depends on the scope of the measure. For measures employed for internal QI, selecting data elements that offer a high degree of standardization between organizations is less of a concern. For quality measures reported to external bodies, data quality, economy of data extraction, and comparability must be carefully balanced. Hospitals struggling to extract and calculate measures for external reporting can benefit enormously from peer learning in QI collaboratives.

7.4.4 Clinician Burden

Simply put, a quality measure has already failed if it requires clinicians' time away from their primary task—delivering patient-centered care and lending eyes, ears, and hands to that task. Documentation is part and parcel of practicing medicine, midwifery, and nursing. However, secondary uses of clinical records data, including quality measures, can begin to impinge upon direct patient care and the success of documentation practices. For example, undue burden is placed on clinicians required to adopt standardized terminologies that are otherwise unnecessary or to complete patient documentation within electronic forms structured solely to facilitate secondary data extraction. Further, recent studies have found that the time clinicians spend doing documentation has increased with implementation of EHRs (Arndt et al. 2017; Payne et al. 2015) and that increased time spent doing computer work (often deemed needlessly complex by clinicians) is contributing to the epidemic of clinician burnout (Epstein 2017; Gawande 2018).

7.5 Identifying and Addressing Common Pitfalls

There are limits to quality measurement and what can be achieved with it. To make best use of measurement-based QI methods, it is essential to acknowledge and remain vigilant about several persistent issues that can derail their effectiveness.

7.5.1 Infrastructure Pitfalls

Documentation and coding issues are rife in quality measurement because it is impossible to fully standardize documentation and coding practices across multiple distributed individuals and sites. For example, the EED algorithm specifies data elements drawn from birth certificate data and billing data (ICD-10 codes). EED quality measures are an instance of data "reuse," meaning data collected for one purpose are transformed and put to another use. Research on data sharing and reuse in the sciences shows that data reuse is extremely difficult (Borgman 2015). Reusing data loses the context of their initial gathering and requires significant effort and resources (Zimmerman 2008; Pine et al. 2016). Improving data quality requires intensive efforts to address emergent data issues along the entire course of the data stream—from clinical charting to coding to data extraction for quality measures (Pine and Mazmanian 2015).

Our previous research on the micro-practices of documentation in hospitals revealed that clinicians often document common procedures incorrectly, for example, documenting an "induction of labor" as an "augmentation of labor" and vice versa, and coders must follow conventions and rules for coding that often prevent them from entering data correctly even if they know that a clinician has not documented correctly in the patient record. Take for example the vignette below:

> The coder "DI" coded a chart for a patient who was induced (labor was started artificially) because her pregnancy had gone on too long. The patient eventually had a cesarean section (surgical birth). When she reached the end of the chart, one of the final documents DI reviewed was the discharge summary, which had been written by a different doctor than the primary doctor who oversaw the birth. For coders, the discharge summary written by a physician is considered the "final diagnosis" and is the most authoritative account. The

discharging clinician is supposed to review all of the patient's charting before writing the discharge summary. In this discharge summary, the discharge doctor wrote that the patient came into the hospital in active labor (not for an induction). The discharge summary did not document a drug to stimulate labor that the patient received during labor or the cesarean section even though previous documentation from the primary doctor recorded giving the drug and doing the surgery. DI had been reviewing the charting piece by piece in Epic and building a preliminary code set in a personal notebook. When DI read the discharge summary, she crossed out induction of labor in the coding notebook (meaning she would not enter a code for this procedure), explaining that the discharge summary is the most authoritative source of data for the coder: "... we go with the final diagnosis, because it was established after study." DI explained that she was certain an induction of labor had occurred, but felt she could not code for it because the discharging doctor did not include a diagnosis that would lead to induction of labor nor note the procedure in the discharge summary. (Pine 2019: 542)

Since the physician discharge note contained incorrect information, the coder could not "code against" the discharge note, even though progress notes and nursing flow sheets indicated the patient had been induced with oxytocin.

Thus, despite advances in ICTs, healthcare organizations are far from being able to leverage data with minimal effort in real time for quality measurement and often need to develop infrastructure to do so. Stakeholders need to take a "sociotechnical" perspective and develop technical and human infrastructures to carry out quality measurement. Human infrastructure for data-driven quality improvement in healthcare includes the following:

- Organizational routines for data collection, management, analysis, reporting, and reflection
- Communication and coordination structures that bridge clinical services, information services, QI, and front-line data workers (clinicians collecting/inputting data, coders, clerks)
- Improvement of data collection and organization *practices* as well as assessment and improvement of data quality
- Explicit and tacit human expertise in constructing, interpreting, and communicating quality measurements

Many hospitals use data tools provided by core measure vendors (companies that calculate measures and transfer results to TJC on behalf of hospitals) as stop-gap infrastructure for quality measurement. Such tools can be very helpful for hospitals struggling to meet exacting standards for calculating and reporting quality measures. However, these vendors do not provide tools for organizational reflection about the results nor offer opportunities to learn from peer organizations or try new measures not required for reporting.

Functional and sustainable data infrastructure fades into the background (Star and Ruhleder 1996), seamlessly supporting patient care. In the absence of functional infrastructure for quality measurement, healthcare organizations and workers struggle, expending enormous effort to engage in quality measurement activities and fill gaps when frequent breakdowns occur. We argue that *there is a need for more infrastructure at the national and regional levels, taking the pressure off hos-*

*pitals to develop infrastructure for quality measurement at the local level and allow-
ing healthcare organizations to capitalize on peer learning and promoting data
integration between hospital data and public data.* The CMQCC MDC, for example, links state hospital discharge data with birth certificate data for all births and
provides member hospitals with a list of all births for a particular time period (e.g.,
monthly) after measure algorithms are applied. Automating certain appropriate processes—such as identifying charts requiring review—considerably reduces hospital
workload.

7.5.2   Methodological Pitfalls

Gaming

The necessary ambiguity in data specifications, coupled with public reporting of
quality measures and implementation of value-based reimbursement, can lead to a
propensity to "game" measures by altering data collection or calculation processes
to intentionally produce a better result. Gaming undermines the utility of quality
measures as both an accountability and a QI tool. Changing the sources of data elements can help ameliorate gaming, since some sources are more resistant to "cooking the books." Hospitals can also reduce gaming by calculating measures based on
the entire population of eligible cases, rather than sampling a subset of cases for a
particular measure.

Balancing Standardization with Local Constraints

Establishing and following uniform specifications is critical in guiding externally
facing hospital quality reporting. Successful quality measurement also depends on
unique local data practices. Each hospital and unit present a different configuration
of personnel, technology, documentation practices, and other resources. As a result,
measurement processes can look quite different from one setting to another. An
ethnographic study of data collection practices around central venous catheter
bloodstream infections found that the counting and calculation procedures used to
procure data varied depending on local context, even though hospitals had received
standardized protocols and data definitions. As a result, numerators and denomina-
tors from different hospitals were never fully comparable (Dixon-Woods et al.
2012). Quality advocates work under the assumption that inaccurate measurement
practices will be reflected in data. But until a measure is collected and rates publicly
reported, it is not obvious if a hospital has set too loose a standard. As sociological
studies of standards reveal, it takes active and ongoing organizational work to make
standards and measures "work" in practice (Timmermans and Epstein 2010).
Deciding on exclusions, collecting, calculating, and presenting data in a way that
enables meaningful comparisons between hospitals cannot be accomplished in a
single reporting period—ongoing effort and refinement of standards are required.

Measures Shift Practice and What We Attend to

How measures are interpreted in practice affects the phenomenon the measures are intended to capture. For example, an unintended consequence of how the EED measure frames the problem of early elective delivery is that some providers and patients alike see 39 weeks as the "ideal" gestational age for a baby to be born. A debate at ACOG's 2016 Annual Clinical Meeting caused considerable dissension when both presenters argued for inducing *all* women at 39 weeks as a way to prevent stillbirth. If the design of the quality measure de facto implies that induction at 39 weeks is a good practice, this produces a problem for women who only go into labor after 39 or 40 weeks, as well as the problems generated by induced labor. Another example comes from local implementations of TJC's quality measure on the percent of babies discharged only on breast milk. To achieve the highest rates of breastfeeding, nursing staff may feel pressured to increase breastfeeding rates even when doing so violates principles of patient-centered care.

Managing Expectations

Advocates of quality measures need to align expectations for the potential as well as likely outcomes. Some stakeholders promoting the EED initiative mistakenly assumed that reducing EEDs would reduce the overall cesarean rate. However, this expectation was unwarranted, since the portion of elective deliveries between 37 and 39 weeks that result in cesarean is similar to cesarean rates after 39 weeks, given the high rate of cesareans in US hospitals. Advocates and users should understand what the primary outcomes of a measurement-based QI program will be; they should create realistic expectations about how measurement-based QI initiatives work in practice.

Recognizing the Limits of Quality Measurement

Directing attention to some care processes and practices via implementing a quality metric inevitably directs attention away from others. While some measure developers work on balancing measures to capture potentially undesirable effects of a given quality measure, there are other unintended consequences less amenable for systematic capture.

Gaps in Measure Availability

There are many areas of maternity care for which vetted quality measures are still unavailable, as advocacy organizations such as Childbirth Connection (http://www.childbirthconnection.org/) have shown. For example, there are no measures that address the full course of care including prenatal visits and tests, coordination of care, intrapartum, and postpartum care. Longitudinal aspects of ongoing morbidity are not captured, including postpartum readmissions and follow-up visits (of the woman and/or infant) via emergency departments or outpatient offices. Patient preferences and patient-centered outcomes, which may be nonclinical but are critical, remain unmeasured. Identifying and filling these gaps are a major goal of maternal quality measure developers. Vedam et al. (2017) developed and validated two scales assessing women's autonomy and roles in decision-making during maternity care and measuring women's experiences of respect and self-determination when interacting with their maternity care providers. While promising, these instruments have yet to be implemented in healthcare systems and evaluated as quality measures. In the 2019–2020 legislative session, the California Dignity in Pregnancy and Childbirth Act (SB-464) was passed and requires every birthing facility in the state to implement an evidence-based, implicit bias program and all healthcare providers in each facility to complete an initial basic training and a refresher course every 2 years.

7.6 Conclusions

The recent focus on measurement-based quality improvement to assess and improve maternity care has yielded important gains. Various initiatives to reduce EED have proven successful, and maternity care quality advocates continue to leverage the power of quality measures to influence health policy and clinical practice and improve outcomes. To make quality measurement more sustainable, measure users must avoid or solve the common pitfalls described above, and measures must be carefully designed to maximize success. Designing quality measures that frame maternity problems in ways that are actionable is crucial, as is using them to facilitate clear actions to move the dial so that effects of QI efforts are visible to those working at the local level. When approaching measures that are difficult to impact, local stakeholders may wish to reframe the problem locally using measures that they develop themselves or adapt national measures so that staff can directly link these measures to shifting practices on the ground.

Acknowledgments We wish to thank Elliott Main, Maureen Corry, Jessica Turon, Crystal Oh, Harshita Beeravolu, Mary Pauline Lowry, Rebecca Bakal, Monica McLemore, and the editors of this volume for their contributions to this work.

Some portions of the analysis of early elective delivery presented here are drawn from a California Maternal Quality Care Collaborative (CMQCC) white paper (Morton et al. 2017).

References

Arndt BG, Beasley JW, Watkinson MD et al (2017) Tethered to the EHR: primary care physician workload assessment using EHR event log data and time-motion observations. Ann Fam Med 15(5):419–426
Borgman CL (2015) Big data, little data, no data: scholarship in the networked world. MIT Press, Boston
CDC, Division of Reproductive Health, National Center for Chronic Disease Prevention and Health Promotion (2018) Perinatal quality collaboratives. Available via CDC. https://www.cdc.gov/reproductivehealth/maternalinfanthealth/pqc.htm. Accessed 14 Apr 2020
Dixon-Woods M, Leslie M, Bion J et al (2012) What counts? An ethnographic study of infection data reported to a patient safety program. Milbank Q 90(3):548–591
Epstein R (2017) Attending: medicine, mindfulness, and humanity. Scribner, New York

Ferlie E, Fitzgerald L, McGivern G et al (2011) Public policy networks and "wicked problems": a nascent solution? Public Adm 89(2):307–324

Gawande A (2018) Why doctors hate their computers. The New Yorker, November 5

Goffman E (1974) Frame analysis: an essay on the organization of experience. Harvard University Press, Cambridge

Janakiraman V, Ecker J (2010) Quality in obstetric care: measuring what matters. Obstet Gynecol 116(3):728–732

Jolivet R, Main EK (2010) Quality measurement in maternity services: Staying one step ahead Retrieved from http://transform.childbirthconnection.org/2011/03/performancewebinar/

Kuhmerker K, Hartman T (2007) Pay-for-performance in State Medicaid Programs: a survey of state Medicaid directors and programs. Commonwealth Fund pub. No. 1018. Available via Commonwealth Fund. https://www.commonwealthfund.org/publications/fund-reports/2007/apr/pay-performance-state-medicaid-programs-survey-state-medicaid. Accessed 14 Apr 2019

Lyons M (2018) The Joint Commission announces new performance measure on unexpected complications in term newborns. Available via TJC. https://www.jointcommission.org/en/resources/news-and-multimedia/news/2018/07/the-joint-commission-announces-new-performance-measure-on-unexpected-complications-in-term-newborns/. Accessed 14 Apr 2019

Main EK, Bingham D (2008) Quality improvement in maternity care: promising approaches from the medical and public health perspectives. Curr Opin Obstet Gynecol 20(6):574–580

Main EK, Oshiro B, Chagolla B et al (2010) Elimination of nonmedically indicated (elective) deliveries before 39 weeks gestational age. March of Dimes. Available from CMQCC. https://www.cmqcc.org/resource/errata-2-83111-elimination-non-medically-indicated-elective-deliveries-39-weeks-gestational. Accessed 14 Apr 2019

Martin JA, Hamilton BE, Osterman MJ et al (2018) Births: final data for 2016. CDC. Available from CDC. https://www.cdc.gov/nchs/data/nvsr/nvsr67/nvsr67_01.pdf. Accessed 14 Apr 2019

Morton CH, Pine KH, Turon J et al (2017) Lessons from the initiative to reduce early elective deliveries in California and the United States (CMQCC White Paper). CMQCC, Palo Alto

National Quality Forum (2009) National voluntary consensus standards for perinatal care 2008: a consensus report, Washington, DC. Available from Quality Forum. https://www.qualityforum.org/Publications/2009/05/National_Voluntary_Consensus_Standards_for_Perinatal_Care_2008.aspx. Accessed 14 Apr 2019

National Quality Forum (2018) Perinatal and reproductive health project 2015–16. Available from Quality Forum. http://www.qualityforum.org/ProjectDescription.aspx?projectID=80680. Accessed 10 Apr 2019

Payne TH, Corley S, Cullen TA et al (2015) Report of the AMIA EHR-2020 Task Force on the status and future direction of EHRs. J Am Med Inform Assoc 22(5):1102–1110

Pine KH (2019) The qualculative dimension of healthcare data interoperability. Health Informatics J 25(3):536–548

Pine KH, Liboiron M (2015) The politics of measurement and action. In: Proceedings ACM CSCW, Seoul

Pine K, Mazmanian M (2015) Emerging insights on building infrastructure for data-driven transparency and accountability of organizations. In: iConference 2015 proceedings. Irvine

Pine KH, Wolf C, Mazmanian M (2016) The work of reuse: birth certificate data and healthcare accountability measurements. In: iConference 2016 proceedings. Philadelphia

Smith H, Peterson N, Lagrew D et al (2016) Toolkit to support vaginal birth and reduce primary cesareans: a quality improvement toolkit. CMQCC. Available at CMQCC. https://www.cmqcc.org/VBirthToolkitResource. Accessed 05 May 2019

Star SL, Ruhleder K (1996) Steps toward an ecology of infrastructure: Design and access for large information spaces. Information Systems Research, 7(1): 111–134

The Joint Commission (2009) Specifications manual for Joint Commission National Quality Core Measures (2010A1). Available from The Joint Research. https://manual.jointcommission.org/releases/archive/TJC2010A1/PerinatalCare.html

Timmermans S, Epstein S (2010) A world of standards but not a standard world: toward a sociology of standards and standardization. Annu Rev Sociol 36(1):69–89

Vedam S, Stoll K, Martin K et al (2017) The mother's autonomy in decision making (MADM) scale: patient-led development and psychometric testing of a new instrument to evaluate experience of maternity care. PLoS One. https://doi.org/10.1371/journal.pone.0171804. Accessed 04 Apr 2019

Wier LM, Andrews RM (2011) The national hospital bill: the most expensive conditions by payer, 2008. HCUP Statistical Brief #107. AHRQ, Rockville. http://www.hcup-us.ahrq.gov/reports/statbriefs/sb108.pdf. Accessed 15 May 2019

Zimmerman AS (2008) New knowledge from old data: The role of standards in the sharing and reuse of ecological data. Science, Technology, & Human Values, 33(5): 631–652

Chapter 8
Unsustainable Surrogacy Practices: What We Can Learn from a Comparative Assessment

Elly Teman and Zsuzsa Berend

8.1 Introduction: Questions About Surrogacy

Our starting point is that transnational surrogacy has spread across the globe in recent decades and controlling or managing it is becoming increasingly difficult. After surrogacy became available to foreigners in India in 2005 and before it was banned there in 2017, much scholarly attention was directed to documenting assisted reproductive practices, and Indian surrogacy became a hot topic for sociological and anthropological research (Markens 2012; Rudrappa 2015; Pande 2014; Deomampo 2016). Critics raised the alarm about outsourcing pregnancy and childbirth to the "Global South" (e.g., Harrison 2016). However, what seems to be happening is that several countries, such as India, Thailand, and Mexico, have banned international couples from accessing surrogacy services, and these bans have redirected assisted reproductive service providers and intended parents (IPs) (Whittaker 2016). Many of the new locations are not in the "Global South" but in Ukraine, Russia, the Czech Republic, and others, and much of the traffic has been flowing toward an already busy destination, the United States.

Since so-called commercial, or compensated, surrogacy has been somewhat distasteful for many people, and critics have painted a picture of exploitation, commodification, and oppression of financially needy surrogates, some countries such as Australia, the United Kingdom, Thailand, and most recently India have tried to ban commercial surrogacy but maintain altruistic surrogacy. However, the difference between commercial and altruistic surrogacy is often illusory, and so-called "altruistic" practices can veil oppression and exploitation (Berend 2016) and be more problematic than compensated surrogacy. It is clear that sustainable solutions

E. Teman (✉)
Department of Behavioral Sciences, Ruppin Academic Center, Emek Hefer, Israel

Z. Berend
Department of Sociology, University of California Los Angeles, Los Angeles, CA, USA

© Springer Nature Switzerland AG 2021
K. Gutschow et al. (eds.), *Sustainable Birth in Disruptive Times*, Global Maternal and Child Health, https://doi.org/10.1007/978-3-030-54775-2_8

will require some regulation to ensure that the rights of all parties involved are balanced and protected in ways that the market cannot provide.

All these developments raise questions about the role of regulation and the social organization of assisted reproductive practices, including surrogacy, in terms of outcomes because they make it clear that banning assisted practices in some countries simply redirects those practices to others. In the following, we compare practices in two countries where surrogacy continues to be practiced legally yet has received less ethnographic attention—the United States (Ragoné 1994; Berend 2016; Jacobson 2016; Markens 2007) and Israel (Kahn 2000; Teman 2010)—in order to illuminate better approaches or solutions to some common problems in surrogacy. Through comparative discussion of our respective research, we aim to highlight findings that can broaden the conversation on sustainable birth practices in other countries where surrogacy is currently practiced, such as the United Kingdom, Greece, Russia, Ukraine, the Republic of Georgia, and Iran.

By "sustainable practices," we mean practices that can be maintained without harming the parties involved; we are not advocating for or against surrogacy itself. Our empirical work in Israel and the United States indicated both similarities and differences in how surrogates and IPs engage in and make sense of surrogacy to meet their needs, as well as how surrogacy practices are organized and regulated by the state and other actors. It is clear that sustainable solutions will require some regulation to ensure that the rights of all parties involved are balanced and protected in ways that the market cannot provide.

Our ethnographic research is grounded in local sociocultural and political contexts; we do not argue that our findings are broadly generalizable to very different countries or settings. By shedding comparative light on practices emergent from our respective fieldwork sites, we can better understand the issues involved and point to what we view as the most central regulatory mechanisms that may shield participants in surrogacy agreements from harm. Given the fragmentation and deregulatory impulses of the medical landscape that have intensified under the Trump presidency in the United States, as well as the limitations of our own data, we cannot in good conscience propose legal, financial, or regulatory policies for surrogacy in the United States or elsewhere. However, we think that our comparison between Israel and the United States may contribute to more informed policies by providing empirical findings that support the beneficial role of regulatory policies adopted in Israel. After a short background on our methods and the legal context in each country, we outline three emergent elements that we believe can minimize harm to those involved in surrogacy: (1) standardization and regulation of contracts as well as clinical practices, (2) mandated screening of surrogates and IPs, and (3) open surrogacy relationships.

8.2   Methods

The research described in this chapter draws from each of our research projects on surrogate motherhood arrangements. While our methods are expanded upon elsewhere (Berend 2010, 2012, 2016; Teman 2010), here we briefly outline these methods and the contexts for our studies. The Israeli study, conducted by Elly between

1998 and 2006, used multi-sited ethnographic research, including in-depth, open-format interviews with 26 Jewish-Israeli gestational surrogates and 35 intended mothers (IMs).[1] Elly updated that study with interviews in the summer of 2016 with 20 Israeli surrogates who had given birth in the past 2 years (Teman 2019).

The American study, conducted by Zsuzsa between 2002 and 2013, consisted of online ethnographic observation of discussion threads on the largest public surrogacy website in the United States (www.surromomsonline.com, henceforth "SMO"), including email exchanges with 35 surrogates recruited from SMO.[2] Founded in 1997, by 2013 SMO had roughly 30,000 members, both IPs and surrogates; many of them posted stories, questions, and advice and engaged in heated debate on critical issues in over 30 forums. Because the overwhelming majority of SMO surrogates live in the United States, we refer to this sample as our US sample. Not all surrogates in the United States participate in the SMO network, although many read the site to gain information or advice.

8.3   The Regulatory Context

The legal and regulatory contexts for surrogacy in the United States and Israel differ greatly, and as a result, there are key differences in how parties are protected in both countries. In the United States, there is no federal law governing surrogacy; every state regulates it differently, and some refrain from regulating it altogether. Regulation pertains only to contracts, if that. For example, while New York, Michigan, and Louisiana ban compensated surrogacy, other states like California allow it, and IPs can establish legal parental rights before the birth (Markens 2007). Surrogacy-friendly state legislation further encourages a commercial market in private surrogacy agencies and fertility clinics that, unlike in Israel, are unregulated in the United States. It makes sense for agencies and clinics to flock to states whose legislation makes it easier for the parties to enter into a surrogacy arrangement. Thus, many different couples and single people, who may not be eligible in Israel based on age, health issues, sexual orientation, etc., are able to become IPs in the United States precisely because it is a lucrative business in a largely unregulated market. Specific surrogacy regulations differ among states, but most of the states that allow compensated surrogacy do not limit who can contract a surrogate or require mandatory contracts or screening, enabling surrogates and IPs to negotiate the conditions of their arrangement either through an agency, a lawyer, or privately (Berend 2016; Teman 2010).

Available statistics on US surrogacy are notoriously unreliable. Agencies have no reporting obligation, independent online matching of IPs and surrogates is on the rise, and fertility clinics report IVF cycles, not surrogate-assisted cases. There are

---

[1] All the names and identifying details have been changed and pseudonyms used.

[2] Since SMO is a public forum, no permission for quoting from threads was necessary.

nonbinding medical guidelines for clinics about embryo transfer practices, and the American Society for Reproductive Medicine recently revised its recommendation, favoring single embryo transfer. However, SMO discussions reveal that many surrogates had more embryos transferred (as a result of the reproductive endocrinologist's recommendation, IP's insistence, or their own desire to get pregnant for the couple) than the previously recommended two maximum.

One example from SMO sheds light on some of the reasons: "After three devastating failed transfers, we are aggressive and transferred five [embryos]." The resulting multifetal pregnancies often require further negotiations about selective reduction (a procedure that reduces the number of embryos in a multiple pregnancy to decrease the risk of preterm delivery or other complications). Surrogates very often say they want to create life, not take it. However, in the earlier days of SMO, they more often discussed their responsibility to the IPs and their desire to make them parents. Increasingly, they articulated their changing sense of responsibility in the following way: "Isn't our responsibility for the babies who cannot speak for themselves? The little embryo entrusted us with its life." Yet multifetal pregnancies can be dangerous for both the surrogate and the babies: SMO stories testify to late pregnancy loss, hospitalization, emergency C sections, and premature, low-birth-weight babies who often spend weeks or months in a NICU and may face multiple developmental challenges and long-term health risks.

Threads on the SMO boards reveal that in this inconsistent regulatory context, agencies, clinics, IPs, and surrogates take it on themselves to mandate screening and come to agreements about compensation, payment schedules, the number of embryos to transfer, and conditions for termination of pregnancy. However, although surrogates increasingly pay attention to contractual details, they also tend to think of the contract as a way not only to protect the parties but also to work out the private relationship between surrogates and IPs: "It's how you all handle the negotiations which will clue you in on your future relationship and communications." Because of how stressful contract negotiations can be, surrogates say it is a good test of a future friendship. SMO threads show that surrogates want more protection for all parties but are wary of regulation, even in the case of clinics: "I truly believe that for that [responsible practices in clinics] to happen … and this can be an ugly word around here … this industry will need better regulation. …But regulation is a totally scary thought."

Conversely, surrogacy in Israel is tightly monitored by the state under a comprehensive law. All surrogacy contracts undertaken in Israel must be centrally approved by a government-appointed committee before couples and surrogates are permitted to proceed. Both surrogates and IPs must be Israeli citizens, share the same religion, and cannot be related to one another. Restrictive regulations prohibit same-sex couples and single men from contracting a surrogate, until recently limiting the option to married, heterosexually paired couples with one shared child or no children, and proven infertility. In 2018 the law was amended to allow single women to contract a surrogate.

The practice is not officially encouraged by the state but viewed as a "last resort" for genetic kinship and is limited in scope to couples in whom the female partner has no womb, has been repeatedly unsuccessful with other reproductive strategies, or is at severe health risk in pregnancy (Teman 2010). Only gestational surrogacy is allowed. So-called traditional surrogacy, in which the surrogate is the biogenetic mother, is not practiced in Israel. Once approved by the committee, contracts are legally valid, the children born are full citizens, and the IPs are recognized as their parents once a parental order is granted following the birth. We argue that our comparison of these very different regulatory contexts reveals the most essential regulatory mechanisms that could limit the most unsustainable practices of surrogacy. These essential mechanisms include regulating surrogacy contracts and clinical practices while allowing open contact between the contracting parties.

8.4 Elements of Sustainable Surrogacy

8.4.1 Standardization and Regulation of Contracts

Standardized and regulated contracts are the first essential element in eliminating unsustainable surrogacy practices; the importance of this element emerges clearly from a comparison of the United States and Israeli regulatory contexts and their consequences on possible harm to participants. The patchwork regulatory scheme in the United States means that contracts are not standardized by states. Many surrogates work out independent ("Indy") arrangements that are not mediated by agencies, mostly to save the often hefty agency fees for their IPs. In Indy arrangements, surrogates negotiate contracts with the help of lawyers paid by the IPs. Some agencies standardize the contract, but even in such cases, surrogates now have more say than they did before to change provisions.

In some cases, surrogates argued for lowering the compensation, saying that the agency-mandated amount was "ridiculously high." Surrogates often battle public suspicion, even accusation that they are "in it" only for the money and want to prove that their real goal is to help. "Most surros were in this to help other couples and not for financial reasons, so if this is true then there really is no reason to keep going higher and higher. I have yet to see a golden uterus. I do feel an experienced surro should be compensated as such, but to me anything beyond $25k is ridiculous and greedy," wrote Molly in 2013.[3]

However, surrogates sometimes insist on adding some safeguards, most notably not putting a cap on reimbursement of lost wages; in difficult pregnancies that require bed rest or frequent medical appointments, such caps could result in net losses for the surrogate and her family. Others, though, choose to forgo certain contractual provisions because they do not want to delay the process or fear that the IPs will not work with them if they perceive the surrogate to be difficult or "money-hungry." As Lori explained on SMO, "I don't want my IPs to feel like I am just

---

[3] All the quotes for the American study are from SMO.

trying to get their money, but I think some of these things [in the contract] aren't fair to me ... but I don't want them to be upset about it."

In some states the contract has no validity. Still, contracts are an important issue for surrogates; they say that the process of negotiating the contracts is how the parties get to raise and discuss all the issues and come to an agreement. If they cannot agree about some key issues, such as selective reduction or reasons for termination of the pregnancy, as well as essential financial provisions, surrogates maintain that it is best to part ways. SMO stories indicate that some surrogates realize too late that the IPs may not agree that a Down syndrome fetus is a healthy and "much loved baby" and ask the surrogate to terminate the pregnancy or selectively reduce a triplet pregnancy. Whether it was the surrogate's mistake to agree to contracts with no clear provisions about these issues is immaterial; she suffers the consequences of such procedures, both physically and emotionally.

Years' worth of stories and advice on SMO notwithstanding, some surrogates cannot imagine that the IPs they "clicked with" who are "desperate to have a child" would terminate a pregnancy for less than a life-threatening condition or would selectively reduce in case of multifetal pregnancy. Because they believe they are "on the same page" with their IPs, some fail to specify in detail the conditions for termination or selective reduction. Surrogates repeatedly urge one another, indicating that the issues persist: "You absolutely must be on the same page as your IPs regarding things like termination and reduction. You can't just sign a contract and think something won't happen to you." Some SMO threads were started with the explicit goal of educating surrogates about the necessity of specifying all these matters.

There are no standard provisions about setting up an escrow account for surrogacy-related expenses. SMO discussion threads reveal cases in which payment stopped or expenses were contested by the couple or the escrow was held by an agency that went out of business and surrogates were left unpaid. Some surrogates have been left with hospital bills because, as the patients, they were the legally responsible party. Most health insurance plans have instituted surrogacy exclusions; thus, IPs often need to buy separate insurance, such as the Surrogate Maternity Contractual Liability Insurance Plan, to cover their contractual obligations to pay the surrogates' medical expenses.

Surrogates know that suing IPs is very costly and time-consuming, and when they were not fully reimbursed for expenses, most women maintain that having closure is more important than getting justice. Laura's argument was fairly typical:

Suing is worthless ... unless you have limitless money to afford the time, cost and energy of a lawsuit ... there isn't much that can be done in regards to the contract. Ironic since everyone says how important contracts are. But it takes hours of legal work, depositions, travel and so on to pursue a case, especially if you decide to throw emotional distress into the mix ... In the end you have to figure out how to make peace with it all.

Conversely, in Israel, although there is no standard contract distributed through the state, the surrogacy committee reviews each contract and asks for revisions and additions—to the degree that lawyers involved in drawing up these contracts now include a set of standard elements they know the committee will request. These include the amount of compensation to the surrogate and the name of the lawyer in charge of distributing the surrogate's fee. Contracts must be submitted together with confirmation that all funds have been deposited in escrow, including funds for psychological counseling for the surrogate and her children up to 6 months following delivery, life insurance for the surrogate, and salary replacement if she has to go on bed rest and to cover childcare, house cleaning, and maternity clothes.

Even if a surrogate feels uncomfortable with these provisions, the committee requires them, and many surrogates end up signing contracts that include protections or benefits that they might have forgone had they not been required. As Hanna said: "Everything that you write in the contract makes you feel really greedy, and there are some standard things. Like if the lawyer tells you that from the 38th week you get a cleaning person to come once a week on the couple's bill, it makes you say, 'Wait, I feel uncomfortable taking more money from them.'"[4]

Israel's medical system covers all maternity-related expenses as well as the costs of IVF. However, such practices are best understood in the context of Israel's nationalist and pronatalist policies. Contracts specify the number of embryos surrogates are willing to have transferred, as well as the conditions under which the contract will dissolve, namely, after six embryo transfers are attempted or after a year and a half has passed since the first transfer is attempted. Surrogacy contracts are submitted to the regulatory committee for review and are signed by the surrogate and the couple in the presence of the committee after both surrogates and IPs are medically and psychologically screened. Couples reported in interviews that the committee asked for revisions and additions to the contract up to seven times before it was approved. Other couples reported that they were asked to add last-minute corrections while they were standing in front of the committee for the final review and signing. Surrogates meet with two members of the committee privately before contract signing and are asked about details of the contract to make sure they are fully aware of and understand what they are signing.

Israeli surrogates described feeling as though they were being "tested" by the committee and compared the interview to exams for entering university or an elite military unit. Hadas said: "They investigated me there for something like three hours." Hanna explained that the committee made her rethink and subsequently reaffirm her choice to become a surrogate: "The committee really checks that you are not doing this out of some kind of desperation. What wound is this sitting on? They really sit there and dig into you. It makes you think, is this really what I am choosing to do?" Raz felt the committee had tried to dissuade her from becoming a surrogate:

> And then comes the most stressful part when you are sitting in front of the committee and you feel like they are trying to make you fail, so you won't do it, not supportive but the opposite. They ask you questions and they give you all the answers for why you shouldn't do it. A thousand and one reasons … On the one hand, I understand they want me to be aware of it all, but on the other hand, it gave me a bad feeling, like why do I have to go through all this?

---

[4] All the quotes from Israeli surrogates are from Elly's interviews.

While the Israeli approach to regulating contracts may be too unwieldy for the more individualistic and libertarian ethos in the United States, we argue that regulating surrogacy and implementing some standards within contracts are crucial to protecting all parties involved. Contractually specifying IPs' financial obligations and setting up mandatory escrow accounts would help protect surrogates from not being compensated, as well as from making unwise decisions for fear of being seen as "greedy." Mandating that IPs cover health insurance and life insurance for the surrogate for the period following contract signing through to 6 months after the birth could mitigate cases where surrogates ended up in financial jeopardy because of out-of-pocket surrogacy-related medical expenses.

Health and employment issues related to the pregnancy may be unpredictable and never fully preventable, but risks can be reduced with regulation. Moreover, setting limits for clinics on embryo transfer and specifying all the reasons for termination of pregnancy would protect surrogates, help prevent some conflicts between IPs and surrogates, and would lead to better health outcomes for the babies created through this process. Our comparative findings show that better regulated practices protect all parties, especially the babies who have no say and are the most vulnerable.

8.4.2 Mandated Screening of Intended Parents

The second element essential to eliminating unsustainable practices is regulation regarding *the screening of IPs and not just surrogates*. Mandatory physical and psychological evaluation of both surrogates and IPs can screen out people who are not fit to become surrogates or to be parents via surrogacy, yet only the former screening is done somewhat seriously in the United States. Most agencies include some background checks to ensure that IPs do not have criminal records but usually do not go farther than that. Lack of comprehensive screening of IPs has resulted in some problematic outcomes in cases such as when twins were handed over to a 62-year-old single man who subsequently was visited by social workers because concerned neighbors reported his failure to care for the girls. Another case involved an unmarried couple in their late 50s and early 60s who failed to show up to claim triplets, conceived with donor gametes. The surrogate took them home, cared for them, and, after going to court, gained custody and put the babies up for adoption.

A third, recent case involved a 50-year-old single deaf man who wanted the California surrogate to abort all fetuses in a triplet pregnancy. He later changed his mind and wanted her to selectively reduce the triplets to twins, because he claimed he was not able to care for triplets financially. The surrogate refused, and after a prolonged legal battle, the intended father was granted custody. It may be difficult to be certain who is or is not eligible for contracting with a surrogate as decisively in the United States as in Israel. Nevertheless, regulation may address some of the issues, such as how many embryos to transfer and who is responsible for the babies once they are born, that arise when it is mostly up to surrogates to decide with whom they are willing to work. Some surrogates are willing, even eager, to work with anyone who wants a baby; for surrogates, saying that anyone who wants a child is unfit for parenthood is problematic—who is to decide? However, not fully screening IPs can lead to poor social and health outcomes and protracted legal battles that do not serve the best interests of surrogates, IPs, or babies.

In Israel, both surrogates and IPs are screened, and IPs must submit a file to the committee that includes documents attesting to their, and the surrogate's, clean criminal record, a full medical history, and the result of recent medical tests showing that they are all healthy, disease-free, and not substance abusers. Screening procedures maintain that there will be a genetic connection between the baby and one of its parents; the sperm is provided by the intended father and the egg by the intended mother (IM) or an anonymous donor. The IM must be 22–45 years old if using her own eggs and 22–51 years if using donor eggs. Single women—permitted to contract a surrogate since the law changed in 2018—must use their own eggs since they are using donor sperm.

The screening of Israeli IPs maintains surrogacy as a "last resort" rather than a free-market option. The committee is quickest to accept applications from IMs who had a hysterectomy or were born without a uterus, as well as in cases in which the IM has a life-threatening disease or a condition that could endanger her during pregnancy. In cases of unexplained infertility or pregnancy loss, the committee requires that the IM has tried to conceive through IVF at least seven times or had a similar number of miscarriages (Teman 2010). The committee requires the surrogate and IPs to undergo in-depth psychological evaluation, including intelligence tests and interviews with a psychologist to test their mental stability and suitability for the surrogacy process. While the screening committee has been criticized by some for limiting surrogacy participants, serving as a mechanism of symbolic control (Teman 2016), it does prevent some of the problems we have documented in the United States.

8.4.3 The Open Surrogacy Relationship

The third element that our data suggest is that surrogacy be an open arrangement in which there is direct, unmediated communication between surrogates and IPs. *A striking similarity that emerges from each of our ethnographic findings in Israel and the United States is that most of the compensated surrogates nevertheless view surrogacy as a "gift relationship" with IPs—in the anthropological sense that involves trust, reciprocity, and mutual obligations (Mauss 2016 [1925]). This gift relationship, in their view, transcends the contractual relationship.* Because of the small sample size in the Israeli study and a large but self-selected group of SMO surrogates in the United States, we do not wish to overgeneralize our findings, but we can say with confidence that in both countries, most paid surrogates think of surrogacy as far more than a business transaction and do not view the baby as a commodity. The following response to an IM's question on the SMO boards about the surrogate-IP relationship is typical of the ongoing relationship with the IPs' family that many surrogates seek:

[What] I can tell you from my experience is that not every surrogate has the same expectations of a relationship after the baby is born. I think the majority of emotional pain comes from the surrogates who were unaware that their relationship with the IPs and their child would end when the pregnancy was over … if your intention is not to continue the relationship after the birth … make certain that is known to the surrogate … She may choose to not be your surrogate. Respect her enough to be honest.

Zohar, an Israeli surrogate whose IPs cut off contact shortly after the birth, expressed how intentions can change during the process, leading to disappointment:

At first you go into this because of the money issue, and then at some stage it stops being the money and it's about her–"you'll hold a baby, you'll become a mother." I remember going to the store and seeing the tiny shoes and saying to myself that I hope she will need to buy those tiny shoes soon, that she will have a reason to buy those tiny clothes, that she'll have a reason to be up all night ….The moment it was over, she called me for a few days to see how I felt because of the cesarean and that was it. Unfortunately, it really hurt me, there was no more contact …. I had hoped there would be some kind of relationship … If I do it again, I will choose a couple that I am sure will stay in contact afterwards.

Our findings from the United States and Israel indicate that surrogates are happier when they have contact with the IPs both during the pregnancy and after delivery, as well as being able to formulate a trusting, rather than a transactional, relationship. Central to both satisfaction and trust is that surrogates and IPs should have the opportunity to discuss and clarify their expectations about the nature and duration of their relationship, have informed consent about the process and its procedures, and have realistic expectations. Further, we have found that surrogates are happiest when there is some clarity about the future of the relationship after the birth. Surrogacy does not have to result in a lifelong friendship, and most surrogates expect diminished contact in the post-birth period, but they are more satisfied when it happens gradually. More importantly, they do not wish to be lied to, misled, or unceremoniously "dumped" after the birth.

Surrogates may wish to form a friendship based on trust with their IPs and may hope for gratitude and appreciation of their contribution as a gift. Yet closeness, trust, and gratitude cannot be enforced, and even surrogacy relationships that begin with trust may end with disappointment or feelings of betrayal. A surrogate who was promised updates but did not receive any after the birth posted the following: "I feel so used and betrayed … I know it is their family and right to do this but it still hurts because I thought I was super clear with them about what I wanted/needed." Another surrogate whose IPs failed to deliver on their pre-birth promises wrote: "I'm a good judge of people … but how can you get the know the real person through lies? … They simply tell you what you want to hear … It was hard the first few months after birth. I felt as if I was dying."

Although regulatory intervention cannot ensure trust or friendship, surrogates and IPs can try to limit the harm that occurs during the process and after the birth through explicit communication. Discussion and support networks may be beneficial for both surrogates and IPs as they learn about potential "red flags," common ambiguities, and provide real-life examples of mistakes and lessons learned.

Discussing problems with fellow surrogates can help those entering negotiations to be more aware and more discerning.

While surrogates may read and hear about wonderful relationships and may expect such a journey, there will always be couples who promise ongoing friendship but do not intend to stay in touch or might originally intend to but change their minds later. Regulation cannot meaningfully address relationship issues because most surrogates want genuine appreciation and friendship, not court-mandated emails or pictures. It appears that fully protecting the parties from disappointments is not a realistic aim, but more open communication between them can help mitigate some harm.

8.5 Summary and Conclusion: A Call to Rethink US Surrogacy Regulation

We end with a fervent call to rethink regulation in the United States. Recent developments in the global surrogacy arena, specifically in Thailand and India, magnify this need. In both countries, inadequate or nonexistent regulation has led to troubling practices. In Thailand, the lack of regulation led to multiple controversies, including the trafficking of Vietnamese women who served as surrogates for Taiwanese couples, as well as two notorious cases in which the lack of IP screening went awry (a Japanese billionaire contracting multiple Thai surrogates and fathering 15 babies, as well as an Australian IP who was revealed to be a convicted pedophile).

These controversies led eventually to Thailand banning commercial surrogacy in July 2014. Rather than adopting a cohesive regulatory mechanism as in Israel, the Thai government now restricts surrogacy to altruistic arrangements between a heterosexual couple (one of whom must be Thai) and a female Thai relative as their surrogate (Whittaker 2016). The banning of commercial surrogacy in March 2017 in India did not seem to be a sustainable solution either, for as Rudrappa (2015) warns, the ban led infertility clinics to shuttle Indian surrogates across international borders in efforts to avoid the ban, making the women wholly dependent upon agencies and clinics, vulnerable and at risk while far from home. Christina Weis (2017: 242) documented similar risks and hardships involved in both the "agency-imposed immobility" and the commuting surrogacy arrangements in Russia, whereby surrogates travel often from afar to St. Petersburg clinics, and their movements as well as contact or lack thereof with IPs are strictly regulated by the agency that recruited them. If surrogates violate the agency-imposed restrictions that separate them from their children and partners during their pregnancies, they can be held financially responsible for miscarriages or other medical issues (Weis 2017: 244).

What model might work in the United States to minimize unsustainable practices? While Israel has successfully regulated surrogacy for 20 years now, its model of centralized state regulation may not be feasible in a larger country like the United

States, where it might be interpreted as an intrusion on privacy and individual agency as well as interference with states' rights. Regulating surrogacy through federal regulations and the courts could, however, improve the landscape of US surrogacy, because it would prevent the current situation where people simply go to another state with less regulation to avoid rules in their own states. Yet US federal bureaucracy is not set up to implement mandatory screening of surrogacy contracts, IPs, or surrogates, let alone fertility clinics, as carefully as in Israel.

Moreover, at this time in US history, any attempt to pass federal legislation on surrogacy would be impeded by a variety of factors: US state-by-state regulation is rooted in other legal practices and in a long-standing philosophy of states' rights, and the free-market model for agencies and clinics is also connected to other complex structural issues. The fertility industry is hugely lucrative; attempts to change the framework for its operation would most likely meet powerful opposition. At the time of our writing (November 2019), the neoliberal state in the United States is powerfully bolstered by recent successful deregulatory legislation.

What is clear in light of recent developments throughout the world is that as countries such as India, Thailand, Nepal, and Mexico close their doors to foreign or commercial surrogacy, the United States continues to be the central magnet for international surrogacy travel. It is therefore *increasingly urgent for regulation to address unsustainable practices before the US surrogacy market grows exponentially* and before more surrogates, IPs, and babies pay the price of the free-market model of surrogacy. If surrogacy continues to be practiced, there are regulatory possibilities that can make it less problematic that policymakers should consider and act upon as we have detailed above and reiterate here: (1) standardization and regulation of contracts and clinical practices; (2) mandatory screening of IPs; and (3) encouraging open communication between the parties. Our findings indicate that the degree of contact should be decided by the parties with the help of expert legal professionals, and surrogates should not be misled about the nature of the relationship.

References

Berend Z (2010) Surrogate losses: understandings of pregnancy loss and assisted reproduction among surrogate mothers. Med Anthropol Q 24(2):240–262

Berend Z (2012) The romance of surrogacy. Sociol Forum 27(4):913–936

Berend Z (2016) The online world of surrogacy. Berghan Books, London

Deomampo D (2016) Transnational reproduction: race, kinship and commercial surrogacy in India. NYU Press, New York

Harrison L (2016) Brown bodies, white babies: The politics of cross-racial surrogacy. NYU Press, New York

Jacobson H (2016) Labor of love: gestational surrogacy and the work of making babies. Rutgers University Press, New Brunswick

Kahn SM (2000) Reproducing Jews: a cultural account of assisted conception in Israel. Duke University Press, Durham

Markens S (2007) Surrogate motherhood and the politics of reproduction. University of California Press, Berkeley

Markens S (2012) The global reproductive health market: U.S. media framings and public discourses about transnational surrogacy. Soc Sci Med 74:1745–1753

Mauss M (2016 [1925]) The tgift, translated by Guyer JI. Hau Books, University of Chicago Press, Chicago

Pande A (2014) Wombs in labor: transnational commercial surrogacy in India. Columbia University Press, New York

Ragoné H (1994) Surrogate motherhood: conception in the heart. Westview Press, Boulder

Rudrappa S (2015) Discounted life: the price of global surrogacy in India. NYU Press, New York

Teman E (2010) Birthing a mother: the surrogate body and the pregnant self. University of California Press, Berkeley

Teman E (2016) Surrogacy in Israel: state-controlled surrogacy as a mechanism of symbolic control. In: Sills ES (ed) Handbook of gestational surrogacy: international clinical practice & policy issues. Cambridge University Press, Cambridge, pp 165–173

Teman E (2019) The power of the single story: surrogacy and social media in Israel. Medical Anthropology 38(3):282–294

Weis CC (2017) Reproductive migrations: surrogacy workers and stratified reproduction in St Petersburg. PhD dissertation, De Monfort University

Whittaker A (2016) From 'Mung Ming' to 'Baby Gammy': a local history of assisted reproduction in Thailand. Reprod Biomed Soc Online 2(C):71–78

Part II
Sustainable Maternity Solutions in Latin America

Chapter 9
Childbirth in Chile: Winds of Change

Michelle Sadler, Gonzalo Leiva, and Ricardo Gómez

In 2017, Chile's IMR (infant mortality ratio; infant deaths/1000 live births) was 6/1000 (UNICEF 2018), and its MMR (maternal mortality ratio, maternal deaths/100,000 live births) was 13/100,000 (WHO 2019). These figures are better than the average for Latin American and the Caribbean, where the IMR averaged 15/1000, and the MMR was 74/1000 in 2017 (UNICEF 2018; WHO 2019). They are undoubtedly excellent indicators, but they hide big gaps in access and quality of healthcare between private and public health facilities. Further, there are extremely high routine interventions during childbirth, as indicated by a national cesarean section rate of 50% in 2015 (INDH 2016). In the country, there are no out-of-hospital options for birth that are recognized by the health system and thus covered by health insurance.

In 2016, 99.7% of births were attended by health professionals in hospitals (DEIS 2018), where the hegemonic model of practice is the technocratic model of childbirth (Davis-Floyd 2001). A study conducted in nine major regional maternity hospitals, with primiparous and multiparous women who were admitted to the labor ward with 2–3 cm of cervical dilatation and whose physiologic labor was a minimum of 4 h, reported the following interventions: 91% had medically induced/augmented labors, 55% had continuous fetal intrapartum monitoring, 56% had episiotomies, and 80% delivered in the lithotomy position (Binfa et al. 2016). These high rates of interventions are harmful and against national and international guidelines (MINSAL 2008; WHO 2018).

M. Sadler (✉)
Faculty of Liberal Arts, Universidad Adolfo Ibáñez, Santiago, Chile

Medical Anthropology Research Center, Universitat Rovira i Virgili, Tarragona, Spain
e-mail: michelle.sadler@uai.cl

G. Leiva · R. Gómez
Center for Perinatal Diagnosis and Research, La Florida Hospital, Santiago, Chile

Faculty of Medicine, Pontificia Universidad Católica de Chile, Santiago, Chile

© Springer Nature Switzerland AG 2021
K. Gutschow et al. (eds.), *Sustainable Birth in Disruptive Times*, Global
Maternal and Child Health, https://doi.org/10.1007/978-3-030-54775-2_9

As elsewhere in Latin America, obstetric interventions are high in both public and private health facilities, but the rate of cesareans is much higher in private hospitals. In 2015, the cesarean rate was 41% in public hospitals and 69% in private hospitals (INDH 2016). This difference relates to the organization of care in each system (Angeja et al. 2006; Murray 2000) and the perverse financial incentives in the private domain leading doctors to conduct routine cesareans (Murray 2000; Sadler and Leiva 2016). In public facilities, the workload is organized and paid according to shifts. Professional midwives (called *matronas*) are the main caregivers for low-risk pregnancies and births, but they are supervised by on-duty obstetricians—who manage high-risk cases, instrumental deliveries (such as forceps), and cesareans. In private facilities, obstetricians are the main care providers for all women throughout pregnancy and delivery, though midwives also attend most births. The midwife stays with the mother throughout, while the obstetrician usually only comes in toward the end. The payment scheme operates per client, which means that shorter labor and elective cesarean increase the providers' and hospitals' profits (Murray 2000; Sadler and Leiva 2016).

The high rate of cesareans in the private sector is especially worrying given the rising privatization of childbirth. During the last decade, the number of births in the private sector grew from 21% to 32% (Sadler and Leiva 2016). This trend is driven by the deficiencies and inequities of the public health system, such as hospital infrastructure deficit, low privacy in patient care, impersonality in the treatment of patients, unfavorable working conditions, and low level of wages (Goic 2015). As elsewhere in the world, these factors lead to some marginalized women lacking access to lifesaving interventions, receiving care that is "too little too late" (TLTL), while many women are receiving unnecessary interventions too early in labor or "too much too soon" (TMTS) (see Miller et al. 2016).

Regarding women's perceptions of care, the study by Binfa et al. (2016) indicated that women across many different regions did not feel heard, did not receive information, and were not considered in decision-making regarding procedures or interventions and in some cases felt mistreated (Binfa et al. 2016). Other studies have shown that cases of abuse and disrespect can be frequent, especially in public health. For example, a survey conducted by the Chilean Observatory of Obstetric Violence showed that in 43% of childbirth experiences in public hospitals, and 17% in private clinics for the period 2014–2017 (sample of 5697 births), women reported they had been criticized or repressed by health professionals for expressing emotions and/or pain during labor and birth (OVO Chile 2018).

Nevertheless, it is important to recognize that during the last decade there have been important efforts to improve the quality of maternity care in Chile. In 2007, a comprehensive program for children and their families, especially those most vulnerable, called "Chile Grows with You" [*Chile Crece Contigo*] was launched, with the mission of accompanying, protecting, and supporting all children and their families in the public healthcare sector. The program placed strong emphasis on promoting personalized care for women and their families during pregnancy and birth (MIDEPLAN 2009), including the Ministry of Health's *Manual for Personalized Attention in the Reproductive Process*. The intention was to create a woman-centered model of birth that would promote the psychological health of mothers and the physiologic processes of labor while minimizing the use of routine interventions (MINSAL 2008). These policies and recommendations have helped to improve some practices—mainly those that constitute indicators of goals from the "Chile Grows with You" program (such as the presence of a companion during labor and birth and skin-to-skin contact with the newborn). Thus, while we appreciate improvements in isolated indicators, we regret to note that there has not been a profound nationwide paradigm shift toward the humanization of care during labor and birth.

Thus, despite the government's efforts, many women in Chile still do not receive evidence-based care. In practice there are problems such as insufficient health staff, inadequate infrastructure, lack of autonomy given to midwives to manage physiologic labors, and insufficient collaboration within health teams. Health professionals lack training in a midwifery or humanistic model of care, and women are not adequately informed about physiologic birth during antenatal care (Binfa et al. 2016). Universities have not adapted or updated their health curricula accordingly.

Yet there are several ongoing processes and experiences that hint at a crack in the system and allow us to predict times of change. We will refer first to the history and impact of childbirth activism in the country and then to recent changes regarding birth territories.

9.1 Childbirth Activism

In the year 2000, the "1st International Conference for the Humanization of Birth" took place in Fortaleza, Brazil, with almost 2000 attendees, including around 60 delegates from Chile. RELACAHUPAN (the Latin American and Caribbean Network for the Humanization of Childbirth) was founded at the Fortaleza meeting with the commitment to advance the right of every woman to access adequate information on childbirth and to promote the "rediscovery of what is normal during the reproductive and neonatal cycle" (Vera 2010: 233, our translation). Soon after the conference, the Chilean branch of RELACAHUPAN was born. In the same year, a landmark seminar on "Humanized Childbirth" took place in Santiago, Chile, organized by the Women's Health Program of the Ministry of Health and the University of Chile.

"Humanized childbirth" became the slogan for a series of actions in Latin America, and Chile intended to put normal birth on the agenda, given rising rates of obstetric interventions and abusive care (Bohren et al. 2015; Freedman et al. 2014). From 2007 onwards, the concept of "obstetric violence" (OV) broke onto the Latin American agenda, giving emphasis to the gender violence component of the problem (Sadler et al. 2016). The concept was coined in the Venezuelan "Organic Law on the Right of Women to a Life Free of Violence" (República Bolivariana de Venezuela 2007), where it was codified as one of the 19 kinds of punishable forms of violence against women. It brought a dramatic shift in the discourse and tone of the discussion, as well as a sense of urgency to the cause. To date, Argentina (2010), Bolivia (2013), Panama (2013), and Mexico (2014) have integrated obstetric violence—or broader concepts such as "violence against reproductive rights" in the case of Bolivia—into their laws (Williams et al. 2018).

In Chile, as mentioned above, the first decade of this new century arrived with a governmental push to reduce routine and nonevidence-based interventions in childbirth and place the woman at the center of care (Miller et al. 2016). As experiences of personalized birth took place within maternity units across Chile, there was great resistance to shifting standards of care. The main argument against change was the threat that it might compromise the positive health indicators that Chile already boasted. Yet it was absurd to believe that reducing routine unnecessary interventions while promoting respectful care could jeopardize the exceptional maternal health outcomes in Chile (Sadler and Leiva 2016). In this scenario, childbirth activism has been key to informing women and denouncing abuses.

The goals of childbirth organizations in Chile during the last 20 years have been similar to those in other Western countries: questioning medical interventions in birth; promoting natural labor and delivery; advocating for birth settings and practices that respect women's and families' agency; and advocating for the right to make informed choices (Akrich et al. 2014). It is necessary to consider that in Chile, "choice" is very constrained given the lack of options within the technocratic model of childbirth (Davis-Floyd 2001, 2018) and the asymmetry of knowledge, experience, and authority between women and their providers. Since 2010, a new wave of young activists got involved in these issues and founded several new organizations. The National Coordinator for Rights in Childbirth was born in 2016, gathering 13 organizations working on the topic. It aims to coordinate actions around the following issues: respect during childbirth, adequate unbiased information and consent about procedures, alternatives to medicalized birth, implementation of evidence-based practices, and legal support after having experienced obstetric violence (OV).

During March 2017, one of these organizations—the Chilean Observatory of OV—launched an online survey on experiences of childbirth promoted through social media, which received 11,400 responses. In June 2018 the results were published, showing a steady improvement in standards of care since the 1970s to date. Although the quality of care has been improving, the study confirms the persistence of very high rates of unnecessary interventions and of abuse and disrespect in maternity care throughout the country, as well as ongoing huge gaps between public and private standards of care (OVO Chile 2018). The results of the survey were used as the basis for launching a working group on "respected childbirth," convened by two congresswomen and civil society organizations working on the topic. The first objective of this group was to generate a bill on respected birth as a continuation of two earlier projects presented since 2015 that are still "sleeping" in congress. The project was submitted to congress on October 2, 2018.

This "evidence-based activism" (Rabeharisoa et al. 2014) implies that knowledge is no longer simply a resource for grounding political claims but can become a vehicle of activism. Patient knowledge and experiences can change the evidence that is available to policy makers and government organizations, who can then act on behalf of those very patients. Put another way, credentialed knowledge and experiential knowledge are articulated together rather than being opposed against one another (Rabeharisoa et al. 2014). These organizations and groups have provoked a "shift in the space of rationality, dialogue, and arguments" by framing the debate in ways that have shown the "deep disagreement as to basic premises in factual, methodological, or conceptual matters" (Villarmea et al. 2015: 183, 169).

Evidence-based activism around childbirth in Chile and Latin America has influenced a growing demand, both in public and private hospitals, for normal physiologic labor and respectful care. The health sector is responding with a growing offer of hospital birthing options as well as a growing midwifery cadre to attend home births. While the options for respectful care during childbirth are more prevalent in the private health sector, they require midwives and obstetricians trained in these practices who are not yet fully integrated in both public and private sectors. Yet even within the public sector, there is change, as our innovative case study from La Florida hospital suggests.

9.2   Territories of Birth: The Case of La Florida Hospital

During the last decade, several projects for humanized childbirth have developed throughout the country within public maternity units. The few initiatives that have been successful have taken place in hospitals classified as Level 1 (< 600 births) or Level 2 (600–1200 births) (Ministerio de Sanidad y Política Social de España 2009). Attempts to implement the model in larger hospitals did not succeed because those trying to do so were unable to convince the entire healthcare staff, and midwives were not given autonomy to offer physiologic care for low-risk births (Sadler 2009). Despite the proven effectiveness of midwifery care models in reducing cesarean rates and unnecessary interventions, and in improving maternal and newborn outcomes as well as maternal satisfaction and well-being, there has been resistance to midwifery care in Chile (McLachlan et al. 2012; Miller et al. 2016; Sandall et al. 2016; Stapleton et al. 2013).

Yet, again, there is change. In May 2016, the maternity of La Florida Hospital—a Level 4 maternity unit as it deals with more than 2400 births per year (Ministerio de Sanidad y Política Social de España 2009)—began to implement a new, humanistic childbirth model on the southeast side of Santiago, Chile's capital. This hospital's obstetrics and gynecology unit has been responsible for around 3000 births per year since the opening of its emergency unit in 2015,[1] while the hospital provides services to families that attend one of the nine primary healthcare centers of La Florida, the third most populous community in the country.

---

[1] Based on Monthly Statistical Records of the Center for the Responsibility (CR) of Women, La Florida Hospital.

The La Florida "Safe Model of Personalized Childbirth" attempts to improve consumer satisfaction, reduce excess and unnecessary interventions (including cesareans), and improve maternal, fetal, and newborn outcomes. This model was initiated in response to a health audit of the maternity unit conducted in 2015 that included an analysis of elective and emergency surgeries—the cesarean rate was 44%—as well as of unnecessary interventions. The emphasis on "safety" aims to communicate that reducing maternal morbidity and mortality is a fundamental objective of respectful care. It also responds to a false assumption among Chilean health providers that normal birth is dangerous and that supporting normal physiologic labor produces worse rather than improved maternal and newborn outcomes.

The program was driven by the heads of the obstetric and midwifery units of the Center for Responsibility of Women (which houses the delivery unit) and managed by a midwife experienced in the humanistic model of childbirth (Davis-Floyd 2001) and familiar with the relevant research in evidence-based care. New clinical protocols were developed with the joint participation of the heads of all health units involved, who then familiarized their extended staff with these protocols during clinical meetings. This process attempted to integrate the entire maternity staff into the new protocols rather than simply allowing program managers to run the model separately. The inclusion criteria for women to access this model of care and the new delivery rooms were defined as women without pathology or with low-risk conditions such as mild anemia, noninsulin-dependent gestational diabetes, intrahepatic cholestasis of pregnancy, polyhydramnios, prolonged pregnancy, previous cesarean, and chronic or gestational hypertension without preeclampsia. The protocol was based on the evidence-based *Guidelines for Mother–Baby Friendly Birthing Facilities* developed by the International Federation of Gynecology and Obstetrics (FIGO) in 2015. The goal for 2020 is to join the *International Childbirth Initiative (ICI): 12 Steps to Safe and Respectful Maternity Care*, a merger of the 2015 *FIGO Guidelines* and the 2008 *International MotherBaby Childbirth Initiative* (IMBCI) (Davis-Floyd et al. 2010)—by fully implementing the 12 Steps of the ICI—a global human rights based and quality of care initiative (Lalonde et al. 2019).

The La Florida "Safe Model of Personalized Childbirth" aims to achieve humanized care via one-to-one continuous care where one midwife is available for each birthing woman. Communication between midwives and obstetricians is both verbal and written, and the protocols specify that the obstetrician only intervenes in situations of cardiotocographic (electronic fetal monitoring) traces that are judged to be "non-reassuring" or "abnormal" (according to the classification by NICE 2014), which represent a minority of cases. Currently, around 85% of births in this model are attended by midwives.

Laboring women are sent home if they present at the hospital before reaching the active stage of labor (defined as starting at 6 cm dilation), with the exception of those who turn up at the maternity three times and who are then registered into the hospital but not in the maternity unit. Once women are in active labor, they are registered into the maternity and attended in the four private birthing rooms following the "Safe Model of Personalized Childbirth" or in other rooms following the traditional-interventionist model, depending on their risk factors and room availability.

Of the 3201 births that occurred within the model from May 2016 to November 2019, there was significant improvement compared to all obstetric outcomes in the hospital for 2018 and compared to the country's indicators for 2018 (Table 9.1). From 2016 to 2019, the unit had a cesarean rate of 6% compared to the entire hospital's cesarean rate of 26%, which has been the lowest institutional cesarean rate in Chile since 2016. Other notable outcomes for the same period in the unit include 0.7% third-degree perineal tear; 16.5% episiotomies; an average of 90 min of uninterrupted skin-to-skin contact after birth; and a 67% breastfeeding rate during the first hour after birth.

La Florida Hospital's "Safe Model of Personalized Childbirth" has been recognized as a pillar of safe delivery and respectful care within Chile, and the hospital has been visited by the Minister of Health as well as used as an example of the path that maternity units across Chile should take. In 2017, it won the INNOVA Health award from the South East Metropolitan Health Service, in the "User Satisfaction" category.

9.3   Home Birth

Beginning in the nineteenth century, Chile tried to professionalize birth attendance to decrease maternal mortality by training skilled midwives and obstetricians and transferring birth from home to hospital. Over the course of the twentieth century, traditional midwives were progressively denied the authority to practice at home (Zárate 2007). The degree of skilled or professional birth attendance increased from 61% in 1957 to 99% in 1990 (Koch et al. 2012) and has remained above 99% since

Table 9.1 Compared obstetric outcomes

	La Florida Hospital, Safe Model of Personalized Childbirth, births from May 2016 to Nov. 2019 (N = 3201)[a]	La Florida Hospital, total births 2018[a,b] (N = 3151)	Chile, public health 2018 (DEIS 2019)
Cesareans	6%	26%	42%
Apgar <7 at 5'	0.4%	1.2%	1.1%
Companion labor/delivery	96.9%	89%	68.4%
Skin-to-skin contact for >30 min	86.7%	80%	75.1%
Blood transfusion rate	1.6%	2.1%	No data

[a]Based on Monthly Statistical Records of the Center for the Responsibility of Women, La Florida Hospital

[b]The 3151 total births of 2018 include the 1080 births that occurred in the Safe Model of Personalized Childbirth during that year. (Data for 2019 for entire maternity not available yet)

then, with almost all births taking place in hospitals and no regulated out-of-hospital alternatives. Although home birth is unregulated and not covered by health insurance, it is not illegal, and around 0.3% of births occurred at home in 2016 (INE 2017). The Health Code (Article 117) regulates the practice of midwifery but not its "territory"—a gap that allows midwives to attend home births despite health authorities being against it. The Health Code states that:

> The professional services of midwives include the care of normal pregnancy, birth and puerperium, and the care of the newborn, as well as activities related to breastfeeding, family planning and the execution of actions derived from the diagnosis and medical treatment and the duty to care for the best administration of health resources for the patient. (MINSAL 1997, our translation)

The debate around home birth became public in 2013, after the media dramatized a story of a home birth transfer that had complications. The health minister at the time and the president of the National College of Midwives both declared themselves against home birth but willing to promote integrated birthing rooms within hospitals to give women more respectful and higher-quality care. The discourse against home birth implied that it is a risk to human health and doesn't allow for obstetric emergencies while emphasizing that labor and delivery can have unforeseen events (El Mercurio 2013). In focusing the debate on the place of birth rather than on the model of care, the discussion left the hegemonic technocratic model intact, positioning childbirth as so inherently dangerous that it requires more, not less, obstetric control (Ramírez 2015). An important newspaper referred to the trend of home birth as controversial and made several inaccurate statements. These included that birth has unpredictable complications requiring a professional in the context of a hospital facility, while an expert in maternal health stated that there were no reported models of home birth abroad with good maternal outcomes (Alarcón 2013). This latter statement ignores the wide population-based studies comparing planned home birth with planned hospital birth in North America and Europe that have found comparable newborn and maternal outcomes, far fewer interventions, less maternal morbidity, and fewer and shorter NICU stays for newborns (Anderson et al. 2021; de Jonge et al. 2009; Janssen et al. 2009; Johnson and Daviss 2005; NICE 2014).

Home birth midwives, who had recently organized themselves as "Maternas Chile," responded by defending their practices and denouncing the obstetric abuse and excessive interventions in hospital births that have been damaging to mother and newborns (Schüller 2013). There have been no official changes in the government position on home birth, which is rising steadily in Chile in response to birth activism and the excessive interventions of hospital-based births (Márquez 2019; Ramírez 2015; Reischmann et al. 2015). The growing public discussion in the media and news about high rates of unnecessary interventions, obstetric violence, and cesareans in Chile has had a huge impact on a new generation of families who value autonomy, informed consent, and respectful care in childbirth. Numerous stories of families who experienced disrespectful care and unnecessary routine interventions, despite having overtly rejected them, are raising awareness that facility-based providers override patient concerns about interventions. Given the absence of midwifery-led birth centers in Chile, home birth is a growing trend that guarantees midwifery care (Márquez 2019; Ramírez 2015; Reischmann et al. 2015).

Maternas Chile began working as a small group of midwives who gathered to share their experiences; by July 2018 the group had 27 members from 8 cities across Chile. It has been given legal status as a trade association and has developed a set of evidenced-based midwifery protocols based on the *Guidelines for Home Births* in Barcelona (Collegi Oficial Infermeria de Barcelona 2010), the UK's NICE (2014) clinical guidelines, and the local experiences of Chile's home birth midwives. The group has developed their own patient consent forms, hospital transfer forms, and birth outcome data forms so that they can systematically study the outcomes for home births. During 2016, home birth midwives were given access to birth certificates after 2 years of resistance from the Chilean Civil Registry. The members of Maternas Chile are currently analyzing data on their perinatal outcomes, scheduling training programs for new midwives entering the association, and reviewing their protocols.[2]

The only available indicators about home birth in Chile were published in a thesis of midwifery students who analyzed retrospective data from Maternas Chile midwives for 491 home births in 2 of the most populated regions of Chile (Metropolitan and Valparaíso) from 2003 to 2014. They reported a continuous rise in the number of home births attended by these midwives, from less than 20 per year in 2003 to around 30 per month in 2017. They characterized women who have home births as belonging mainly to the middle-upper socioeconomic level, with 70.7% of their sample having completed university studies. Given that home birth is not covered by health services or insurances, it is affordable only to upper-income families. The authors reported excellent outcomes for the sample: transfer to hospital 8.6%, episiotomies 2.2%, perineal tears 32.2% (of which 99.4% were first degree and 0.6% were second degree), neonatal complications 2%, and maternal complications 1.6% (Reischmann et al. 2015). These results contrast with the poor outcomes and poor treatment that many women receive during institutionalized childbirth.

9.4   Final Words

The encouraging processes and initiatives we have presented show how consumers, academics, clinicians, and policy makers are collaborating to bring about profound and sustainable changes in the landscape of childbirth in Chile. Why do we call them sustainable? Sustainability, as defined by the World Commission on Environment and Development (1987), is development that meets the needs of the present generation without compromising the ability of future generations to meet their needs. How are we protecting the present and caring for future generations through childbirth? Women- and family-centered childbirth can be found in

---

[2] Information from personal communications with Maternas Chile midwives.

societies that are able to put human beings first, attending to the integral needs of mothers and babies far beyond the technical aspects of care that privilege providers at the expense of mothers or bureaucratic institutions at the expense of midwives and other caregivers. Respectful childbirth empowers women, families, and providers, leaving all groups better prepared to care for the newborns who represent the future generations of caregivers. Further, the midwifery model of care empowers health providers, who feel part of a profound caregiving experience that connects them to mothers and the wider family and community. It protects the future health of communities and saves scarce resources that can be used for other healthcare needs. As an example, the 2016 Public Expenditure Review in Chile conducted by the World Bank identified excess annual expenses of US \$9.2 million related to cesarean section (MINSAL 2018).

In Chile, we observe a growing awareness of the importance of protecting the normal physiology of childbirth and respectful care from within the health sector and from consumer groups. The model of midwifery and respectful care that is being implemented in La Florida Hospital is being touted as an example to follow. While few women and families once sought out home birth, it too is now a growing trend across the country, with organized midwives practicing with evidence-based protocols and tracking their outcomes. Obstetric abuses that seemed invisible have been placed in the media spotlight, and there are concerted efforts to raise awareness around and end obstetric violence in Chile, with a group of congresswomen and civil organizations working for a bill on respectful childbirth to be approved in Congress.

While promising, these advances are not enough. The national norms regarding childbirth, such as the "*Manual for Personalized Attention in the Reproductive Process*" (MINSAL 2008), need to be updated and given the status of clinical guidelines because until now they have been taken merely as recommendations, and not protocols, by health professionals around the country. This would need to go hand in hand with a mandatory inclusion of the personalized model of childbirth in the health curricula and training programs within universities, medical, and midwifery schools. Another important next step is to redirect resources within health services and institutions toward midwifery care and toward respectful care for women. Public maternity units need more resources to reach the one-to-one continuous model of care, in which one midwife cares for each woman, which has been the standard in the private healthcare sector.

Health authorities and the College of Midwives are opposing home birth despite the fact that there are no other out-of-hospital alternatives to institutional deliveries. The lack of choice regarding birth territories constitutes a troubling scenario, in which health authorities insist on improving maternity wards within hospitals and clinics in both the public and private healthcare sectors, instead of expanding the available options by creating birth centers or integrating and regulating home birth. This lack of choice has become even more evident during the COVID-19 epidemic, which has been a concern in Chile in March of 2020. As in the United States, according to Davis-Floyd et al. (2020), the situation has generated an escalating demand for home birth as women feel at risk of infection if they give birth in a hospital, and yet health authorities have been emphatic in denying that option. Responding to media coverage on the increase of home birth in this scenario, the Chilean Society of Obstetrics and Gynecology issued a statement saying that "childbirth in a hospital or clinic turns out to be, regardless of the context, the safest option for the mother and the newborn" (SOCHOG 2020).

Some practices that seemed firmly installed are being threatened: there are reports of public and private maternities prohibiting women from being accompanied at birth and not allowing skin-to-skin contact after birth (OVO Chile 2020). This is happening despite the fact that central health authorities have issued a call not to do so; the updated protocols state that women should always have a companion of their choice, and the separation of newborns from their mothers is only justified in preterm births or maternal deterioration due to COVID-19 (Colegio de Matronas de Chile 2020; SOCHIPE 2020).

It is profoundly concerning that rights that were regulated and had taken years to install can be disregarded so quickly and easily. Organizations such as the Chilean Observatory for Obstetric Violence have issued statements reflecting on these issues and calling for a deeper discussion on birth territories that can protect women's rights during childbirth (OVO Chile 2020). If people infected with COVID-19 are concentrated in hospital, to question whether this is the safest place of birth for low-risk women and their babies becomes urgent and more necessary than ever (Dahlen 2019). Thus, we believe that after this pandemic passes, the winds of change will continue to blow with renewed momentum!

References

Akrich M, Leane M, Roberts C et al (2014) Practising childbirth activism: a politics of evidence. BioSocieties 9:129–152. https://doi.org/10.1057/biosoc.2014.5

Alarcón M (2013) Polémica tendencia, aumentan los partos domiciliarios. El Mercurio. http://impresa.elmercurio.com/Pages/NewsDetail.aspx?dt=04-06-2013%200:00:00&PaginaId=53&SupplementId=2&BodyId=0. Accessed 4 June 2017

Anderson DA, Daviss BA, Johnson KC (2021) What if another 10% of deliveries in the United States occurred at home or in a birth center? Safety, economics and politics. In: Daviss BA, Davis-Floyd R (eds) Birthing models on the human rights frontier: speaking truth to power. Routledge, New York/London. (in press)

Angeja ACE, Washington AE, Vargas JE et al (2006) Chilean women's preferences regarding mode of delivery: which do they prefer and why? BJOG 113(11):1253–1258. https://doi.org/10.1111/j.1471-0528.2006.01069

Binfa L, Pantoja L, Ortiz J et al (2016) Assessment of the implementation of the model of integrated and humanised midwifery health services in Chile. Midwifery 35:53–61. https://doi.org/10.1016/j.midw.2016.01.018

Bohren MA, Vogel JP, Hunter EC et al (2015) The mistreatment of women during childbirth in health facilities globally: a mixed-methods systematic review. PLoS Med 12(6):e1001847. https://doi.org/10.1371/journal.pmed.1001847

Colegio de Matronas de Chile (2020) Matronas y matrones emplazan al Ministro de Salud: "No se olviden de las embarazadas en esta pandemia". https://colegiodematronas.cl/?p=2752. Accessed 12 Apr 2020

Collegi Oficial Infermeria de Barcelona (2010) Guía de asistencia del parto en casa. Collegi Oficial Infermeria, Barcelona

Dahlen HG (2019) Is it time to ask whether facility based birth is safe for low risk women and their babies? EClinicalMedicine 14:9–10. https://doi.org/10.1016/j.eclinm.2019.08.003

Davis-Floyd R (2001) The technocratic, humanistic, and holistic models of birth. Int J Gynaecol Obstet 75(1):S5–S23

Davis-Floyd R and Colleagues (2018) Ways of knowing about birth: mothers, midwives, medicine, and birth activism. Waveland Press, Long Grove

Davis-Floyd R, Pascali-Bonaro D, Davies R et al (2010) The International MotherBaby Childbirth Initiative: a human rights approach to optimal maternity care. Midwifery Today Int Midwife 94(12–14):64–66

Davis-Floyd R, Gutschow K, Schwartz D (2020) Pregnancy, birth, and the COVID-19 pandemic in the United States. Med Anthropol. https://doi.org/10.1080/01459740.2020.1761804

De Jonge A, Van der Goes BY, Ravelli ACJ et al (2009) Perinatal mortality and morbidity in a nationwide cohort of 529 688 low-risk planned home and hospital births. Br J Obstet Gynaecol 116(9):1177–1184. https://doi.org/10.1111/j.1471-0528.2009.02175.x

DEIS, Departamento de Estadísticas e Información en Salud, Ministerio de Salud de Chile (2018) Indicadores Básicos de Salud 2016. http://www.deis.cl/wp-content/uploads/2018/12/IBS-2016.pdf. Accessed 15 Oct 2019

DEIS, Departamento de Estadísticas e Información en Salud, Ministerio de Salud de Chile (2019) Serie A, REM-A24 Atención en Maternidad. http://webdeis.minsal.cl/rem2018/?serie=1&rem=36&seccion_id=370&tipo=3&tipoReload=3&regiones=0&regionesReload=0&servicios=-1&serviciosReload=-1&periodo=2018&mes_inicio=1&mes_final=12. Accessed 15 Nov 2019

El Mercurio (2013) Minsal y Colegio de Matronas en alerta por nuevos casos de partos a domicilio sin regulación. http://www.emol.com/noticias/nacional/2013/05/04/596861/minsal-y-colegio-de-matronas-en-alerta-por-nuevos-casos-de-partos-realizados-en-las-casas.html. Accessed 15 Jan 2017

FIGO (International Federation of Gynecology and Obstetrics), International Confederation of Midwives, White Ribbon Alliance et al (2015) Mother–baby friendly birthing facilities. Int J Gynaecol Obstet 128(2):95–99. https://doi.org/10.1016/j.ijgo.2014.10.013

Freedman LP, Ramsey K, Abuya T et al (2014) Defining disrespect and abuse of women in childbirth: a research, policy and rights agenda. Bull World Health Organ 92(12):915–917. https://doi.org/10.2471/BLT.14.137869

Goic A (2015) El sistema de salud en Chile: Una tarea pendiente. Rev Med Chil 143:774–786. https://doi.org/10.4067/S0034-98872015000600011

INDH, Instituto Nacional de Derechos Humanos (2016) Situación de los derechos humanos en Chile: Informe Anual 2016. http://www.indh.cl/informe-anual-situacion-de-los-derechos-humanos-en-chile-2016. Accessed 28 Jan 2017

INE, Instituto Nacional de Estadísticas Chile (2017) Anuario de estadísticas vitales 2017 http://www.ine.cl/docs/default-source/publicaciones/2017/anuario-de-estadisticas-vitales-2015.pdf?sfvrsn=14. Accessed 25 May 2018

Janssen PA, Saxell L, Page LA et al (2009) Outcomes of planned home birth with registered midwife versus planned hospital birth with midwife or physician. Can Med Assoc J 181(6–7):377–383. https://doi.org/10.1503/cmaj.081869

Johnson KC, Daviss BA (2005) Outcomes of planned home births with certified professional midwives: large prospective study in North America. Br Med J 330:1416. https://doi.org/10.1136/bmj.330.7505.1416

Koch E, Thorp J, Bravo M et al (2012) Women's education level, maternal health facilities, abortion legislation and maternal deaths: a natural experiment in Chile from 1957 to 2007. PlosOne 7(5):e36613. https://doi.org/10.1371/journal.pone.0036613

Lalonde A, Herschderfer K, Pascali-Bonaro D et al (2019) The International Childbirth Initiative: 12 steps to safe and respectful MotherBaby–Family maternity care. Int J Gynecol Obstet 146(1):65–73. https://doi.org/10.1002/ijgo.12844

Márquez Y (2019) Parto en casa contemporáneo en Santiago de Chile; percepciones, conocimientos y saberes que se dan en el parto en casa según las mujeres y matronas. Tesis para optar al grado de Magister en Antropología, Universidad de Humanismo Cristiano. http://bibliotecadigital.academia.cl/bitstream/handle/123456789/5006/TMAN%2028.pdf?sequence=3&isAllowed=y. Accessed 20 Oct 2019

McLachlan HL, Forster DA, Davey MA et al (2012) Effects of continuity of care by a primary midwife (caseload midwifery) on caesarean section rates in women of low obstetric risk: the COSMOS randomised controlled trial. Br J Obstet Gynaecol 119(12):1483–1492. https://doi.org/10.1111/j.1471-0528.2012.03446.x

MIDEPLAN, Ministerio de Planificación Gobierno de Chile (2009) Ley 20379: Sistema interesectorial de protección social. https://www.leychile.cl/Navegar?idNorma=1006044. Accessed 20 Feb 2017

Miller S, Abalos E, Chamillard M et al (2016) Beyond too little, too late and too much, too soon: a pathway towards evidence-based, respectful maternity care worldwide. Lancet 388(10056):2176–2192. https://doi.org/10.1016/S0140-6736(16)31472-6

Ministerio de Sanidad y Política Social de España (2009) Maternidad Hospitalaria: Estándares y recomendaciones. http://www.msc.es/organizacion/sns/planCalidadSNS/docs/AHP.pdf. Accessed 23 Feb 2017

MINSAL, Ministerio de Salud Gobierno de Chile (1997) Ley 19536: Concede una bonificación extraordinaria para enfermeras y matronas que se desempeñan en condiciones que indica, en los establecimientos de los servicios de salud. http://www.leychile.cl/Navegar?idNorma=81502. Accessed 10 Jan 2017

MINSAL, Ministerio de Salud Gobierno de Chile (2008) Manual de Atención Personalizada del Proceso Reproductivo. http://web.minsal.cl/portal/url/item/795c63caff4fde9fe04001011f014bf2.pdf. Accessed 19 Mar 2017

MINSAL, Ministerio de Salud Gobierno de Chile (2018) Licitación Pública ID 757-120-L118: DIPLAS 02661, Identificación clínico sanitaria de las intervenciones en los partos naturales y los por cesárea. www.mercadopublico.cl. Accessed 9 Nov 2018

Murray S (2000) Relation between private health insurance and high rates of caesarean section in Chile: qualitative and quantitative study. BMJ 321(7275):1501–1505. https://doi.org/10.1136/bmj.321.7275.1501

NICE, National Institute for Health and Care Excellency (2014) Intrapartum care for healthy women and babies, Clinical Guideline (updated Feb. 2017). https://www.nice.org.uk/guidance/cg190. Accessed 17 Nov 2018

OVO Chile, Observatorio de Violencia Obstétrica (2018) Resultados primera encuesta sobre el nacimiento en Chile. OVO Chile, Santiago

OVO Chile, Observatorio de Violencia Obstétrica (2020) Declaración pública sobre Covid-19 y nacimientos en Chile. http://ovochile.cl/declaracion-publica-sobre-covid-19-y-nacimientos-en-chile/. Accessed 8 Apr 2020

Rabeharisoa V, Moreira T, Akrich M (2014) Evidence-based activism: patients', users' and activists' groups in knowledge society. BioSocieties 9(2):111–128. https://doi.org/10.1057/biosoc.2014.2

Ramírez C (2015) Parto en casa planificado con asistencia profesional: recuperando el protagonismo. Memoria para optar al Título de Antropóloga Social, Departamento de Antropología, Universidad de Chile. http://repositorio.uchile.cl/bitstream/handle/2250/140306/tesis%20carla%20ramirez%20%281%29%20%281%29.pdf?sequence=1&isAllowed=y. Accessed 20 Feb 2017

Reischmann P, Risi C, Serrano N (2015) Evaluación de la atención del parto en casa planificado con asistencia profesional, durante los años 2003–2014. Seminario de grado para optar al grado de licenciado, Escuela de Obstetricia y Puericultura, USACH

República Bolivariana de Venezuela (2007) Ley Orgánica sobre el derecho de las mujeres a una vida libre de violencia. GORBV, Sept. 1738.668. http://virtual.urbe.edu/gacetas/38770.pdf. Accessed 30 Jan 2017

Sadler M (2009) Re-visión del parto personalizado: herramientas y experiencias en Chile. Ministerio de Salud, Santiago

Sadler M, Leiva G (2016) Nacer en el Chile del Siglo XXI: el sistema de salud como un determinante social crítico en la atención del nacimiento. In: Cabieses B, Bernales M, Obach A et al (eds) Vulnerabilidad social y su efecto en salud en Chile. Universidad del Desarrollo, Santiago, pp 61–77

Sadler M, Santos MJ, Ruiz-Berdún MD et al (2016) Moving beyond disrespect and abuse: addressing the structural dimensions of obstetric violence. Reprod Health Matters 24(47):47–55. https://doi.org/10.1016/j.rhm.2016.04.002

Sandall J, Soltani H, Gates S et al (2016) Midwife-led continuity models versus other models of care for childbearing women. Cochrane Database Syst Rev (4):CD004667. https://doi.org/10.1002/14651858.CD004667.pub5

Schüller P (2013) Partos en la casa: matronas defienden práctica y descartan riesgos. Diario La Nación. http://www.lanacion.cl/noticias/site/artic/20130510/pags/20130510173232.html. Accessed 15 Jan 2017

SOCHIPE, Sociedad Chilena de Pediatría Rama de Neonatología (2020) Recomendaciones para la prevención y manejo del recién nacido, Pandemia Covid (Versión 3.0). https://sochipe.cl/v3/covid/27.pdf. Accessed 15 Apr 2020

SOCHOG, Sociedad Chilena de Obstericia y Ginecología (2020) Comunicado Revista Paula. https://sochog.cl/archivos/12969. Accessed 12 Apr 2020

Stapleton S, Osborne C, Jessica T (2013) Outcomes of care in birth centers: demonstration of a durable model. J Midwifery Womens Health 58(1):3–14. https://doi.org/10.1111/jmwh.12003

UNICEF (2018) Levels and trends in child mortality, report 2018: estimates by the United Nations Inter-agency Group for Child Mortality Estimates. UNICEF, New York

Vera G (2010) Relacahupan: 10 años de trabajos, desafíos y logros. Revista Tempus Actas Saúde Coletiva 4(4):233–236

Villarmea S, Olza I, Recio A (2015) On obstetrical controversies: refocalization as conceptual innovation. In: Perona AJ (ed) Normativity and praxis mímesis, Milán, pp 157–188

WHO (2018) WHO recommendations on intrapartum care for a positive childbirth experience. WHO Publications, Geneva

WHO (2019) Trends in Maternal Mortality 2000 to 2017: estimates by WHO, UNICEF, UNFPA, World Bank Group and the United Nations Population Division. WHO Publications, Geneva

Williams CR, Jerez C, Klein K et al (2018) Obstetric violence: a Latin American legal response to mistreatment during childbirth. BJOG 125:125–1211. https://doi.org/10.1111/1471-0528.15270

World Commission on Environment and Development (1987) Our common Future. Oxford University Press

Zárate MS (2007) Dar a luz en Chile, S. XIX: De la ciencia de hembra a la ciencia obstétrica. Dirección de Bibliotecas, Archivos y Museos y Universidad Alberto Hurtado, Santiago

Chapter 10
Humanizing Care at the Maternity Hospital Estela de Carlotto in Buenos Aires: Providers Relearning Their Roles

Celeste Jerez

It was a sunny Saturday morning in October 2017 when our team entered the fourth workshop for pregnant people and their birth companions, called "Integral Preparation for Motherhood" (IPM). The four free IPM workshops are run by the staff of the Maternity Estela de Carlotto (MEC)—a public hospital located in the western suburbs of the Province of Buenos Aires in Argentina.[1] Pregnant women and their companions formed a circle sitting on chairs or exercise balls, as well as on handwoven mats and rugs on the floor.[2] During the meeting, the staff psychologist said something like: "You are sexually active women being pregnant and after giving birth, that is why you leave the MEC with a contraceptive method. In Sexual Health we do not talk about 'patients,' we speak about 'users.' The method you choose and when to use it is your decision, not ours."

During each fourth meeting of the IPM, the social worker invited women who have given birth in the MEC to tell their birth stories, explaining how this can be empowering for others: "The testimony given by women empowers other women, because you can imagine and feel what happens in that moment." Nina, who gave birth at the MEC, explained, "When I was in labor, accompanied by my sister, the

---

[1] In 2017, there were four IPM meetings repeated each month of the year; their topics included (1) prenatal surveillance, danger signs, and going to the hospital; (2) national laws for respectful labor and delivery and family-centered care; (3) newborn care, health, and breastfeeding; (4) and postpartum care, contraception, and sexual and reproductive rights. Most IPM meetings began with 20 min of relaxation exercises, breathing, and stretching for all participants.

[2] In order to safeguard the identity of our 40 subjects, who included pregnant people, their birth companions, and the MEC staff, we have maintained their anonymity and changed names while obtaining informed consent. I use the term "pregnant people" to indicate any person with the possibility to gestate who was pregnant at the time of the research. However, I will also respect the categories used by official documents and by the people interviewed.

C. Jerez (✉)
Research Institute for Gender Studies, School of Philosophy and Liberal Arts, University of Buenos Aires, Buenos Aires City, Argentina
e-mail: celestemjerez@gmail.com

© Springer Nature Switzerland AG 2021
K. Gutschow et al. (eds.), *Sustainable Birth in Disruptive Times*, Global Maternal and Child Health, https://doi.org/10.1007/978-3-030-54775-2_10

midwives were there but they were not there, they were there to support me but not interrupt the moment."

These overheard fragments of a conversation introduce the possibility of "sustainable birth" in the MEC and across Argentina with the following components: free contraception, free care during pregnancy, labor, delivery, and postpartum for everyone and midwives who provide respectful and unobtrusive care. The organizational culture developed by MEC staff is a turning point in the hegemonic, technocratic medical model of birth usually found in Argentina (Davis-Floyd 2001, 2018; Menéndez 1994). This new culture is a qualitative leap against abusive and invasive obstetric care and for the humanization of childbirth, and its existence provides a visible social impact in this region (Blázquez Rodríguez 2005; Fornes 2011; Jerez 2015; Jordan 1993; Sadler 2001). The MEC provides a regional scenario where care providers relearned their roles to avoid medical practices related to obstetric violence, understood as a manifestation of gender violence.[3]

Specifically, I understand "sustainability" in childbirth in Argentina to mean that care providers relearn their roles in a noninterventionist model of childbirth in the public healthcare system in ways that avoid obstetric violence and promote the humanization of care. My theoretical-political framework of this definition of "sustainability" is a feminist perspective on anthropology that analyzes processes of health/disease/care, that is, a focus on sex/gender inequalities in health and a nonessentialized vision of the human body (Esteban 2006). I will describe this relearning of the practitioners' roles within the specific context of the MEC as based on four principles or sets of meaning that promoted sustainable changes over time and that illustrate a specific organizational culture of public healthcare.

10.1 Sustainable Birth Principle #1: The Importance of a Name

The MEC is a public health institution[4] in Argentina built to reduce maternal and neonatal mortality rates and guided by the paradigm of humanized childbirth (Davis-Floyd 2001, 2018), within a framework of programs, initiatives, and national

---

[3] Since 2017, in Buenos Aires we have been running a health research group focused on "obstetric violence in Latin America." Our first publication describes how over the last 10 years, a new legal construct has emerged in the Latin America region that encompasses elements of quality of obstetric care and mistreatment of women during childbirth (Williams et al. 2018). Obstetric violence is understood within the framework of gender violence, through National Law 26,485 (Article 6, Paragraph e). Venezuela (2007), Bolivia (2013), Panama (2013), and Mexico (2014) also have laws prohibiting obstetric violence, though they are rarely enforced.

[4] The healthcare system in Argentina includes three sectors: public, private, and social security. This chapter will focus on the public sector, which is under the umbrella of national and provincial health ministries and includes networks of hospitals and public health centers that provide free care to anyone who needs it.

laws that focus on guaranteeing the integral rights of cis[5] heterosexual women and people who identify as LGTTBIQ.[6] This public hospital symbolizes a government guarantee of healthcare as a human right and access to healthcare for all, regardless of ability to pay, assuring universal coverage of maternal healthcare services as one of the five priority actions for quality maternal care (Koblinsky et al. 2016). MEC's name refers to Argentina's famous human rights activist Estela Barnes de Carlotto, who is the actual president of *Abuelas de Plaza de Mayo*, a group of grandmothers who agitated against the violence, disappearances of thousands of people, and human rights abuses of the last Argentinian dictatorship (1976–1983) for nearly 40 years.[7]

Estela Carlotto's name is connected to the idea of respectful and sustainable birth because her life story is the story of the first women in Argentina who gave their maternity a political sense of struggle, in order to seek justice for the crimes committed by the last Argentine dictatorship.[8] Estela's daughter, Laura Carlotto, a member of Montoneros, a Peronist group in the 1970s, was kidnapped by the last Argentinian dictatorship when she was 3 months pregnant and held in captivity in a clandestine detention center where she gave birth.[9] Her son was given a false identity and raised by a family that illegally appropriated him with the complicity of military doctors. Estela searched tirelessly for her daughter and grandson, and since 1978 she was instrumental in forming the *Abuelas de Plaza de Mayo*, whose members began to systematically search for missing children and grandchildren and to publicly denounce these disappearances, walking around the Mayo's Square (*Plaza*

---

[5] The prefix "cis" is used to designate people who identify with the sex and/or gender assigned at birth, while trans people are people who do not identify with the sex and/or gender that was assigned to them when born.

[6] In Argentina, LGBTTIQ stands for people who identify as: lesbians, gays, bisexuals, transvestites, trans, intersex, and queer. In Argentina, members of this group have promoted the drafting of several laws, including the Equal Marriage and the Gender Identity laws (laws 26,618 and 26,743 respectively) in 2010 and 2012. They have also promoted access to health and labor rights for all Argentinians who identify as LGBTTIQ.

[7] On March 24, 1976, in Argentina began the most cruel civic-ecclesiastic and military dictatorship in the country's history. A government coup was carried out by a military group made up of the commanders of the three armed forces who defeated the constitutional government of President María Estela Martínez de Perón. These atrocious actions were characterized by state terrorism, the constant violation of human rights, the disappearance of 30,000 people (the majority of whom were students, workers, union leaders, and Peronist and leftist party activists), the systematic appropriation of newborns, and other crimes against humanity. The dictatorship ended on December 10, 1983, the day of the government assumption of the elected president Raúl Alfonsín.

[8] According to the former directors of the MEC, Patricia Rosemberg and Cecilia Zerbo, "the organization's name was selected together with the staff, seeking a sense of struggle for human rights related to motherhood, even in situations of adversity. The name highlighted the need to continue the search for social justice in aspects related to our organization in the field of health. The exemplary figure of Estela de Carlotto allows a strong collective identity and also gives us the pleasure of honoring her story" (Rosemberg and Zerbo 2017: 172).

[9] In Argentina, the people who were kidnapped and disappeared were usually taken to a clandestine detention center where they were interrogated under torture for several weeks or months before being released, kept in detention, or executed extrajudicially.

de Mayo) with signs and a white handkerchief on their heads. The *Abuelas de Plaza de Mayo* spearheaded a social and political project that by 2018 had recovered the identities of 127 grandchildren including Guido, Estela's grandson, who was recovered in 2014.

Furthermore, Estela Carlotto's name is also connected to the idea of sustainable birth because it protests the cruelty of detaining young women activists (like Estela's daughter) who were subject to extended detention, torture, and violent childbirths in concentration camps before the government kidnapped their children (Calveiro 1998). By focusing on pregnant women, the dictatorship made childbirth one more step in organized violence against women, with the complicity of military and civil doctors who attended births in horrific conditions.[10] Also, these doctors falsified the birth certificates as "home births," erasing this experience of terror from official narratives (Regueiro 2008).

By naming this public hospital, where humanized birth prevails, for the president of the *Abuelas de Plaza de Mayo*, MEC staff—as part of a public state institution—visibly acknowledged a political reparation for those women detained during the last dictatorship who delivered in horrific circumstances. The name becomes a principle of sustainable birth as it promotes *Abuelas Plaza de Mayo* as one of the fundamental antecedents in our country of women involved in public political activities, in this case collectively denouncing the state violence of the dictatorship.

10.2 Sustainable Birth Principle #2: Reorganizing Complex Childbirth Care

The MEC was founded in 2013 for three primary reasons: (1) to reduce the high maternal and infant mortality in the region; (2) to transform a private birth center focused on the paradigm of humanized childbirth that had operated in the 1980s into a full-fledged public hospital; and (3) to signal a concrete commitment to sexual and reproductive health that arose from municipal, provincial, and national policies. To understand reason 1, let us briefly turn to the demographics of Health Region VII,[11]

---

[10] From December 2017 to August 2018, I conducted fieldwork on the trial for crimes against humanity concerning the Military Hospital in Buenos Aires, where women detained by the last Argentine dictatorship gave birth, their children were born in captivity, and birth records were falsified, with the complicity of both military and civil officers. As part of this investigation, I analyzed the violent and abusive maternity care provided to the kidnapped women in the Military Hospital as a gendered punishment and as a reaffirmation of childbirth as a pathological event. In addition, it was the first trial for crimes against humanity in which the Public Prosecutor's Office specifically called the medical care provided "obstetric violence." To learn more about the case, see the following note from my authorship: https://www.pagina12.com.ar/139982-la-accion-expansiva-de-la-marea-verde (Date of consultation: December 2019).

[11] Buenos Aires Province (307,571 km2 of surface, representing 11.06% of the total of the country) contains 12 health regions composed of 135 municipalities, created in 2006. They are defined as a

where the Moreno municipality is located; these demographics are from 3 years before the MEC opened (Table 10.1).

Before the MEC opened, there was a dearth of hospitals in the region—with 2407 inhabitants per one labor and delivery bed—because there were only two hospitals in all of Health Region VII: the tertiary level National Hospital Prof. A. Posadas and the secondary level Provincial Hospital Mariano and Luciano de la Vega, which were responsible for the 42,000 deliveries in the region in 2010.

This absence of secondary level hospitals meant that many low-risk pregnant people without complications ultimately delivered at tertiary care centers; there was only one center focused on normal deliveries. As a result, normal, uncomplicated births were treated as high-risk deliveries requiring medical intervention, and eventually a decision was made to open the MEC specifically for normal, low-risk deliveries. Besides serving as a secondary level facility, the MEC is a maternal/neonatal hospital that focuses on childbirth attended primarily by midwives, as well as on sexual and reproductive health.[12] It is networked with the 40 primary level healthcare centers within Health Region VII, including the two hospitals named above. The creation of the MEC enabled a new kind of sexual and reproductive healthcare in Moreno that also strengthened and mobilized better referral networks and improved maternal and neonatal outcomes through the entire region.

The creation of the MEC with its focus on normal, low-risk deliveries is sustainable in part because it enables pregnant people to seek their first antenatal screenings and care at primary health clinics while planning a delivery at the MEC.[13] If complications are identified during antenatal screenings or delivery, the user is

Table 10.1 Health Region VII demographics from 2010

	Births annually	Population	Maternal mortality ratio	Infant mortality ratio
Moreno	10,000[a]	452,505	149/100,000	5/1000
Health Region VII	42,000	2,253,772	77/100,000[b]	13/1000
Buenos Aires Province	288,000	15,625,084	44/100,000	12/1000
Argentina	756,000	40,117,096	58/100,000	11/1000

[a]70% of these 10,000 births were in the public health sector, and 30% resulted in cesareans. Trujui, the city where the MEC is located, has some of the highest numbers of pregnancies in Moreno
[b]One of the highest in the entire Buenos Aires Province

network integrated by all the provincial public health establishments that provide healthcare in its three levels of complexity—primary, secondary, and tertiary.

[12] With an area of 5600 square meters, the MEC has 40 beds, 9 offices, laboratory and blood draw services, diagnostic imaging and neonatology, a vaccination room, 3 operating rooms, 4 labor and recovery units, and a residence for people who come from afar to deliver at the MEC.

[13] The "screening" is an obstetric consultation and clinical exam of the pregnant person that evaluates the type of delivery required and risk of complications. In 2016, 72% of the potential deliveries passed through MEC screening.

referred to a tertiary care hospital via agreed-upon referral protocols. Thus, the screening serves to guarantee the humanized care that is the hallmark of the MEC by distinguishing low-risk pregnancies that will not require much, if any, technological intervention. By instituting a set of protocols that identify the complications that require referral to tertiary care, people with normal pregnancies and labor need not suffer interventions not recommended for low-risk pregnancies. The maternity care system also guarantees respectful care during labor and delivery and ensures that low-risk pregnant women can avoid interventions that have little benefit and are not recommended for routine use, such as episiotomies, inductions, etc. (Miller et al. 2016). The focus on normal and low-risk births in the MEC is ensured by the midwifery staff that attends them in the four units of labor and recovery—specially equipped rooms for respected childbirths.

In 2016, midwives represented 22% of the MEC's leased positions—the largest professional group in the MEC staff. Ensuring that childbirth care in the MEC is primarily provided by midwives constitutes a commitment to quality care and differential access according to the level of intervention needed for each delivery (Renfrew et al. 2014). In summary, the MEC care model is sustainable because it ensures low or no intervention in normal physiologic births attended by midwives. Furthermore, its existence as a second level healthcare center, along with the screening process, consolidates a model of division of care according to the complexity of childbirth, promoting better referral networks within primary, secondary, and tertiary level hospitals.

In 2016, after 3 years of existence, the MEC showed very promising quality indicators, even though it still only deals with a very low percentage of deliveries in Health Region VII (Table 10.2):

10.3   Sustainable Birth Principle #3: Providers as Protagonists of the Paradigm Shift

The MEC model of care is part of a broader attempt by the Ministry of Health to humanize childbirth through the "Safe and Family-Centered Maternities" (*Maternidades Seguras y Centradas en la Familia*) (MSCF) program founded in

Table 10.2 MEC health quality indicators, 2016

	MEC	Argentinian Health System (2016)
Number of deliveries	1633	728,035
Accompaniment chosen by the pregnant person during labor, delivery, postpartum	96%	36%
Use of oxytocin	1.5%	Not found
Cesarean rate	13.4%	32%
Episiotomies performed in primiparous women	14.2%	61%
Babies admitted to the NICU	3.1%	6%
Neonatal deaths	0	4716

2010. Endorsed by the Pan American Health Organization (PAHO) and UNICEF, the MSCF initiative has promoted improved outcomes by favoring the minimum interventions necessary in pregnancy, labor, delivery, and the postpartum period, through ten implementation strategies (Larguía et al. 2011):

1. Recognize the MSCF policy within the institution
2. Provide prenatal support and care for women and their families
3. Respect the decisions of pregnant women and their families in labor and delivery
4. Prioritize joint healthy mother and newborn care with postpartum participation of the family
5. Facilitate the inclusion of mother, father, and any family in the neonatal intensive care units (NICU)
6. Allow mothers to stay or sleep near their newborns while they are in the NICU
7. Have hospital volunteer staff
8. Organize postpartum care for healthy newborns and at-risk newborns that prioritize family inclusion
9. Actively work to promote breastfeeding
10. Receive and provide cooperation with other institutions that relate to sexual and reproductive health

These strategies center the pregnant woman as the protagonist of the entire maternity care process and focus on quality of care, cost-effectiveness, and sustainability and replicability. The report on the impact of the MSCF initiative in 14 hospitals made by UNICEF Argentina, 4 years after it was launched in the country (2010–2014), shows that 60% progress was made toward the general objectives of the initiative.

MEC's paradigm of humanized birth was instituted in workshops conducted over the first 4 months of 2013 (January–April) before the MEC opened its doors to the public. Because the MEC practitioners came from other hospitals where the technocratic model of birth had prevailed, the objective was to retrain these staff members to work within the humanistic model of birth. As Andrés, who managed this initial training at the MEC, noted, "The first months here, we started a process of training about the importance of respectful care and we designed the services ourselves. That took a lot of work, a lot of months of working body-to-body with providers."

During this initial training in 2013, all MEC practitioners were exposed, without hierarchical distinctions, to academics from national universities and the national Ministry of Health, activists who had worked on gender and sexual identity, and community members who could explain the evidence-based practices that improve outcomes for pregnant people and newborns. There were also sessions on the difficulties of changing clinical practices and the psychology of resistance within groups to the challenges of promoting a new care paradigm. MEC practitioners themselves were involved in developing and illustrating their interdisciplinary protocols of care and in planning the services they would provide. The staff discussed how they could best promote and provide humanized care in this new setting, connected with primary and tertiary level health clinics in Health Region VI, developing the valuable skill of identifying and receiving the uneventful pregnancies and referring the complicated ones (Campbell et al. 2016).

By asking the MEC care providers to unlearn and abandon the technocratic model that they had initially been trained in to begin to practice in a humanistic fashion, the MEC directors guaranteed that their efforts would be sustainable and persist into the future. By asking staff to recognize that they now had a new role in a new model of care, they allowed staff to feel themselves to be the protagonists of the learning process, rather than being "schooled" or criticized for practices they had learned under the traditional technocratic model of care. By allowing staff to have power and experience transformation rather than imposing a new type of care in a top-down manner, they enabled a transition that was empowered by the staff themselves rather than forced upon them. The self-affirming nature of this process of change percolated through all levels of the staff, thereby ensuring its success and sustainability. One of the MEC neonatologists described how challenging it was to modify her interventionist practices: "When there is a birth in the 'respectful labor and delivery rooms,' I watch, I do not need to go in and intervene, but I just approach, observe, and wait. I have learned that waiting is a valuable part of my work." This neonatologist and all other MEC practitioners now understand that waiting and not intervening can be more valuable than jumping to intervene.

10.4   Sustainable Birth Principle #4: Childbirth in a Sexual and Reproductive Healthcare Setting

The MEC opening in 2013 came 3 years after the founding of MSCF. The MSCF initiative described above resulted from a political shift toward promotion of greater sexual and reproductive rights in Argentina between 2002 and 2015, including laws that protect and promote the rights of cis heterosexual women and LGTTBIQ communities.[14] In this sense, MEC practitioners were trained to be protagonists in their own transformation based on a sexual and reproductive rights paradigm, including practices against gender and obstetric violence, and an inclusion of all gender identities and of sexual diversity.

One of the main objectives of the MEC was to generate an organizational culture focused on rights, especially sexual and reproductive rights. In concrete practice, this guarantee of social rights means not only the right to reject the invasive treatments that form part of what Davis-Floyd (1993, 2001, 2018) has called "the technocratic model of birth" but also the right to information and access to a variety of

---

[14] Sexual Health and Responsible Procreation Law (Law 25.673, of 2002); Respected Birth, Rights of Parents and Children during the Birth Process (Law 25,929, of 2004); Integral Sexual Education (Law 26,150, of 2006); Integral Protection to Prevent, Punish and Eradicate Violence against Women (Law 26,485, of 2009); Equal Marriage (Law 26,618 of 2010); and Gender Identity (Law 26.743 of 2012. In 2015 Article 11 was regulated; it requires access to integral health for trans people through active training for health professionals), among others.

contraceptive methods, as the first person quoted in this chapter reflected, in which anyone who has given birth in the MEC leaves with a contraceptive method. This guarantee of social rights includes legal abortions[15] and a range of sexual health services that promote rights based on gender equity and sexual diversity in the same setting.[16] In relation to these objectives, the members of the Interdisciplinary Sexual Health Team, composed of 15 practitioners (as of 2017), function as counselors in pre- and post-abortion. A member of this team told me:

> Today we wonder why we call the institution "Maternity" when in fact we do tasks that are specifically linked to sexual and non-reproductive health … Maybe we can change our name so that it is consistent with the tasks we do and stop emphasizing only maternity— that is not the only thing we work on. In addition, it would seem that we propose mother- hood as a destination, and it is not so.

MEC staff spoke about humanizing childbirth while avoiding thinking of mater- nity as a destination and proposing a model of sexual and nonreproductive care. I understand that the MEC includes a nondeterministic, non-essentialized vision of the body, promoting the rights of cis women and LGTTBIQ communities by guar- anteeing safe obstetric practices for all parents, regardless of their sexual orienta- tion, and promoting medical practices related to nonreproductive rights, gender identity, and sexual diversity (Jerez 2015). They attempt to guarantee contraception and abortion, avoid reproducing the mandate of compulsory maternity, and offer vasectomies to cis heterosexual men and trans people.

Maria, a trans woman who had worked on behalf of LGTTBIQ rights in Moreno, asked for a vasectomy in 2016. In her case, MEC respectful care included using the name and gender pronouns she had chosen as well as fostering discussions about cis-heteronormative bias in clinical histories through MEC providers. Further, les- bian women who came to the MEC for colposcopies—a procedure used after an abnormal pap smear to examine the cervix—have been able to share their sexual identity with MEC practitioners, integrating it into the comprehensive sexual health medical practice. During a MEC workshop called "We Want to Live: International Day of NO Violence against Women, Transvestites and Trans People," a trans activ- ist gave a presentation called "Institutional Violence towards the Trans Community." Her presentation generated a discussion among MEC staff, who expressed a wish to be trained in trans issues and in setting up a sexual diversity office at the MEC. One

---

[15] In Argentina, in 2012 there was a trial called "F.A.L." (the initials of a 15-year-old pregnant girl) that clarifies the interpretation of Article 86 of the penal code regarding the non-punishability of abortions through two causes: in all types of rape and if life is at risk or the health of the pregnant person. Based on this fact, in 2012, the National Health Ministry established a protocol for the care of legal abortions, called "Protocol for the integral care of people with the right to legal termination of pregnancy" (2015 MINSAL), which points out two reasons why it is legal to practice abortions in public health centers: the health reason and the rape reason.

[16] According to the difficult political panorama of adjustment of public policies carried out by President Mauricio Macri and the governor of the Buenos Aires Province, María Eugenia Vidal (2015–2019), the Ministry of Health (MOH) reduced contraceptives overall, eliminated inject- ables, and stopped subsidizing vasectomies without a scalpel. This was a clear sign of the progress of conservative policies in the Latin American region.

psychologist noted, "Trans men approach us, and yet we often do not have the tools to understand their surgical reassignment." Juan, a liaison management coordinator, supported having trans activists train the MEC staff.

MEC promotes sustainable birth by creating an institutional framework that guarantees sexual and reproductive rights for all people, including contraceptive methods, and regardless of gender identity or sexual orientation. This framework includes guaranteeing the rights of lesbians to have gynecological consults; assuring legal abortions and contraceptive methods; offering training for all MEC staff to improve their care for trans people; and guaranteeing respectful delivery for all pregnant people, regardless of sexual orientation and gender identity. In the same setting, these practices create an organizational culture that integrates sexual and reproductive rights with parental rights around respectful childbirth care.

10.5 Conclusion: A Humanized Model to Deepen and Expand

The case of the MEC as a public health institution illustrates how practices related to the guarantee of humanized delivery prevent the reproduction of obstetric violence (Jerez 2015). Through a feminist perspective in anthropology, I have shown that the MEC achieves its goals to promote the sexual and reproductive rights of cis heterosexual women and LGTTBIQ people because it consolidated its model of care through a careful and sustained process of definitions that can be summarized as follows:

1. The MEC built a political-social identity based on the collective memory of Estela de Carlotto and her role in the human rights movement of Argentina.
2. It made a commitment to reduce maternal and infant mortality in the region by including the MEC in a system of transfer and referral among primary care centers and secondary and tertiary care hospitals, focusing on the care of low-risk deliveries by midwives in rooms especially designed for low or no intervention.
3. It retrained medical staff in a humanized model of care by making providers protagonists in their own transformations.
4. It guaranteed the rights of cis heterosexual women and LGTTBIQ people by offering integrated sexual and reproductive rights across the entire institution.

These four principles or sets of meaning promoted sustainable changes in MEC practitioners, who relearn their roles in a noninterventionist, humanistic model of childbirth in the public healthcare system that avoids obstetric violence. These sustainable changes can be exported to other institutions and regions in the country. The MEC is already training other medical staff at other public hospitals in Argentina, with help from the Argentinian Ministry of Health and UNICEF, to replicate the successes that have been achieved.

Acknowledgments This chapter is the result of 9 months of fieldwork at the MEC (May 2017– January 2018) and was part of my doctorate in social anthropology, which includes a feminist and intersectional analysis. This fieldwork was also part of the ninth UBANEX project at the University of Buenos Aires, an annually subsidized research action program, directed by Monica Tarducci PhD. Our team included students and the following feminist researchers: Claudia Cernadas Fonsalías, Valeria Fornes, Marlene Russo, Mayra Valcárcel, and myself, all anthropologists from the University of Buenos Aires (UBA) belonging to the *Colectiva de Antropólogas Feministas* (CAF). I would like to thank the MEC staff and the directors. I also deeply thank Robbie Davis-Floyd for inviting me to write this chapter and for her careful edits.

References

Blázquez Rodríguez M (2005) Aproximación a la antropología de la reproducción. AIBR Revista de Antropología Iberoamericana 42:1–22

Calveiro P (1998) Poder y desaparición: los campos de concentración en Argentina. Ediciones Colihue SRL, Buenos Aires

Campbell OMR et al (2016) The scale, scope, coverage, and capability of childbirth care. Lancet 388(10056):2193–2208

Davis-Floyd R (1993) The technocratic model of birth. In: Hollins S et al (eds) Feminist theory in the study of folklore. University of Illinois Press, pp 297–326

Davis-Floyd R (2001) The technocratic, humanistic, and holistic paradigms of childbirth. Int J Gynecol Obstet 75:5–23

Davis-Floyd R (2018) The technocratic, humanistic, and holistic paradigms of birth and health care. In: Davis-Floyd R and colleagues (eds) Ways of knowing about birth: mothers, midwives, medicine, and birth activism. Waveland Press, Long Grove, p 3–44

Directorate of Systematized Information (2019) Ministry of Health of the province of Buenos Aires, Buenos Aires. http://www.ms.gba.gov.ar/sitios/infoensalud/estadistica/. Accessed 30 Nov 2019

Esteban ML (2006) El estudio de la salud y el género: las ventajas de un enfoque antropológico y feminista. Salud colectiva 2(1):9–20

Estela de Carlotto Maternity Institutional Report (2016) Vital statistics. Dept systematized evaluation of the Safe and Family-centered Maternity Initiative 2010–2014. Final Report UNICEF, Argentina

Fornes V (2011) Parirás con poder... (pero en tu casa). El parto domiciliario como experiencia política contemporánea. In: Feliiti K (ed) Madre no hay una sola. Experiencias de maternidad en la Argentina. Ediciones Ciccus, Buenos Aires, pp 133–154

INDEC Institute (2010) National population, household and housing census. Buenos Aires

Jerez C (2015) Partos "humanizados," clase y género en la crítica a la violencia hacia las mujeres en los partos. Tesis de Licenciatura. Facultad de Filosofía y Letras, Universidad de Buenos Aires, Buenos Aires

Jordan B (1993) Birth in four cultures: a cross-cultural investigation of childbirth in Yucatan, Holland, Sweden and the United States, 4th edn. Waveland Press, Prospect Heights

Koblinsky M et al (2016) Quality maternity care for every woman, everywhere: a call to action. Lancet 388(10057):2307–2320

Larguía AM et al (2011) Maternidad segura y centrada en la familia (MSCF), conceptualización e implementación del modelo. http://www.unicef.org/argentina/spanish/GUIA_MSCF.pdf. Accessed 15 July 2018

Menéndez E (1994) La enfermedad y la curación ¿Qué es medicina tradicional? Alteridades 7:71–83

Miller S et al (2016) Beyond too little, too late and too much, too soon: a pathway towards evidence-based, respectful maternity care worldwide. Lancet 388(10056):2176–2192

National Directorate of Maternity and Children (2016) Organization of the monitoring of high risk premature newborns. National Ministry of Health Argentina, Buenos Aires

Regueiro S (2008) Inscripciones como hijos propios: construcción de identidad y parentesco de niños desaparecidos. In: Paper presented at the IX Congreso Argentino de Antropología Social, Facultad de Humanidades y Ciencias Sociales, Misiones National University, Argentina, 5–8 August

Renfrew MJ et al (2014) Midwifery and quality care: findings from a new evidence-informed framework for maternal and newborn care. Lancet 384(9948):1129–1145

Rosemberg P, Zerbo MC (2017) Propuesta de gestión de políticas públicas orientadas a garantizar derechos raíces: Maternidad Estela De Carlotto. Mora 23(1):170–177

Sadler M (2001) El nacimiento como acontecimiento médico. Werkén 2:113–124

Second national report of epidemiological survey SIP-Argentina Management (2018) National Ministry of Health, Argentina

Williams CR, Jerez C, Klein K et al (2018) Obstetric violence: a Latin American legal response to mistreatment during childbirth. BJOG Int J Obstet Gynaecol. https://doi.org/10.1111/1471-0528.15270

Chapter 11
Luna Maya Birth Centers in Mexico: A Network for Femifocal Care

Cristina Alonso, J. M. López, Alison Lucas-Danch, and Janell Tryon

11.1 Luna Maya: History and Context

Luna Maya Birth Center provides a model of community-informed maternal and family health care in two very different communities in Mexico: Mexico City and San Cristóbal de Las Casas in Chiapas, near the Guatemalan border. The flexibility of the Luna Maya model allows for the integration of international best practices and guidelines into a traditional culture of care that has been informed and determined by women in the communities it serves. The growth and success of Luna Maya's model of care is due to a humanistic and femifocal approach that goes well beyond ordinary community-based midwifery care, by connecting women, children, and families throughout their lives. The Luna Maya model offers a full scope of practice including: well-woman care, gynecological care, pregnancy care, abortion care, childbirth care, and postpartum care. Luna Maya is sustained by a network of providers that includes midwives, midwife apprentices, lactation consultants, childbirth educators, physicians, acupuncturists, body workers, therapists, and educators in yoga, movement, and child development classes. Luna Maya provides an

C. Alonso (✉)
MPH, CPM, Luna Maya, Mexico City, Mexico
e-mail: cris.alonso@gmail.com

J. M. López
School of Pharmacy and Clinical Sciences, University of Bradford, Bradford, UK
e-mail: j.lopez@bradford.ac.uk

A. Lucas-Danch
MPH, MSW, Ojai, CA, USA
e-mail: AlisonDanch@gmail.com

J. Tryon
MPH, Brooklyn, NY, USA
e-mail: janell.tryon@gmail.com

environment where both women and midwives are empowered in caregiving that can sustain women's health.

Founded in 2004, Luna Maya has survived funding cuts, legal battles, and the war on drugs, despite heavy social and government emphasis on the dangers of childbirth, midwifery, and especially out-of-hospital birth. In this chapter, we will explore aspects that make Luna Maya sustainable as an institution that include, though are not limited to:

1. Emphasis on a femifocal model of care that empowers and promotes women's needs and health within the community.
2. Quality of care based on human rights that cares for staff and patients in collaborative and participatory fashion.
3. Commitment of staff, who find sanctuary in working in a woman-centered space.
4. Clear values, mission, and programmatic focus.

In this chapter, we describe how caring for women and meeting their needs, listening to their voices, and applying informed consent in every step of health care provides a sustainable environment where both staff and women can learn and feel listened to and honored for who they are. Our institutional values are clear: *"We believe access to care is a human right,"* and guide decisions and interactions. In a country affected by disproportionate levels of gender-based and structural violence, an ongoing drug war, systematic obstetric violence, and sexual harassment, the sustainability of Luna Maya lies in the community and staff choosing to maintain a safe space for women. This safe space is created by the circular decision making at annual and monthly meetings, and by constant addition of staff and volunteers who actively shape the sustainability of Luna Maya as a holistic, femifocal, and community-based model of care.

Since its opening in 2004, Luna Maya has broadened the very meaning of midwifery for women in Mexico. Given the high rate of maternal mortality, the poor quality of maternity care, and the history of government repression of the Maya peoples in Chiapas, it was clear that women needed a humanized intervention that would help them access affordable and respectful maternity care. The Luna Maya model of care has been both humanistic and holistic (see Chap. 1 for a description of the technocratic, humanistic, and holistic models of care) from its beginning and has consistently tried to address the broader psychosocial needs of its clients and their children through a variety of complementary therapies and child development tools.

11.2 The Landscape of Maternal Health in Mexico

In 2015, Mexico's national maternal mortality ratio (MMR) of 38/100,000 live births was a disappointment to the policy makers and frontline providers who had worked diligently to improve Mexico's maternal health standards (WHO et al. 2015). While Mexico's MMR varies widely across its 32 districts/federal entities, it is highest in the districts with the highest rates of Indigenous inhabitants as well as those with the highest rates of poverty, such as Chiapas (Gay and Billings 2009).[1] In 2013, Chiapas had an MMR of 68/100,000—the second highest in the nation—while its IMR (infant mortality ratio: infant deaths/1000 live births) of 18 was the highest (INEGI 2013; Alonso et al. 2018). Chiapas is one of the top five most marginalized states in the country, with the highest recorded unemployment levels and the lowest rate of female educational attainment of all 32 federal states in Mexico.

An evaluation of MacArthur-funded interventions around maternity care across Mexico highlighted the need for a fundamental transformation in maternity care, including "instituting a midwifery model of care; improving quality of care; and continuing to report and analyze causes of maternal deaths" (Gay and Billings 2009). After Mexico's professional midwifery schools were closed in the 1960s, facility-based deliveries had been in the hands of general physicians, obstetricians, and medical interns, whose technocratic, medicalized model of birth resulted in a 47% cesarean rate in 2015.

The medicalization of birth in Mexico, as elsewhere in Latin America, has become an alarming public health problem with severe consequences for mothers, newborn, families, and providers. There are ample indications of dysfunctionality in maternity care, including multiple reports of abusive care and obstetric violence, inappropriate or overused interventions, and failure to provide needed interventions (Castro and Erviti 2014; GIRE 2015; Miller et al. 2016). Women in Chiapas are caught between two difficult choices: to birth at home with family members under the care of traditional midwives, or to birth in a highly medicalized hospital where one out of two women has a cesarean. In short, women in Chiapas embody the difficult choices between "too much too soon" (TMTS) maternity care and "too little too late" (TLTL) care (Miller et al. 2016).

Birth centers such as Luna Maya provide a physical sanctuary and a bridge between TMTS and TLTL. Professional midwives provide respectful care that avoids the overuse of non-evidence-based routine interventions, many of which have been shown to lead to poor maternal and perinatal outcomes (Miller et al. 2016). Further, at a time when institutionalized birth is normative, mothers at Luna Maya receive a full scope of care that integrates informed consent, humanity, respect, and continuity of care for women and their families. This model works *with* medicine, not against it, in an environment where women are becoming discouraged and are increasingly avoiding obstetric care, even when needed, because of well-founded fears of abuse and maltreatment (Sialubanje et al. 2015; Sarker et al. 2016; GIRE 2015). According to results from the 2016 national survey on dynamics around domestic relationships (ENDIREH 2016), 33.2% of women reported obstetric violence in their births and only 9% consented to a cesarean, though many more

---

[1] As Graciela Freyermuth noted (2006), "maternal mortality in Mexico has an Indigenous face. Official statistics demonstrate that Indigenous women have three times higher risk than non-Indigenous women of dying because of causes related to maternity," which contributes to the doubling of the MMR in regions where a large percentage of the overall population is made up of Indigenous communities (Gay and Billings 2009).

had one (Frias and Castro 2017). Luna Maya provides a bridge that respects traditional values and incorporates/adapts traditional methods of intrapartum and postpartum care for women.

It is this bridge that is the cornerstone of the sustainability of Luna Maya.
Although Luna Maya was shut down by health authorities in 2011 because it did not
conform to the regulatory framework for obstetric hospitals and Mexico lacks regulation for birth centers, the community demanded it be revived. Despite adverse
political conditions, Luna Maya returned to Chiapas and expanded to Mexico City.
Staff attribute their motivation to continue providing women-centered out-of-
hospital birth care and education to the perseverance and support of the community,
first in Chiapas, and now in our recently opened Luna Maya Mexico City birth center.

11.3   Luna Maya Vision and Mission: Empowering Women and Communities

Because of the historic and institutionalized denial of human rights to Indigenous
communities, the Indigenous women of the Chiapas region have been a critical
starting point for enhancing a rights-based approach to women's health. Luna
Maya's community-based, femifocal model seeks to challenge the government-
sponsored model of maternity care that is negligent of Indigenous communities'
health concerns. The Luna Maya model is wary of the antenatal and intrapartum risk
associated with hospital emergency obstetric care that disregards the reproductive
rights, consent, or agency of Indigenous women. This government model of healthcare ignores Indigenous forms of healing in the pursuit of biomedical solutions
(Pelcastre-Villafuerte et al. 2014). Luna Maya seeks to transcend the chasm between
biomedicine and traditional medical knowledge systems by empowering women
and traditional midwives to better understand the normal physiology of pregnancy,
labor, and delivery, while also acknowledging the importance of emergency obstetric care when indicated. Luna Maya supports local practices during labor and delivery, such as asking the mother to choose what family members will accompany her
during labor and delivery, the use of herbs and heat during labor, the drinking of
maize milk (*atole*) to improve the laboring woman's strength, and other healing
services that traditional midwives historically provided in Chiapas. This emphasis
on a community model of care has created a safe space where Indigenous women
report feeling represented and heard.

Luna Maya charges fees for services and subsidizes these fees with grants and
crowdfunding. In addition, women will have to pay for labs and ultrasounds with
other providers or obtain them at the local public hospital where these services are
free. Forty percent of our clients are Indigenous women who pay as they can, over
50% are mestizo women, and around 10% are foreigners. Luna Maya carries out a
socio-economic survey of all clients who request a discount on payment and is sensitive to the neighborhood and community the family belongs to as a strong indicator

of income. Luna Maya can accept private insurance—which most people in Chiapas do not have. Luna Maya respects and empowers mothers and midwives to respect and assert Indigenous cultural values and norms. For example, current international recommendations state that women should access care in the first trimester and should receive care every month, yet in Chiapas it is common for Indigenous women to access care only in the third trimester. Indigenous cultural norms suggest that women should have their baby "positioned" by a traditional or empirical midwife in the last months of pregnancy. Local norms also encourage women to give birth at home unless complications or emergency delivery are foreseen. Women who seek care in public institutions are often scolded, threatened, and told they will lose their Conditional Cash Transfer benefits if they do not attend a certain amount of prenatal visits or if they give birth outside the hospital (Murray de Lopez 2018; Lovera 2018).

In an effort to compromise, regardless of weeks of gestation, Luna Maya has developed a policy that allows women to give birth with our midwives as long as they have had at least one prenatal exam. Our staff midwives accompany women who are in active labor and have not received any prenatal care to the hospital because they are considered to be out of the scope of practice for out-of-hospital midwives. Although most birth center and midwifery protocols require more than one prenatal visit, this open-door policy allows women to feel comfortable and welcome while also respecting the midwives' preference that a woman visit the antenatal clinic at least once before labor begins. By holding to a model of care that empowers and respects both mothers and midwives, Luna Maya birth centers are both autonomous and sustainable.

After a century of slow progress, some midwives in Mexico are establishing autonomous physical spaces for their birthing practices that are outside of and independent of government control, in which they can avoid the obstetric violence and racist treatment that Indigenous and other women often suffer in government facilities. There is copious evidence that the midwifery model of care for low-risk and some high-risk women leads to improved maternal and neonatal outcomes, fewer interventions, lower costs, improved quality of care, and more humanized birth than obstetric or technocratic models of care (Renfrew et al. 2014; ten Hoope-Bender et al. 2014; Benatar et al. 2013; Greulich et al. 1994). Nevertheless, midwives continue to be systematically dominated, disenfranchised, and subordinated by a model of care that privileges obstetricians and risk factors while exacting oppressive surveillance of those midwives who have little choice but to work within the obstetric model of care. Global research demonstrates that many midwives feel exhausted, burnt out, and unable to provide quality midwifery care within hierarchical hospitals where obstetric protocols dominate and separation of mind and body is pervasive (WHO 2016; Filby et al. 2016). By maintaining midwifery autonomy, Luna Maya both engenders high-quality care for mothers and provides its midwives with the opportunity to practice their skills in caring, nurturing, and empowering women across their reproductive lifespan.

Self-care has been an essential value and aspect of sustainability for Luna Maya. Early on, founder Cristina Alonso began an apprenticeship education program to educate midwives to work in the Luna Maya model. Some former apprentices have moved on to open other practices, while others have stayed on. Self-care for the staff is continuously assessed in the following ways:

- Weekly case review meetings with midwives and apprentices
- Bi-weekly study groups & monthly staff meetings
- Annual operating and visioning meeting
- Flexible vacation policy
- Annual circular staff evaluation, where staff identify desired areas of growth
- Staff given free or at cost access to Luna Maya health services including massage, acupuncture, herb baths and steams, herbal products, medical care, flower remedies, and therapists
- Continued education for clinical and administrative staff
- Group therapy and mediation in times of crisis, bad outcomes or when in need
- Inclusion of rituals to celebrate anniversaries, students' graduations, birthdays, holidays, and other important moments
- Clinical sabbaticals available for midwives after 4 years of employment

As one of our midwifery apprentices, Kay,[2] describes:

> Our team believes in what they do. Although, sadly, loving and respectful care is a luxury in Mexico, Luna Maya provides it. Although we charge for services, profit is not our main objective, but the values that the organization defends and protects. And the women see and feel these values in action. Our team has very well trained and professional people. Systemic violence and inappropriate use of power are cultural problems that are reproduced at every level in the vast majority of Mexican health care facilities, thereby providing us with an opportunity to offer real alternatives. Many women and families know the model and they are excited to defend and promote it.

And Ana, another apprentice and mother of two babies born at Luna Maya, notes: "Luna Maya is sustainable because of those of us who work here with all our hearts to achieve our mission statement, making sure that all women have safe and dignified care."

11.4 Creating a Femifocal Model: Beyond Full Spectrum Care

In this chapter, we have described our Luna Maya model as "femifocal" to indicate a focus on all people who identify as female, regardless of whether they are mothers or not. Luna Maya invokes the term *femifocal* to conceptualize the multiplicity of female experiences and the ability to honor and respect every woman who approaches Luna Maya. "Femifocal" recognizes that a woman is at the center of her own social, political, and cultural ecology, rather than seeing her solely as a biological machine needing medical attention (Davis-Floyd 2001, 2018a; Lucas and Tryon

---

[2]All people discussed in this chapter have been given pseudonyms and identifying details have been changed to protect their identities.

2014; Alonso et al. 2018). Femifocal care allows for women to always find a reason to visit Luna Maya, making sustainability also based on the array of services. It is common to hear women talking in reception, waiting spaces or even the kitchen about their birth stories and health—even if their baby is now 10 years old. Storytelling and space-sharing create a community of women who find strength and empowerment through being the protagonists of their health and life; while building friendships in the hallways and rooms of Luna Maya with other women who share their values.

Femifocal care encompasses the spectrum of reproductive care and beyond. Rather than allowing abortion debates to lead to a care stalemate, Luna Maya seeks to depoliticize this debate by committing to a femifocal vision that seeks a broader and more inclusive movement for all women and their various health goals. Currently, the Luna Maya birth centers may be the only two in Mexico that provide gynecologic and abortion care in addition to birth-related midwifery services.

11.4.1   Sustainable Femifocal Care in Action: Case Studies

Deborah first came to Luna Maya after lying in the local hospital for two nights. She had begun to miscarry an 8-week pregnancy and her husband had taken her there. Because of the legal and ethical controversy around abortion care in Chiapas, where abortion is only legal in cases of rape and risk to maternal or fetal health, the medical team had put Deborah on an IV with antibiotics and waited. After two days in the hospital with no resolution, her father-in-law called the Luna Maya midwives and asked if they could treat her. Deborah left the hospital on a Sunday afternoon and came to Luna Maya, where the midwives performed a manual vacuum aspiration, placed an IUD, prepared Bach flower remedies, and the therapist treated her for the shock and trauma of having been accused of causing the miscarriage by the hospital nursing staff.

Three years later, Deborah became pregnant again and birthed her first child in water in her home attended by the midwives. She birthed a second child at home three years later. She came to our infant massage classes when the children were little, and then to our Monday child development classes. Deborah and her husband had a difficult relationship. Full of tension and passion, they would separate for months at a time. Deborah would often come to Luna Maya asking for a well-woman care consultation, but really just to cry and be listened to by her midwives. When her husband would leave, the mothers from the child development class would help her with childcare and provide a supportive environment.

Deborah's story provides an insight into the continuum of care that Luna Maya provides as it serves as a space to integrate life events. There, Deborah was able to receive clinical, therapeutic, and community support over the course of many years. Luna Maya was available to meet Deborah's physical and emotional needs in an integrated and humanized manner.

Angelica had been in labor for three days. The traditional midwife in attendance was out of ideas on how to help her, and one of her friends decided to call the Luna Maya midwives to see if they could help to prevent a cesarean at the local hospital. The midwives arrived and found the baby was facing the wrong direction (posterior) and therefore couldn't fit through the pelvis. They helped rotate the baby and 20 minutes later she birthed a happy, healthy little boy. Three years later, she attended Luna Maya's care from the beginning of her pregnancy. This time her husband, who was in the US during her first pregnancy, was present and caught the baby himself. Angelica sells fruit at the market and her sisters are now looking forward to getting married so they can have their babies with Luna Maya. Recently, Angelica's sister-in-law gave birth to her first baby at home on a dirt floor with the Luna Maya midwives and her mother tending to the fire on the anafre *(small aluminum grill where corn is roasted that must be tended during birth to keep the birth room warm).*

Although Angelica had not received prenatal care from the Luna Maya midwives, there are several neighborhoods in San Cristóbal where traditional midwives and/or family members can seek a second opinion prior to a transport. Occasionally, the midwives will determine that the mother must be transported to the hospital and will go with the woman to advocate for her rights. Often, the woman is dehydrated or the placenta is retained and our midwives can provide appropriate intervention outside of the hospital. This story exemplifies how a community-based midwifery practice extends to all family members, empowering them to be advocates for maternal health. It also underscores the significance of client-based care and client advocacy. Intercultural integration, informed consent, and client-directed care allow women in marginal communities to feel safe, heard, and supported in their decisions. As one mother explained:

> *The midwives are calm and patient, they take their time to explain everything. I feel like all my doubts are dispelled. In my first pregnancy I went to the hospital and I had to wait five hours to see the doctor. They scolded me and asked me why I hadn't come sooner. They only saw me for 15 minutes and I felt sad and confused after I left. This time I'm happy to come to the visits--sometimes they take an hour and the midwives listen to my fears.*

This testimony summarizes the community's support for the compassionate and full-spectrum care provided at Luna Maya.

11.5   Sustainability for Luna Maya

Luna Maya has become a sustainable institution through the following principles and practices, which, we propose could be replicated in other birth centers and obstetric units across Mexico:

1. **Femifocal care**: Emphasis on a social and women-centered model of care promoted by the community. Luna Maya's providers are committed to delivering femifocal care that fully supports a woman's agency to determine how, when, and whether to enter motherhood or not.
2. **Integrated care:** Luna Maya's model of care promotes a wider view of biosocial health in which midwifery care is integrated with family planning, newborn and infant care, pediatric care, nutrition, well-woman care, sexual health, and gynecologic care (Pathmanathan et al. 2003). A vision and practice that sees women as multi-layered, complex, and socially embedded understands that not

all women want or need the same course or type of care. Quality of care is based on human and women's rights and also includes caring for staff.

3. **Humanized care**: Luna Maya practices a humanized midwifery model that reintroduces the emotional and human aspects of the birth experience. It emphasizes a rights-based approach to reproductive, maternal, and sexual care that is free from abuse, obstetric violence, negligence, disrespect, humiliation, and other forms of mistreatment (GIRE 2014; Bohren et al. 2015; Freedman et al. 2014; Vogel et al. 2015).

4. **Informed consent-based care**: Informed and respectful care specifically seeks to prevent psychological abuse, lack of information, lack of respect for women's decisions, humiliation, or stigmatization.

5. **Client-directed care**: In every aspect of service provision, the clients of Luna Maya have the capacity to guide their own care. Women thus emerge from the process deeply transformed, not just as mothers but also as agents of health and power. Women who have birthed at Luna Maya often later train as doulas, provide postpartum support to other mothers, and participate in ongoing workshops and trainings, creating a community of women who relate to Luna Maya on many levels.

6. **The strength and commitment of the staff,** who find sanctuary in working in a woman-centered space.

7. **Continuity of care and provider**: Luna Maya commits to providing its clients with care from the same provider or team of providers, from the first prenatal appointment to the last postpartum visit and beyond (Benatar et al. 2013; Sandall et al. 2013). We of Luna Maya define this continuity of care to extend to reproductive, family planning, gynecological, birth-related, pediatric, and alternative healing services, so that the same team of providers tends to the various aspects of women's well-being and health. This emphasis on continuity of care seeks to avoid fragmentation of the woman and her experiences. This model prevents midwives' burn-out, as care is relationship-based and occurs through mutual decision making, thereby nourishing both the providers and the client. Midwives do not scold or punish women for their decisions, nor are midwives themselves scolded or punished for women's decisions and outcomes. Weekly case review allows for a deep understanding of the woman's situation and choices as well as creating a unified plan of action and team position in collaboration with the woman.

8. **Self-care for both women and staff**: One-hour visits, home visits, herb baths, kindness, and humor are examples of how the midwives relate to and care for their clients and for each other. The same principles are expressed within staff interaction and engagement. Staff are deeply committed and in annual evaluations express their satisfaction with working at Luna Maya. Monthly gatherings, celebrations, and closeness of the team allow for Luna Maya's values to be carefully applied within the team, ensuring support, kindness, and respect at all levels. The need for mutual nurturing and care among staff members exists worldwide, yet has been under-appreciated by social scientists and development workers (see Walsh 2009). One of our staff midwives, Andrea, explains:

I believe what makes Luna Maya sustainable is its human capital. Each woman who works in Luna Maya is aligned with the mission and vision. It's much more than "work," but service to all women, to the country, to humanity. And the leadership has been able to sustain the midwives throughout failure and try new things. We are always supported in our personal development.

9. **Holistic care**: Luna Maya's model of care is holistic because it weaves physical, mental, spiritual, emotional, and social health into every provider–client interaction. Drawing from the WHO definition of health, Luna Maya views health as inclusive of physical, mental and social well-being and not merely the absence of disease (Davis-Floyd 2001, 2018a; Glasier et al. 2006). As programs, activities, and new collaborators are proposed, they must relate to and represent our core values. Staff revise these values constantly to ensure relevance and application. Maintaining programmatic focus allows Luna Maya staff and community to be clear about what Luna Maya does and does not do. Luna Maya does not shift its goals despite shifts in funding priorities, although this has meant that some years we have had to resort to crowdfunding to subsidize services.

10. **Women's healthcare across the life-course**: Luna Maya provides for care across the life-course for women, by acknowledging that sexual, reproductive, gynecological, and maternal health are often inextricably linked. Luna Maya defines *full spectrum care* as providing a continuum of reproductive services for women including childbirth, well-woman, family planning, and abortion care.

11.6 A Vision Forward: Integrating Birth Centers into a Network

Luna Maya has developed and grown since 2004 to a model that has learned hard lessons and created qualitative success despite specific rejection and mobbing[3] from the government. We recently described our process and methodology in a manual and online course in Spanish called *How to Open a Midwifery Center* targeting Mexican and Latin American providers. Our goal is to encourage others and show them how to replicate our midwifery center model, and thereby to create a critical mass able to advocate for the inclusion of birth centers in Latin American healthcare systems. Opening and maintaining birth centers in Latin America presents numerous challenges that include:

1. Lack of midwifery schools that educate in the midwifery and out-of-hospital/community birth models.
2. Lack of funding and capital available for midwives to open a birth center.

---

[3] Mobbing is defined as workplace bullying where harassment occurs on the part of a number of people, institutions, community members, or peers through rumors, innuendos, intimidation, humiliation, discrediting, or isolation.

3. Free obstetric care in hospitals, which competes directly with private services.
4. Poverty alleviation programs that obligate women enrolled in them to birth in hospitals.
5. The fact that, although users are willing to pay for services, economic crises and un- and under-employment make cost recovery extremely difficult.
6. Lack of regulation of birth centers and specific bullying from the government against midwives, which makes keeping birth centers open a challenge.
7. Lack of access to birth certificates for some out-of-hospital birth providers, which presents a significant challenge for midwives and parents.
8. Lack of regulation of midwives, which makes advertising, transport, and formal negotiations with health officials difficult.

In 2017, to strengthen political presence and advocacy, Luna Maya founded the Mexican Network of Midwifery Centers (*Red de Casas de Partería Mexico*: casas-departeria.org). As health systems begin to look critically into using resources and evaluating impact, evidence-based decisions will be essential. The safety of regulated birth centers has been well established in high resource countries (Stapleton et al. 2013; Alliman and Phillippi 2016; Birthplace in England Collaborative Group 2011). Although the birth center model is being implemented in low resource settings, there is little formal research on maternal or neonatal outcomes in such settings.

Quantitative data collected in the MANA Stats research database for Luna Maya shows a 10% cesarean rate compared to the current national cesarean rate of 46%, and a 95% exclusive breastfeeding rate at last postpartum visit (usually 6 weeks). No maternal deaths have occurred, nor any severe maternal morbidity in the last decade. However, Luna Maya remains outside of and unrecognized by the Mexican health care system. In the case of emergency transports, the midwives encounter discrimination, harassment, blame, and lack of communication with medical staff. Families are often told that the emergency was caused by the midwife, even when the transport is timely and for justified clinical reasons. This harassment severely delays access to emergency care and leaves the families feeling confused and at fault. Lack of communication between midwives and the receiving hospitals further restricts the capacity of hospital medical staff to make sound clinical decisions, as they often lack the patient's medical history and a detailed picture of the events that precipitated the transfer.

Midwifery care works best within a network of care providers that includes emergency services. A better recognition of autonomous midwifery care that includes Luna Maya's birth centers would alleviate the current situation where Indigenous women often delay transport due to fear or lack of resources. Given that the landscape of maternity care in Mexico is currently characterized by too many cesareans (TMTS), too little quality and labor and delivery wards that are over-capacity and under-resourced (TLTL), health policy makers must better integrate autonomous models like Luna Maya. Such integration will help relieve some of the pressures on the existing health care system, while ensuring that autonomous midwives receive the "mutually accommodative" (Davis-Floyd 2018b) backup care they need. The key to sustainable birth in Mexico lies with the integration of femifocal and family-centered birthing spaces that push the entire system to honor women, intercultural diversity, and humanized, high-quality care for all.

References

Alliman J, Phillippi J (2016) Maternal outcomes in birth centers. J Midwifery Womens Health 00:1–31

Alonso C, Lucas-Danch A, Murray de Lopez J et al (2018) Lessons from Chiapas: caring for indigenous women through a femifocal model of care. In: Schwartz D (ed) Maternal health, pregnancy-related morbidity and death among indigenous women of Mexico and Central America: an anthropological, epidemiological and biomedical approach. Springer, Berlin

Benatar S, Garrett AB, Howell E et al (2013) Midwifery care at a freestanding birth center: a safe and effective alternative to conventional maternity care. Health Serv Res 48(5):1750–1768. https://doi.org/10.1111/1475-6773.12061

Birthplace in England Collaborative Group (2011) Perinatal and maternal outcomes by planned place of birth for healthy women with low risk pregnancies: the birthplace in England national prospective cohort study. Br Med J 343:7400

Bohren M, Vogel J, Hunter E et al (2015) The mistreatment of women during childbirth in health facilities globally: a mixed methods systematic review. PLoS Medicine 12(6):e1001847

Castro R, Erviti J (2014) 25 years of research on obstetric violence in Mexico. Revista CONAMED 19(1):37–42

Castro R, Frías SM (2020) Obstetric violence in Mexico: results from a 2016 national household survey. Violence Against Women 26(6–7):555–572. https://doi.org/10.1177/1077801219836732

Davis-Floyd R (2001) The technocratic, humanistic, and holistic models of birth. International Journal of Gynecology & Obstetrics 75(1):S5–S23

Davis-Floyd R (2018a) The technocratic, humanistic, and holistic paradigms of birth and health care. In: Davis-Floyd R et al (eds) Ways of knowing about birth: mothers, midwives, medicine, and birth activism. Waveland Press, Long Grove, pp 3–44

Davis-Floyd R (2018b) Homebirth emergencies in the US and Mexico: the trouble with transport. In: Davis-Floyd R et al (eds) Ways of knowing about birth: mothers, midwives, medicine, and birth activism. Waveland Press, Long Grove IL, pp 283–322

Filby A, McConville F, Portela A (2016) What prevents quality midwifery care? A systematic mapping of barriers in low and middle income countries from the provider perspective. Plos One 11:e0153391. https://doi.org/10.1371/journal.pone.0153391

Freedman L, Ramsey K, Abuya T et al (2014) Defining respect and abuse of women in childbirth: a research, policy and rights agenda. Bull World Health Organ 92:915–917

Frias S, Castro R (2017) Violencia obstétrica en México, resultados de la ENDIREH. Paper presented at the Primer Congreso de Violencias de Género contra las Mujeres, UNAM-CRIM, December 2017. Available via: https://www.crim.unam.mx/congresoviolencias/sites/default/files/Mesa%202_Castro%2C%20Fr%C3%ADas.pdf

Gay J, Billings D (2009) Evaluation of The MacArthur Foundation's work in Mexico to reduce maternal mortality. MacArthur Foundation. Available via: https://www.macfound.org/media/files/MACARTHUR-EVAL-MEXICO-MM.PDF

Glasier A, Gülmezoglu AM, Schmid GP et al (2006) Sexual and reproductive health: a matter of life and death. Lancet 368(9547):1595–1607

Greulich B, Paine LL, McLain C et al (1994) Twelve years and more than 30,000 nurse-midwife-attended births: The Los Angeles County and University of California women's hospital birth center experience. J Nurse Midwifery 39:185–196

Grupo de Información en Reproducción Elegida (2014) Omisión e Indiferencia. Derechos Reproductivos en México. Available via: http://informe.gire.org.mx/
Grupo de Información en Reproducción Elegida (2015) Niñas y mujeres sin justicia, Derechos Reproductivos en México. Available via: https://gire.org.mx/838-2/
INEGI (2013) Conjunto de Datos, Mortalidad general. https://www.inegi.org.mx/sistemas/olap/Proyectos/bd/continuas/mortalidad/MortalidadGeneral.asp
Lovera S (2018) Prospera en México prohibe la partería tradicional. Periodismo de Investigación, April 19, 2018, p 66. Available via: http://www.pagina66.mx/prospera-en-mexico-prohibe-la-parteria-tradicional/
Lucas AB, Tryon J (2014) The Luna Maya model of care: a femifocal family care birth center. Tuftscope Interdisciplinary Journal of Health, Ethics, and Policy Medford, MA 14:22–29
Miller S, Abalos E, Chamillard M et al (2016). Beyond too little, too late and too much, too soon: a pathway towards evidence-based, respectful maternity care worldwide. Lancet (London, England) 388(10056):2176–2192. https://doi.org/10.1016/S0140-6736(16)31472-6
Murray de López J (2018) When the scars begin to heal: narratives of obstetric violence in Chiapas, Mexico. International Journal of Health Governance, Special Edition on Maternity Care Governance in a Global Context 23(1):60–69
Pathmanathan I, Liljestrand J, Martins J et al (2003) Investing in maternal health: learning from Malaysia and Sri Lanka (English) Health, nutrition, and population series. World Bank, Washington DC. Available via: http://documents.worldbank.org/curated/en/367761468760748311/Investing-in-maternal-health-learning-from-Malaysia-and-Sri-Lanka
Pelcastre-Villafuerte B, Ruiz M, Meneses S et al (2014) Community-based health care for indigenous women in Mexico: a qualitative evaluation. Int J Equity Health 13(1):2
Renfrew MJ, McFadden A, Bastos MH et al (2014) Midwifery and quality care: findings from a new evidence-informed framework for maternal and newborn care. Lancet 384(9948):1129–1145
Sandall J, Soltani H, Gates S et al (2013) Midwife-led continuity models versus other models of care for childbearing women. Cochrane pregnancy and childbirth group. Cochrane Database Systemic Review 9:CD004667
Sarker BK, Rahman M, Rahman T et al (2016) Reasons for preference of home delivery with traditional birth attendants (TBAs) in rural Bangladesh: a qualitative exploration. PLoS One 11(1):e0146161. https://doi.org/10.1371/journal.pone.0146161
Sialubanje C, Massar K, Hamer D et al (2015) Reasons for home delivery and use of traditional birth attendants in rural Zambia: a qualitative study. BMC Pregnancy Childbirth 15:206
Smith-Oka V (2013) Managing labor and delivery among impoverished populations in Mexico: cervical examinations as bureaucratic practice. American Anthropologist 115. https://doi.org/10.1111/aman.12046
Stapleton SR, Osborne C, Illuzi J (2013) Outcomes of Care in Birth Centers: demonstration of a durable model. J Midwifery Womens Health 00:1–12
ten Hoope-Bender, de Bernis L, Campbell J et al (2014) Improvement of maternal and newborn health through midwifery. Lancet 384(9949):1226–1235
Vogel J, Bohren M, Tuncalp O et al (2015) How women are treated during facility-based childbirth: development and validation of measurement tools in four countries- phase 1 formative research study protocol. Reprod Health 12:60
Walsh D (2009) Small really is beautiful: Tales from a Freestanding Birth Center in England. In: Davis-Floyd R, Barclay L, Daviss B et al (eds) Birth models that work. University of California Press, Berkeley, pp 159–186
WHO, UNICEF, UNFPA, World Bank Group and the United Nations Population Division (2015) Trends in maternal mortality: 1990 to 2015, estimates by WHO, UNICEF, UNFPA, World Bank Group and the United Nations Population Division
World Health Organization (2016) Midwives voices, midwives realities report 2016. Available via: https://www.who.int/maternal_child_adolescent/documents/midwives-voices-realities/en/

Chapter 12
Reconstructing Referrals: Overcoming Barriers to Quality Obstetric Care for Maya Women in Guatemala Through Care Navigation

Kirsten Austad, Anita Chary, Jessica Hawkins, Boris Martinez, and Peter Rohloff

This chapter describes Guatemala's Indigenous Maya traditions of home birth and midwifery. Home birth has long been integrated into Maya religious and cultural life as an important rite of passage into motherhood with spiritual significance, and a time for sociality and reciprocity among Maya women (Berry 2010; Cosminsky 1982; Paul 1975). Despite drastic reductions in home births in most Latin American countries, nearly half of all births in Guatemala still occur at home with traditional midwives (Ministerio de Salud Pública y Asistencia Social (MSPAS) 2015).

Scholars, health care providers, and policymakers widely code pregnancy and childbirth as "unsafe" for Maya women (Berry 2010). Maternal mortality rates in Guatemala are three times higher among Maya women than among non-Indigenous

Authors Kirsten Austad, Anita Chary have equally contributed to this chapter.

K. Austad
Center for Research in Indigenous Health, Wuqu' Kawoq|Maya Health Alliance, Tecpán, Guatemala

Department of Family Medicine, Boston University School of Medicine, Boston, MA, USA
e-mail: kirsten@wuqukawoq.org

A. Chary (✉)
Center for Research in Indigenous Health, Wuqu' Kawoq|Maya Health Alliance, Tecpán, Guatemala

Department of Emergency Medicine, Massachusetts General Hospital, Brigham And Women's Hospital, Boston, MA, USA
e-mail: anita.chary@mgh.harvard.edu

J. Hawkins
Center for Research in Indigenous Health, Wuqu' Kawoq|Maya Health Alliance, Tecpán, Guatemala

Berkeley School of Public Health, University of California, Berkeley, CA, USA
e-mail: jessica@wuqukawoq.org

© Springer Nature Switzerland AG 2021
K. Gutschow et al. (eds.), *Sustainable Birth in Disruptive Times*, Global Maternal and Child Health, https://doi.org/10.1007/978-3-030-54775-2_12

women (Avila et al. 2015). There are several reasons for this disparity, which relate to the "three delays" model of obstetric emergencies (Thaddeus and Maine 1994). First, Maya women delay decisions to seek obstetric care given strong cultural preferences to deliver at home, economic constraints, and perceptions of poor-quality care in biomedical settings (Berry 2010). Second, delays in reaching biomedical institutions occur because the majority of Maya women live in rural areas with poor transportation infrastructure and thus little or no means to access biomedical institutions in emergencies (Glei and Goldman 2000). Third, when Maya women do reach public biomedical institutions, they face delays in receiving adequate health care due to lack of resources and to discrimination (Berry 2010; Cerón et al. 2016; King et al. 2015).

This chapter describes an important but underexplored contributor to the "third delay" in emergency obstetric referrals of Maya women: institutional bureaucracy. We define "institutional bureaucracy" as "systems and techniques of administrative control as well as the individuals who operate them or operate within them" (Chary et al. 2016, p. 306), and consider this concept within clinical settings. Our ethnographic data demonstrate how health care bureaucracy can delay and prevent appropriate clinical care while contributing to ongoing obstetric violence. We additionally address a viable and sustainable solution to this predicament.

Our analysis also calls into question the sustainability of universal institutional delivery, a global development priority, as a means to reduce high maternal mortality rates in rural or other low-resource settings. This chapter highlights hospital resource constraints and bureaucratic processes that would only worsen with increased patient volume. We understand "sustainability" as the strategic use of resources to meet human needs while promoting ecological harmony and balance. A sustainable model of birth recognizes and deploys local expertise and innovates around local resource limitations to creatively push the boundaries of possible health care outcomes. We cannot accept or ignore the high maternal mortality and obstetric violence that Maya women encounter. We present a new model of maternity care that improves health outcomes while respecting robust local practices of home birth within a health care system plagued by severe resource limitations.

B. Martinez
Center for Research in Indigenous Health, Wuqu' Kawoq|Maya Health Alliance, Tecpán, Guatemala

Department of Internal Medicine, Saint Peter's University Hospital, Rutgers University, New Brunswick, NJ, USA

P. Rohloff
Center for Research in Indigenous Health, Wuqu' Kawoq|Maya Health Alliance, Tecpán, Guatemala

Division of Global Health Equity, Brigham and Women's Hospital, Boston, MA, USA

We begin with contextual information about maternal mortality in Guatemala and our involvement in providing obstetric care to Maya women for more than a decade. We then recount a case study illustrating how institutionalized racism and bureaucracy produce adverse maternal outcomes. We present a sustainable model of health care navigation that offers safer institutional birth for Maya women and then re-imagine our case study had care navigation been available.

12.1   Guatemala and Maternal Mortality

Guatemala is a multi-ethnic nation comprised of 23 Indigenous groups, the majority of whom are Maya and represent 45% of the national population (MSPAS et al. 2017). Centuries of Spanish colonialism and state-sponsored genocide of Maya people (1960–1996) have resulted in enduring political and economic marginalization of Maya communities. Most Maya individuals (79%) live in poverty (Central Intelligence Agency 2016) have poor access to biomedical health care (Chary and Rohloff 2015) and face disparities in health outcomes (MSPAS et al. 2017).

The burden of maternal mortality Maya women face has been a pressing public health concern for decades. In the latter half of the twentieth century, as part of broader international initiatives to incorporate local healers into biomedical health systems, the Guatemalan government and international health agencies focused on training traditional Indigenous midwives to identify and manage obstetric complications in home deliveries. While the MMR (maternal mortality ratio, maternal deaths/100,000 live births) dropped from 220 to 140 between 1994 and 2005, Guatemala remained far from meeting its Millennium Development Goals target MMR of below 70 (WHO 2015). As a result, public health policy shifted away from training traditional midwives toward emphasizing obstetric care in public hospitals (King et al. 2015). Consequently, midwife training programs in Guatemala now largely function to encourage midwives to refer women to biomedical facilities (King et al. 2015; Gobierno de Guatemala and MSPAS 2013; MSPAS 2015).

These policy changes have increased the rate of referrals of Maya women to government-run health facilities during pregnancy and delivery. To support the push to institutional deliveries, the Ministry of Health adopted policies encouraging care provision in Mayan languages and welcoming traditional midwives for patient accompaniment (MSPAS 2011). However, no formal implementation plan ensures compliance with these guidelines. In reality, most services are not available in Indigenous languages, Maya cultural preferences are ignored, and traditional midwives continue to be mistreated and/or excluded when accompanying patients (Stollak et al. 2016; King et al. 2015). For these reasons, many Maya women still refuse referrals to institutional obstetric care. Those who do follow up on referrals often experience mistreatment, institutional bureaucracy, and poor-quality biomedical care. We turn to these themes in more detail following a brief description of our methodology.

12.2 Methodology

These data draw from our collective experiences as anthropologists (AC, JH) and health care providers (KA, AC, BM, PR) working with the Wuqu' Kawoq/Maya Health Alliance (MHA), an NGO providing free high-quality medical care for Indigenous Guatemalans in Mayan languages. MHA has 14 years of experience in community-based maternal and child health services in rural Guatemala, predominantly in the regions of Chimaltenango, Sololá, and Suchitepéquez. Care is primarily delivered by Indigenous nurses and supervised by physicians in NGO clinics and during home visits. Because MHA is one of the few biomedical organizations offering care in Mayan languages in these areas, we often attract patients who have little contact with and/or severe misgivings about the public health system.

As a part of our maternal-child work, we collaborate with a local network of nearly 50 traditional midwives in our catchment area. To facilitate this collaboration, fully described elsewhere (Stroux et al. 2016), traditional midwives utilize a mobile health phone application that provides decision support to guide home prenatal visits and reduce delays in care by facilitating communication with our doctors and nurses. We began supporting referrals for institutional delivery by coordinating transportation and providing financial support for women with an obstetric emergency identified by collaborating traditional midwives. However, some women nonetheless refused referral due to fears of hospital care, including fears of mistreatment and forced sterilization. One such case that led to maternal death is described below. This woman's story, among others, inspired our specialized obstetric care navigator program that now provides accompanied referrals for Maya mothers. From April 2017 to 2018, we assisted with nearly 300 accompanied obstetric referrals to public biomedical institutions, with over 90% of women completing their referrals.

MHA clinicians and anthropologists review high-risk obstetric cases and adverse maternal outcomes with the NGO care team, conduct interviews with patients' family members and health care providers, and participate in maternal morbidity/mortality debriefings with departmental administrators of the Ministry of Health regarding patients whom we have referred. Here, we draw on these interviews and our experiences during the maternal death reviews and debriefings. Our analyses are further informed by over 200 semi-structured interviews we have conducted with Maya women, midwives, and other obstetric care providers over the past ten years in Chimaltenango and Suchitepéquez (Chary 2010; Chary et al. 2013a, b). Informed consent was obtained from all participants. Ethics approval was granted by the MHA Institutional Review Board. All names of individuals used herein are pseudonyms.

12.3 Telma

Telma,[1] a 35-year-old Kaqchikel-speaking mother of three, lived in a rural village 2 h from the nearest city. Thirty-three weeks into her pregnancy, she developed a severe headache and dizziness and sought out her traditional midwife Luisa. Luisa recognized the signs of preeclampsia, a potentially life-threatening high blood pressure disorder, and accompanied Telma to our clinic. Blood pressure readings and laboratory data confirmed severe preeclampsia. Our clinical team recognized that Telma required urgent hospitalization to control her blood pressure with intravenous medication, steroids to hasten fetal lung maturation, and induction of labor to prevent severe complications and maternal or neonatal death. Telma and her husband Pablo listened intently, nodding as our staff explained in Kaqchikel the gravity of the situation. However, Telma declined hospitalization. Her rationale was clear: "If I go to the hospital, I'm going to die there."

Telma relayed stories of family members and neighbors who sought care from public hospitals and left sicker and poorer than when they had arrived. Similar perceptions have been described throughout rural Guatemala (Berry 2010; Cerón et al. 2016; Rööst et al. 2004). In part, these perceptions result from conflicting sets of therapeutic expectations among Indigenous patients and non-Indigenous providers (Berry 2010). However, negative perceptions are also based on the realities of long wait times for both outpatient and emergency care, frequent lack of medications, understaffing, and inadequate facilities (Chary and Rohloff 2015; Garces et al. 2015).

While Telma refused hospitalization, she did request that we treat her high blood pressure. During daily subsequent home visits, Telma's blood pressure continued to rise, and we reiterated our strong recommendation of hospitalization with induction of preterm delivery given the significant risks to her health. After much persuasion, Telma finally agreed, and the team provided her with the referral documentation required for hospitalization.

However, when Telma and Pablo arrived at the hospital, the security guard did not allow them to enter. Instead, he brought over a young, non-Indigenous nurse, to whom Telma gave the referral documents. The nurse did not even bother to open the envelope containing the documents. Rather, while standing outside the hospital fence, she took Telma's blood pressure, declared it normal (blood pressure fluctuation is common in women with preeclampsia) and informed Telma that she could not see a doctor. Telma and her husband felt defeated. Yet because they had been socialized to defer to authorities and lacked the Spanish fluency to insist upon clinical assessment, they returned home.

Over the following days, we made multiple subsequent attempts to contact Telma and Pablo by telephone but received no answer. We saw her again only after Luisa, concerned by Telma's lack of response, made an unscheduled home visit and, upon hearing her story, brought Telma back to see our medical team. Emotionally

---

[1] Pseudonym; all names and identifying details of the people in this chapter have been changed.

exhausted, Telma recounted her hospital rejection and allowed us to take her blood pressure again; it was severely elevated. Telma politely thanked us for our concern but felt going to the hospital again would be futile. She restated that submitting to hospital care was tantamount to death or invisibility and reiterated her wish to give birth at home as she had planned. She lovingly took the hand of her four-year-old daughter, who had been clinging to her leg, and walked home to prepare lunch. We watched her leave the clinic, feeling helpless to provide her with life-saving medical care.

A few days later, Telma's husband called to inform us that Telma and their newborn son had died. He recounted through tears how Telma awoke during the middle of the night with an excruciating headache. Panicked, she asked her husband to use the little money they had to pay a private car to transport her back to the hospital, where hospital staff belatedly made the diagnosis of severe preeclampsia. They induced labor, but the newborn suffered severe consequences of preeclampsia and prematurity and died of respiratory failure. Telma became very ill on her second postpartum day and was transferred to a larger hospital in Guatemala City. Nurses and physicians explained to Pablo that Telma was gravely ill, but his Spanish was insufficient to understand their explanations of why she died. When we participated in the formal maternal death review conducted by the Ministry of Health, medical records revealed that Telma had undergone a postpartum curettage for persistent bleeding, which likely led to infection and death from septic shock. Daily progress notes revealed that the attending medical team's recommendations to monitor her infection with laboratory studies and treat her with antibiotics were never carried out.

12.4   Hospital Bureaucracy and the Failure of Systems of Care

While the Guatemalan constitution theoretically guarantees citizens free government-sponsored health care, because of funding shortages, many basic services such as lab tests and medications are not provided at primary or even secondary level facilities like the hospital in Guatemala City (Chary and Rohloff 2015). Resource-limited public hospitals must rely on patients' family members to obtain lab tests, supplies, and medications at better-stocked private clinics and pharmacies. Many of our patients refer to the tasks of obtaining these tests and supplies as "chores" (Chary et al. 2016), which often prove insurmountable, as they were for Telma's husband. In order to obtain tests and medications for Telma, Pablo would have had to first use public transportation to navigate the auxiliary medical facilities within the dangerous and unfamiliar capital city. Even if he had found the entire list of supplies requested by the inpatient medical team, the total cost would have exceeded his annual income. He did not know that he could have approached hospital social workers about obtaining discounts on certain items, such as imaging studies and medications. And even if he had known about the discounts, he lacked the literacy and Spanish fluency to negotiate the maze of paperwork and long lines to receive them; no Kaqchikel interpreters were available.

Telma's and Pablo's experiences resonate with scholarly observations about how institutional bureaucracy impedes access to social services (Auyero 2012; Gupta 2012; Hetherington 2011; Petryna 2002). Telma's story illustrates two features of institutional bureaucracy that delay and prevent emergency obstetric care. The first is what Lipsky (1980) refers to as "street-level bureaucracy," or how an institution's frontline workers, such as security guards, clerks, and junior nurses, create and implement institutional policies by controlling access points and intake procedures. Telma's efforts to receive timely obstetric care were thwarted precisely by these street-level bureaucrats—a hospital guard and a nurse.

We have met numerous Indigenous patients seeking urgent obstetric care similarly turned away by such gatekeepers. For instance, a hospital security guard turned away Silvia, a 30-year-old mother of four, who was feeling unwell from several days of vaginal bleeding from a first-trimester miscarriage. When she collapsed at home the next day from continual bleeding and could not be roused, her family rushed her back to the hospital where she was admitted. She received fluids, a blood transfusion, and surgical evacuation of her uterus for an incomplete miscarriage. Silvia attributed being turned away at her first visit to her "dark skin" and "Indigenous clothing." As another example, while performing clinical rotations in public health facilities, we have witnessed secretaries and nurses deny Maya women urgent obstetric care for forgetting to bring records of their prenatal visits, laboratory exams, or ultrasounds.

Street-level bureaucrats represent the first contact for patients seeking emergency care in most Guatemalan facilities, yet they lack medical expertise to triage and they perpetuate bias and exclusion. This dynamic is particularly important in obstetrics, given the need for quick decisions in life-threatening situations. To some extent, street-level bureaucrats are merely following hospital protocols when they ask for patients' appointment cards, medical records, or referral letters to grant entry. However, their interpersonal interactions and implicit biases create a policy of routine exclusion of Indigenous women that exists outside of the official administrative structure.

Medical errands ("chores") are a second form of institutional bureaucracy that limits access to quality obstetric care. Laboratory supplies and potentially life-saving antibiotics were not available to Telma at the hospital due to stockouts, and Pablo was unable to navigate Guatemala City to obtain them. This situation is not uncommon. For example, another patient of ours, Delmi, whose midwife referred her to the hospital, recounted being frightened by a doctor who told her that she needed an urgent cesarean section to save her and her baby's lives. The doctor's urgency, however, seemed to dissipate as he informed Delmi and her husband that they would first need to purchase and bring to the hospital medical supplies such as intravenous fluids, needles, and surgical gloves before he would perform her surgery. Such tasks are nearly impossible for impoverished, non-Spanish speaking Maya patients.

Notably, not all medical errands have a biomedical indication. For example, several public facilities require women with even low-risk pregnancies to obtain one or more ultrasounds as a prerequisite for routine prenatal care appointments or institutional delivery. While the biomedical rationale behind this prerequisite is unclear, the ultrasound requirement effectively functions as a denial of care for the many women who cannot afford the exam's cost.

Such experiences can be understood within a framework of obstetric violence. Activists—many based in Latin American countries—developed the concept in the 2000s to denounce the disrespect, mistreatment, and physical abuse toward laboring women (Bohren et al. 2015; Bowser and Hill 2010). The original definition of obstetric violence in Venezuelan law in 2007 emphasized health care personnel's dehumanization of parturients, medicalization of childbirth, and infringements on women's autonomy (Pérez D'Gregorio 2010). Scholarly discussions of obstetric violence have recently drawn on the concept of disrespect and abuse of women in childbirth, which Freedman et al. (2014) conceptualize as rooted in both individual behaviors and system deficiencies; these are mutually reinforcing in limiting availability, accessibility, and quality of care, and in normalizing violence. Importantly, as Dixon (2015, p. 447) describes, there are multiple registers of obstetric violence, including "tangible and acute violent act[s]" as well as "chronic and systemic violence" that make women vulnerable to biomedical appropriation of their bodies and reproductive lives.

Our data highlight the bureaucratic components of obstetric violence. Public hospitals as bureaucracies are simultaneously ensconced in hegemonic political-economic structures and operated by individual agents. As street-level bureaucrats disproportionately turn Indigenous pregnant women away from hospitals, racial discrimination becomes institutional policy. As protocols, paperwork, and medical errands delay care disproportionately for Indigenous women, Maya mothers and neonates die—and the deaths are often blamed on traditional midwives. Techniques of institutional bureaucracy become inseparable from racial discrimination and facilitate obstetric violence.

12.5   A Solution: Patient Accompaniment and Care Navigation

What might have been done to avert the deaths of Telma and her son? While there are no simple solutions to overcoming the barriers to obstetric care that Maya women face, if Telma had received emergency obstetric care when she first presented with preeclampsia symptoms, she and her son might have survived. Having learned from Telma's experience, we now offer Maya mothers "obstetric care navigators"— local women bilingual in Spanish and Kaqchikel who are trained to provide accompaniment during hospital referrals. Care navigators constitute a powerful means to overcome the institutional bureaucracy that impedes access to obstetric care.

Our model of obstetric patient navigation builds on two trends in global health care delivery. The first, *patient accompaniment*, engages community members to reduce patient-side barriers to care. It can increase uptake of health care provision and improve patient outcomes, as the NGO Partners in Health has shown in Haiti (Behforouz et al. 2004). The second, *care navigation*, employs individuals to help patients longitudinally traverse a continuum of health care services, especially in oncological care (Freeman 2013). Our model further recognizes that patient navigators provide Indigenous patients with a kind of *cultural capital*—a term used by Bourdieu (1977) to describe the cultural competencies and assets that allow for advancement within certain institutions. In Guatemalan hospitals, these competencies include literacy, Spanish language fluency, self-confidence to advocate for one's needs and perspective, awareness of institutional rules and protocols, and familiarity with the urban geography of auxiliary medical facilities (Chary et al. 2016).

Since 2010, our organization has operated a patient navigator program to facilitate care for rural Mayan-speaking patients with complex chronic medical conditions requiring specialized services. The patients using our patient navigator program range from children with congenital heart defects requiring surgical repair to adults with cancer needing chemotherapy. Patient navigators coordinate the logistics of and transport to appointments and interpret between Spanish and Mayan languages during clinical encounters. Most importantly, patient navigators are equipped with the cultural capital required in Guatemalan hospitals: they are literate, young, technologically savvy, and receive specific training on the policies of Guatemalan health care institutions, as well as interpersonal and situational skills for dealing with bureaucracy (Chary et al. 2016). Patient navigators keep track of and fulfill any prerequisites for care—such as obtaining lab tests, medications, medical supplies, and required paperwork—often performing medical errands on behalf of patients and their families. Our program has grown exponentially, and over 1000 patients have used navigators thus far (Chary et al. 2016).

A recent large-scale study of Indigenous women using facility-based care in Guatemala indicated that the two strongest predictors of satisfaction with care were: (1) being allowed accompaniment and (2) feeling that the care had been respectful (Colombara et al. 2016). As MHA became known for collaborations with traditional midwives and care navigation, we piloted *obstetric* care navigation to improve Indigenous women's health outcomes and satisfaction with hospital-based obstetric care (Austad et al. 2017). We trained four patient navigators in obstetrical referral, who take turns being on call for our traditional midwifery network. When a midwife refers a patient, the navigators quickly coordinate transport, facilitate hospital entry, complete bureaucratic hospital procedures, and provide language interpretation, in addition to critical emotional support that is currently lacking during institutional deliveries in the public sector in Guatemala. To monitor the program's success, we track the volume of obstetric referrals in our collaborating midwives' cohort, the referral completion rate, the length of time required to complete each referral, and patient/family satisfaction with obstetric care navigation.

The hospital resource constraints and bureaucratic procedures we describe herein preclude the sustainability of universal institutional delivery in Guatemala and other low- and middle-income countries. Rather than promote universal institutional delivery, we hope that patient navigators, deployed selectively for women with high-risk pregnancies, will improve maternal and neonatal outcomes while promoting four goals key to a more sustainable model of birth in Guatemala:

(1) Women who prefer home births have a reduced risk of adverse outcomes with access to timely and efficient referrals to emergency obstetric care through our patient navigator network.

(2) Patient navigators improve hospital birth experiences, reducing the pervasive aversion to hospital care as women's positive experiences spread through word of mouth.

(3) Bilingual care navigators allow non-Indigenous biomedical providers to have more positive and meaningful communication with Indigenous women.

(4) Obstetric care navigators demonstrate respectful maternity care for hospital staff, including techniques to support women during labor that they otherwise would not learn.

In these four ways, our care navigation program models a growing recognition that "the right amount of care needs to be offered at the right time, and delivered in a manner that respects, protects, and promotes human rights" (Miller et al. 2016, p. 2176).

Publication of results and lessons learned, including barriers faced, will be shared once the pilot project is completed. Looking forward, we see a number of potential paths toward sustainability for the obstetric care navigator program. This pilot program was designed to be easily scalable to allow other NGOs or Ministries of Health to deploy the strategy focally in areas of high maternal mortality at a reasonable cost. Nearly all of our care navigator reimbursement derives from pay-for-performance scales based on referral volume and success rate, allowing programs to titrate the number of referrals accepted to funding level. Alternatively, communities could organize themselves to train and support obstetric care navigators to serve expecting mothers in their village on a volunteer basis or funded by a small fee paid by pregnant women, creating paid job opportunities for Indigenous women.

The new role of obstetric care navigator complements the work of traditional midwives who, despite official policies of inclusion for a number of years, continue to face racial discrimination and exclusion in public hospitals (MSPAS 2011). The verbal abuse our collaborating midwives face when attempting to accompany their clients to a hospital has made most of them reluctant to take on the care navigator role. They are keenly aware that they lack the necessary cultural capital to do so. The presence of obstetric care navigators in hospitals and the proliferation of care provided in Mayan languages, facilitated by their presence as interpreters, may slowly change hospital norms fueled by underlying racial biases against Indigenous women that negatively impact both patients and traditional midwives.

The long-term goal is a fundamental change in institutional biases to allow traditional midwives themselves to accompany their clients to hospital deliveries. We hope that patient navigators act as the wedge that pushes maternity wards to honor the official policies of inclusion, and that these navigators will help midwives to one day feel empowered to enter the labor and delivery wards and take over most of the tasks currently filled by obstetric care navigators. Notably, however, some of our collaborating traditional midwives have commented that creating a separate role for accompaniment is preferred, as it allows them to focus on community-based prenatal care and low-risk deliveries.

Ultimately, broader social changes are necessary to yield substantial and sustainable reductions in maternal mortality among Maya communities. Such changes include increased government spending on rural health care and infrastructure, improved racial bias training of health care personnel, shifting hospital norms to decrease disrespectful and abusive medical treatment, and inclusion of Maya people in higher education and medical training programs. Obstetric care navigators offer a sustainable and interim solution that empowers Maya women and their midwives to obtain successful obstetric referrals.

12.6   Telma's Story Retold

While there is nothing we can do to change Telma's outcome, her legacy galvanized us to propose obstetric care navigation as a sustainable strategy to improve maternal health among rural Maya women in Guatemala. We now retell Telma's story as we imagine it would have unfolded had she received obstetric care navigation services.

Thirty-three weeks into Telma's pregnancy, her traditional midwife Luisa became concerned that Telma had preeclampsia. After many instances of mistreatment in the hospital, Luisa decided to call the MHA midwife line for support regarding hospital evaluation for Telma. An MHA physician reviewed the case, including automatic blood pressure readings sent from a smartphone, and confirmed the diagnosis. Telma initially refused when Luisa recommended hospital evaluation. But, when our obstetric care navigator Merida visited Telma and patiently explained each step of the journey, Telma and her husband agreed and headed to the city in an MHA car. To facilitate prompt care, they first went to a reliable private laboratory to obtain the necessary tests and ultrasound the public hospital required of all women with preeclampsia.

At the hospital, Merida explained Telma's problem in fluent Spanish to a security guard, with whom she had developed a cordial working relationship while accompanying prior patients. When the triage nurse took Telma's blood pressure and found it normal, Merida reviewed with the triage nurse the referral letter documenting the numerous elevated blood pressure readings in the past hours. The nurse agreed that Telma should be evaluated. When a doctor came to take Telma's history, Merida presented the referral letter and the lab results confirming the diagnosis of severe preeclampsia. The doctor informed Telma that she would need to be admitted. Merida interpreted the doctor's comments from Spanish to Kaqchikel, allowing

Telma to ask if she would need an operation or whether the baby could be born "normally."

When Telma began labor and hospital staff asked Pablo to wait outside, Merida remained with her, providing comfort and reassurance. Merida advocated for Telma by suggesting alternative labor and birthing positions and provided frequent updates to Pablo. Telma's baby boy survived despite multiple complications of prematurity. When Telma had persistent postpartum bleeding, the doctors gave her husband a list of equipment and medications they would need to "clean her uterus" of the remaining placenta. Because her husband was frightened and unfamiliar with the busy city streets, Merida went with him to a nearby pharmacy she worked with frequently and purchased all the necessary supplies so that Telma's treatment was not delayed. Timely antibiotics resolved Telma's developing uterine infection, and Merida drove the growing family back to their rural home. Telma and her baby received a house call from an MHA nurse a few days later to check her blood pressure and ensure the baby was feeding well. While Telma would have preferred a home birth, she was thrilled with her four-year-old daughter's joy upon seeing her mother and baby brother arrive home.

References

Austad K, Chary A, Martinez B, Juarez M, Martin YJ, Ixen EC, Rohloff P (2017) Obstetric care navigation: a new approach to promote respectful maternity care and overcome barriers to safe motherhood. Reprod Health 14(1):148. https://doi.org/10.1186/s12978-017-0410-6

Auyero J (2012) Patients of the state: the politics of waiting in Argentina. Duke University Press, Durham. https://doi.org/10.1215/9780822395287

Avila C, Bright R, Gutierrez JC et al (2015) Guatemala health system assessment. Health Finance & Governance Project Abt Associates Inc., Bethesda

Behforouz HL, Farmer PE, Mukherjee JS (2004) From directly observed therapy to accompagnateurs: enhancing AIDS treatment outcomes in Haiti and in Boston. Clin Infect Dis 38(Supplement 5):S429–S436. https://doi.org/10.1086/421408

Berry NS (2010) Unsafe motherhood: Mayan maternal mortality and subjectivity in post-war Guatemala. Berghahn Books, New York

Bohren MA, Vogel JP, Hunter EC et al (2015) The mistreatment of women during childbirth in health facilities globally: a mixed-methods systematic review. PLoS Med 12(6):e1001847. https://doi.org/10.1371/journal.pmed.1001847

Bourdieu P (1977) Outline of a theory of practice (trans: Nice R), 1st edn. Cambridge University Press, Cambridge. https://doi.org/10.1017/CBO9780511812507

Bowser D, Hill K (2010) Exploring evidence for disrespect and abuse in facility-based childbirth: report of a landscape analysis. USAID, Washington, DC

Central Intelligence Agency (2016) The world factbook: Central America: Guatemala. https://www.cia.gov/library/publications/resources/the-world-factbook/geos/gt.html

Cerón A, Ruano AL, Sánchez S (2016) Abuse and discrimination towards indigenous people in public health care facilities: experiences from rural Guatemala. Int J Equity Health 15(77):77. https://doi.org/10.1186/s12939-016-0367-z

Chary A (2010) Contextualizing blame in mothers' narratives of child death in rural Guatemala. In: Paper presented at the American Culture Association & Popular Culture Association Conference, St. Louis, MO, 31 March–3 April

Chary A, Rohloff P (eds) (2015) Privatization and the new medical pluralism: shifting healthcare landscapes in Maya Guatemala. Lexington Books, Lanham

Chary A, Kraemer Díaz A, Henderson B, Rohloff P (2013a) The changing role of Indigenous lay midwives in Guatemala: new frameworks for analysis. Midwifery 29(8):852–858. https://doi.org/10.1016/j.midw.2012.08.011

Chary A, Messmer S, Sorenson E et al (2013b) The normalization of childhood disease: an ethnographic study of child malnutrition in rural Guatemala. Human Organ 72(2):87–97. https://doi.org/10.17730/humo.72.2.f2014210742702r2

Chary A, Flood D, Austad K, Moore J et al (2016) Navigating bureaucracy: accompanying Indigenous Maya patients with complex health care needs in Guatemala. Human Organ 75(4):305–314. https://doi.org/10.17730/1938-3525-75.4.305

Colombara DV, Hernández B, Schaefer A et al (2016) Institutional delivery and satisfaction among Indigenous and poor women in Guatemala, Mexico, and Panama. PLoS One 11(4). https://doi.org/10.1371/journal.pone.0154388

Cosminsky S (1982) Childbirth and change: a Guatemalan study. In: MacCormack CP (ed) Ethnography of fertility and birth. Academic Press, New York, pp 205–230

Dixon LZ (2015) Obstetrics in a time of violence: Mexican midwives critique routine hospital practices. Med Anthropol Q 29(4):437–454. https://doi.org/10.1111/maq.12174

Freedman LP, Ramsey K, Abuya T et al (2014) Defining disrespect and abuse of women in childbirth: a research, policy and rights agenda. Bull World Health Organ 92(12):915–917. https://doi.org/10.2471/blt.14.137869

Freeman HP (2013) The history, principles, and future of patient navigation: commentary. Semin Oncol Nurs 29(2):72–75. https://doi.org/10.1016/j.soncn.2013.02.002

Garces A, McClure EM, Hambidge KM et al (2015) Trends in perinatal deaths from 2010 to 2013 in the Guatemalan Western Highlands. Reprod Health 12(2):S12. https://doi.org/10.1186/1742-4755-12-s2-s14

Glei DA, Goldman N (2000) Understanding ethnic variation in pregnancy-related care in rural Guatemala. Ethn Health 5(1):5–22. https://doi.org/10.1080/13557850050007301

Gobierno de Guatemala, Ministerio de Salud Pública y Asistencia Social (MSPAS) (2013) Ley para la maternidad saludable. MSPAS, Guatemala City

Gupta A (2012) Red tape: bureaucracy, structural violence, and poverty in India. Duke University Press, Durham. https://doi.org/10.1215/9780822394709

Hetherington K (2011) Guerrilla auditors: the politics of transparency in neoliberal Paraguay. Duke University Press, Durham. https://doi.org/10.1215/9780822394266

King N, Chary A, Rohloff P (2015) Leveraging resources in contemporary Maya midwifery. In: Chary A, Rohloff P (eds) Privatization and the new medical pluralism: shifting healthcare landscapes in Maya Guatemala. Lexington Books, Lanham, pp 123–140

Lipsky M (1980) Street level bureaucracy: dilemmas of the individual in public services. Russell Sage Foundation, New York. https://doi.org/10.1177/003232928001000113

Miller S, Abalos E, Chamillard M et al (2016) Beyond too little, too late and too much, too soon: a pathway towards evidence-based, respectful maternity care worldwide. Lancet 388(10056):2176–2192. https://doi.org/10.1016/s0140-6736(16)31472-6

Ministerio de Salud Pública y Asistencia Social (MSPAS) (2011) Guía para la implementación de la atención integral maternal y neonatal. MSPAS, Guatemala City

Ministerio de Salud Pública y Asistencia Social (MSPAS) (2015) Primera encuesta sobre el trato durante la atención del parto en los servicios de salud del MSPAS 2014–2015. MSPAS, Guatemala City

Ministerio de Salud Pública y Asistencia Social (MSPAS), Instituto Nacional de Estadística, ICF International (2017) VI Encuesta nacional de salud materno infantil (ENSMI) 2014–2015. Ministerio de Salud Pública y Asistencia Social. MSPAS, Guatemala City

Paul L (1975) Recruitment to a ritual role: the midwife in a Maya community. Ethos 3(3):449–467. https://doi.org/10.1525/eth.1975.3.3.02a00050

Pérez D'Gregorio R (2010) Obstetric violence: a new legal term introduced in Venezuela. Int J Gynecol Obstet 111(3):201–202. https://doi.org/10.1016/j.ijgo.2010.09.002

Petryna A (2002) Life exposed: biological citizens after Chernobyl. Princeton University Press, Princeton. https://doi.org/10.2307/j.ctt7rtb3

Rööst M, Johnsdotter S, Liljestrand J, Essen B (2004) A qualitative study of conceptions and attitudes regarding maternal mortality among traditional birth attendants in rural Guatemala. BJOG Int J Obstetr Gynaecol 111(12):1372–1377. https://doi.org/10.1111/j.1471-0528.2004.00270.x

Stollak I, Valdez M, Rivas K, Perry H (2016) Casas maternas in the rural highlands of Guatemala: a mixed-methods case study of the introduction and utilization of birthing facilities by an indigenous population. Glob Health Sci Pract 4(1):114–131. https://doi.org/10.9745/ghsp-d-15-00266

Stroux L, Martinez B, Coyote Ixen E et al (2016) An mHealth monitoring system for traditional birth attendant-led antenatal risk assessment in rural Guatemala. J Med Eng Technol 40(7–8):356–371. https://doi.org/10.1080/03091902.2016.1223196

Thaddeus S, Maine D (1994) Too far to walk: maternal mortality in context. Soc Sci Med 38(8):1091–1110. https://doi.org/10.1016/0277-9536(94)90226-7

WHO (2015) Trends in maternal mortality: 1990 to 2015 estimates by WHO, UNICEF, UNFPA, World Bank Group and the United Nations Population Division. WHO Publications, Geneva

Part III
Sustainable Maternity Solutions in Low- and Middle-Income Countries

Chapter 13
A Sustainable Model of Assessing Maternal Health Needs and Improving Quality of Care During and After Pregnancy

Mary McCauley and Nynke van den Broek

13.1 Background

This chapter focuses on improving maternity care in the context of the sustainable development goals (SDGs), which are most broadly oriented towards improving health and well-being, rather than reducing maternal deaths, as was the focus of the MDGs. This chapter will review how concepts of *quality of care* can be used to improve antenatal, intrapartum and postpartum care in a sustainable fashion by improving the safety, effectiveness and experience of care within existing health-care systems. This chapter will also discuss evolving definitions for maternal morbidity, while closing with some key policy implications and remaining challenges for ensuring sustainability.

13.2 Introduction

SDG 3 aims to ensure that women have a universal right to health and well-being that requires that all women have an equal chance to "survive and thrive" during and after pregnancy (UN 2015a). Regarding maternity care, this SDG goal grants all women equal rights to have a healthy and desired pregnancy and childbirth (UN 2015a, b). However, this goal is far from being achieved as women across the globe face numerous barriers to accessing high-quality maternity care because of socio-economic inequalities, structural violence and marginalization that harm their physical, mental and emotional health and well-being (UN 2015b).

M. McCauley (✉) · N. van den Broek
Liverpool School of Tropical Medicine, Centre for Maternal and Newborn Health,
Liverpool, UK
e-mail: marymccauley@doctors.net.uk

© Springer Nature Switzerland AG 2021   187
K. Gutschow et al. (eds.), *Sustainable Birth in Disruptive Times*, Global
Maternal and Child Health, https://doi.org/10.1007/978-3-030-54775-2_13

Despite significant progress in reducing maternal mortality, an estimated 303,000 women died due to pregnancy-related complications in 2015, which equates to roughly 830 women dying every day (WHO et al. 2015). Most (99%) of these deaths occur in low- and middle-income countries (LMIC) (WHO et al. 2015). Related to these maternal deaths are the annual toll of 2.5 million neonatal deaths and 2.6 million stillbirths, 1.3 million of which occur intrapartum (WHO et al. 2015; Frøen et al. 2016). Many of these maternal and perinatal deaths were preventable if evidence-based measures and interventions had been followed (WHO 2015a).

Complications during pregnancy and childbirth are a leading cause of death, disability and ill-health among women of reproductive age (WHO 2015a, 2016; Graham et al. 2018). Yet maternal mortality accounts for a small fraction of the overall burden of poor maternal health (Chou et al. 2016). Maternal deaths are merely the "tip of the iceberg" with a variety of maternal morbidities representing part of the underlying iceberg (Liskin 1992). By concentrating only on why women are dying, we risk overlooking many major and minor complications or conditions that women suffer during and after pregnancy (Chou et al. 2016). Historically, maternal mortality and morbidity have been studied in isolation from one another, even though their direct causes overlap. To achieve further global reductions in maternal mortality and achieve improved maternal health, it is clear that a more comprehensive and sustainable approach is needed that addresses the continuum of care and quality of care (PMNCH 2011; Firoz 2013; McCauley et al. 2018).

13.3   Progress on Improving Maternal Health

Given the timing of maternal deaths during or immediately after labour and delivery and the inconsistent evidence of how much antenatal care reduces maternal mortality, the efforts around reducing maternal mortality have been directed at intrapartum interventions. Between 1990 and 2015, these efforts resulted in an uptake of skilled birth attendance from 57% to 74% (Campbell et al. 2016). Further, a renewed emphasis on improving antenatal and postnatal care has resulted in an increase in one or more antenatal visits from 65% to 83% and an increase in the WHO-recommended four or more antenatal visits from 37% to 64% (Campbell et al. 2016). The relatively low number of antenatal visits may constitute a series of missed opportunities to address the physical and psychosocial needs of women in an integrated manner. The provision of high-quality maternity care would improve the recognition of some risk factors or conditions associated with maternal morbidity and mortality, as well as the timely management of such conditions to avoid progression to more severe complications, thereby reducing adverse outcomes for both mother and baby.

For women who do access healthcare services, some do receive high-quality care but more than often many experience one of two extremes: too little, too late (where women receive care that is not timely or sufficient); and too much, too soon, marked by over-medicalization and excessive use of unnecessary interventions (such as unnecessary caesarean section; routine induced or augmented labour; routine continuous electronic fetal monitoring; routine episiotomy; and routine antibiotics postpartum) (Miller et al. 2016). Both extremes represent maternal health care that is not grounded in evidence (Miller et al. 2016). Many women, especially those living in low- and middle-income countries receive poor quality care, access to evidence-based care is often inadequate; there is lack of equipment, supplies and medicines; inadequate numbers of skilled, motivated and empathic healthcare providers; and lack of interfacility referrals (Miller et al. 2016).

13.4   Maternal Health Indicators and Definitions

A maternal death is "the death of a woman while pregnant or within 42 days of termination of pregnancy, irrespective of the duration and site of the pregnancy, from any cause related to or aggravated by the pregnancy or its management but not from accidental or incidental causes" (WHO 2012). The MMR (maternal deaths/100,000 live births) represents the risk of dying from childbirth and pregnancy-related causes, yet it does not include maternal morbidity. In 2015, the MMR in LMIC countries (239) was 20 times that found in high-income countries (12) (WHO et al. 2015). These large disparities reflect inequality in access to and quality of emergency and routine care for women during and after pregnancy between women with low- and high-income and those women living in rural versus urban areas.

13.5   Severe Acute Maternal Morbidity

Severe acute maternal morbidity (SAMM), also known as "maternal near miss", refers to a woman who nearly died but survived a complication that occurred during pregnancy, childbirth or within 42 days of termination of pregnancy, or without residual morbidity (Say et al. 2009). SAMM data are vital to better estimate whether or not essential and emergency obstetric care is provided or available. It is assumed to be a better indicator for designing, monitoring and evaluating maternal health programs than maternal mortality alone, as it represents a wider group of women at risk of complications. Previously, research on maternal morbidity has focused on SAMM, which is usually assessed at secondary or tertiary healthcare levels using internationally accepted criteria (Tunçalp et al. 2013; van den Akker et al. 2013).

13.6   Maternal Morbidity

An international group of experts working with WHO havehas defined non-severe maternal morbidity as "any condition that is attributed to or aggravated by pregnancy and childbirth which has a negative impact on the woman's wellbeing and/or functioning" (Firoz et al. 2013). Until recently, this type of maternal morbidity, which is recognized at the primary level by provider or mothers themselves, has been poorly documented (Zafar et al. 2015).

Early calculations estimated that for every maternal death, 20 to 30 more women suffer maternal morbidity (Ashford 2002). More precise mathematical modelling of available data suggests that of the 136 million women who give birth each year, roughly 1.4 million women experience SAMM, 9.5 million experience other complications and 20 million suffer from long-term morbidities or disabilities (WHO 2015b).

A recent study was the first of its kind to assess the prevalence of maternal morbidity in four LMIC settings (McCauley et al. 2018). This descriptive observational cross-sectional study assessed physical (infectious and medical/obstetric), psychological and social morbidities in 11,454 women in India (2099), Malawi (2923), Kenya (3145) and Pakistan (3287). Almost three out of four women had more than one symptom (73.5%), abnormalities on clinical examination (71.3%), or laboratory investigation (73.5%). In total, 9% of women had an infectious disease (HIV, malaria, syphilis, or chest infection) and 23.1% had signs of early sepsis. Overall, 47.9% of women were anaemic, 11.5% had other medical or obstetric conditions, 25.1% had psychological morbidities (depression, thoughts of self-harm) and 36.6% had social morbidity (domestic violence, substance misuse) (McCauley et al. 2018).

The study concluded that, despite women reporting that they are satisfied with their health, there is evidence of morbidity from a variety of physical and psychosocial causes. This study also demonstrates that maternity care needs to account for women's broader psycho-social well-being. It recommends that current antenatal and postnatal care packages need to be adapted and improved to provide comprehensive, holistic care in ways that meet a woman's health needs (McCauley et al. 2018). Furthermore, routine screening for depression and domestic violence should be implemented in order to improve maternal health and reduce maternal morbidity (McCauley et al. 2020).

13.7   Quality of Maternity Care

While uptake or utilization of healthcare has increased, there has not been a concomitant increase in the quality of that maternity care. It is widely acknowledged that maternity care in LMIC as well as high-income settings often is not evidence-based (Miller et al. 2016), is not respectful (Freedman et al. 2014, Bohren et al. 2015), not mother-baby-family friendly (Lalonde et al. 2019), and either unavailable or of sub-standard quality (Campbell et al. 2016). Yet due to the push for meeting SDGs, healthcare providers are expected to provide both more and better care, even as these goals may be at odds with one another. Most healthcare providers in LMIC are trying to expand maternity care within healthcare systems that face shortages of staff, equipment, essential medicines and infrastructure. In many cases, the scope of practice of healthcare providers (especially at the primary care level) has increased, such as with "task shifting". Current pre-service training often does not fully equip healthcare providers for their newly expanded roles and competencies. The lack of competency-based, in-service trainings available to providers reduces provider morale and complicates the continuity of care that is expected both within and beyond the clinic.

National confidential inquiries into the causes of and factors associated with maternal and newborn deaths, as well as smaller scale studies assessing quality of healthcare provision, have identified that poor-quality care contributes to high levels of maternal and neonatal death (Fauveau and de Bernis 2006; Althabe et al. 2008). There is also a relationship between uptake and coverage of care and quality of care. We know that women's awareness of poor quality of care or abusive care can deter women from accessing care even when it was affordable and available nearby (Bohren et al. 2015; Campbell et al. 2016). This fact was highlighted by Fathalla almost 20 years ago, when he emphasized, "The question should not be why do women not accept the service that we offer, but why do we not offer a service that women will accept" (Fathalla 1998).

Quality of care is an important consideration in international initiatives, and global leaders have agreed to collaborate by aligning efforts, which will reduce the burden of data collection and reporting for countries and improve linkage of results with decision making. New tools for the assessment of quality of care have been developed and there is international consensus on indicators for quality of care in maternal, newborn and child health (Madaj et al. 2017).[1]

13.8 Evidence-Based Care for Mothers and Babies

Quality of care has improved due to a shift towards evidence-based medicine that is defined as: "The conscientious, explicit and judicious use of current best evidence in making decisions about the care of individual patients" (Sackett et al. 1996). Other terms such as "evidence-based healthcare" or "evidence-based practice" are used to illustrate that quality of care goes beyond individual patient care to inform the delivery of care provided through the wider healthcare system (Miller et al. 2016). Internationally, high-quality independent systematic reviews of interventions that relate to pregnancy, childbirth and up to 30 days following childbirth are published by the Pregnancy and Childbirth Cochrane Group (http://pregnancy.cochrane.org/). In many high-income countries, these reviews are regularly used to develop and update national guidelines and protocols for healthcare. Yet evidence-based practice remains a relatively new concept that needs to be strengthened in many LMIC.

---

[1] Note that for Donabedian (1988), quality of healthcare is measured in terms of (1) structure or inputs: the material, human and intellectual resources needed to provide care; (2) processes: the activities in which these resources are used to provide care; and (3) outcomes: the results of the activities.

13.9 A Culture of Quality Within Maternity Care

Developing a "culture of quality" is an important pre-requisite for (or part of) the implementation of quality improvement methodology. Quality improvement relies on participation and teamwork to solve problems and implement solutions, recognizing that the impact is most powerful when team members draw on the participation, experience and knowledge of all stakeholders. Quality is not the product of an individual, but of staff working together.

Case studies from Honduras and Malawi illustrate how effective quality improvement teams were established in healthcare facilities to improve the quality of obstetric care (Bouchet et al. 2002; Kongnyuy et al. 2008, 2009). The Honduras study revealed that teams were highly motivated and excelled at analysing problems but required more support in developing solutions. Involvement of managers within the quality improvement team and in the maternal death review process helped create a culture of quality and trust that led to improved results. The focus was on finding solutions rather than on the barriers to providing good quality care (Bouchet et al. 2002). Studies in Malawi to improve the quality of skilled birth attendance through the introduction of standards-based audits in emergency obstetric and newborn care have highlighted the importance of establishing active quality improvement teams. These studies stress the importance of local providers agreeing upon standards that define high quality of care in line with current evidence-based medicine and respectful standards of care for mothers and babies.

In Malawi, a standards-based audit was introduced into healthcare facilities using existing national and international guidelines and protocols around postpartum haemorrhage (Kongnyuy et al. 2009). By including all cadres of staff who provide maternal and newborn care in these settings – including obstetricians, doctors, midwives and clinical officers in the development of the standards, ownership and sustainability were promoted. Equally important was the involvement of managers and policy makers in the process, as this facilitated the implementation of recommendations and mobilization of resources where required.

There are a variety of methods to improve the quality of care that are already accepted and used. These include: conducting maternal mortality reviews, neonatal or perinatal death reviews, "near-miss" audits and standards-based audits (Fauveau and de Bernis 2006; Raven et al. 2011). These types of audit or review essentially ask the questions: what was done well, what was not done well and how can care be improved in the future? These kinds of audits and reviews have been widely promulgated across the globe by the WHO following a principle of "no shame, no blame" for mistakes that providers make (WHO 2004). While this principle helps to identify the critical areas in which clinical care or continuity of care is lacking or in need of improvement, it has not always been rolled out as readily as envisioned due to ingrained, bureaucratic obstacles (Lewis 2008; Graham 2009).

Standards are a means of describing the level of quality that healthcare organizations are expected to meet or aspire to. Standards are set with clear objectives, and with structures, processes and outcome criteria. If healthcare providers themselves can evaluate the care they are giving and change their practices that are not evidence-based or reflect poor and abusive care, then standards as well as audits should lead to improved motivation, ownership and sense of responsibility for delivering good quality care. A Cochrane review on audit and feedback concluded that they are most likely to be effective when baseline performance is low, feedback is given more than once, is explicit and includes an action plan (Ivers et al. 2012).

Graham (2009) defined the process of standards-based audit or an "audit cycle" as following five steps: (1) identify the standards for audit; (2) assess current practice and compare against agreed standards; (3) where standards are not met, a root cause analysis is conducted to understand the reasons for this failure and used to identify which changes are needed; (4) actions are implemented; and (5) practice is subsequently re-evaluated (e.g. at 3–4-month interval). Several standards can be audited at the same time, and cycles repeated over time as needed, to encourage an ongoing process of quality improvement.

Initiatives that aim to change practices relating to improved quality of care require integrated programs designed to target the healthcare providers and systems within which care is organized. A systematic approach to evaluation is needed that includes assessment of multiple indicators – both those reflecting processual changes and those reflecting outcomes (WHO 2015a). To strengthen healthcare systems and improve the health of mothers and babies, any proposed program should employ innovative approaches to address the kind of care that women want and expect within their local communities. This strategy will ensure that maternity care is integrated, evidence-based and meets the 12 steps set forth by the *International Childbirth Initiative* (Lalonde et al. 2019; see Appendix to Introduction of this volume).

13.10 Measures for Sustainable Improvements

To sustainably improve maternity care requires the following measures, which are summarized as follows:

- Identify bottlenecks to assess the status of antenatal and postnatal care.
- Assess maternal morbidity during and after delivery.
- Introduction of a quality improvement process at the healthcare facility level.
- Taking a health systems approach.
- Implementation research to assess "what works where and how".

Baseline surveys are needed to better assess the status of availability and quality of antenatal and postnatal care at healthcare facilities in target districts in LMIC settings. A mixed-methods approach should be used to determine: who provides care where, and what is the content and quality of care provided. This approach will lead to the identification of the availability and quality of antenatal and postnatal care packages at primary and secondary levels, and to the assessment of gaps in human resources, consumables and equipment, and infrastructure. In line with the signal functions for Emergency Obstetric Care (WHO 2009), it is important that the international community agrees on the minimum components (or signal functions) of ANC and PNC against which availability can be mapped.

Currently, there is a lack of studies that have used standardized, well-documented and transparent methodologies to assess maternal morbidities that are not life-threatening. Better measures to document and monitor broader maternal morbidity will help inform policy and program decisions and resource allocations to improve maternal health. The development of new tools to comprehensively assess maternal morbidity that can be used at the community level, as well as at higher levels of the health system, is an urgent priority.

The process of standards-based audits can be introduced to develop and strengthen the capacity of healthcare providers and managers as a mechanism for improving care. Healthcare providers should receive in-service "skills and drills"-based training on how to provide mother-baby-friendly and evidence-based integrated care that spans the continuum, including antepartum, intrapartum and postpartum periods. Peer-to-peer learning should be supported by using previously trained healthcare providers to cascade knowledge and skills and share lessons learned. Training packages that are inter-disciplinary and based on evidence-based guidelines and protocols are most effective.

There is a need for programs to address larger and longer-term needs for human resources, infrastructure equipment and consumables, encouraging and enabling change in the healthcare system to ensure reduction in "stock outs" of essential medicines, vaccinations and diagnostic supplies that are essential for quality maternity care. There is a need to build the capacity of healthcare providers in management, leadership and health systems thinking – including in the development, adoption and audit of standards that are pertinent to leading and managing the wider healthcare system.

With advances in health research, studies have been conducted to identify best practices and established guidelines for clinical healthcare. Despite these efforts, significant gaps exist between these guidelines and the actual delivery of healthcare interventions. Implementation research is important to evaluate how health services and health outcomes can be improved through the systematic uptake of research findings into routine program practices. In addition, implementation research generally involves local program managers in the research, thereby facilitating the process of creating local ownership of practices and including research findings into both practices and policy. There is a need to assess the overall effectiveness of programs, including healthcare provider performance, availability and quality of the key components of antenatal and postnatal care, and health outcomes for mothers and babies during pregnancy and in the postnatal period.

In future programs, it will be important to generate the evidence for replicable and scalable intervention packages and solutions to increase their availability and sustainability and improve the quality of care for mothers and babies globally. Sharing lessons learned across and between settings and with stakeholders at national and international levels should be used to proactively inform policy and practice to ensure that maternity care is safe, effective, patient-centred, timely, efficient and equitable.

References

Althabe F, Bergel E, Cafferata ML et al (2008) Strategies for improving the quality of healthcare in maternal and child health in low- and middle-income countries: an overview of systematic reviews. Paediatr Perinat Epidemiol 22:42–60

Ashford L (2002) Hidden suffering: disabilities from pregnancy and childbirth in less developed countries. Population Reference Bureau, MEASURE Communication, Washington DC

Bohren MA, Vogel JP, Hunter EC et al (2015) The mistreatment of women during childbirth in health facilities globally: a mixed-methods systematic review. PLoS Med 12(6):e1001847; discussion e1001847. https://doi.org/10.1371/journal.pmed.1001847

Bouchet B, Francisco M, Ovretveit J (2002) The Zambia quality assurance program: successes and challenges. Int J Qual Health Care 14:89–95

Campbell O, Calvert C, Testa A et al (2016) The scale, scope, coverage, and capability of childbirth care. Lancet 388:2193–2208

Chou D, Tunçalp Ö, Firoz T et al (2016) Constructing maternal morbidity – towards a standard tool to measure and monitor maternal health beyond mortality. BMC Pregnancy Childbirth 16:45. https://doi.org/10.1186/s12884-015-0789-4

Donabedian A (1988) The quality of care. How can it be assessed? J Am Med Assoc 260(12):1743–1748

Fathalla M (1998) Preface. Paediatr Perinatol Epidemiol 12(S2):vii–viii

Fauveau V, de Bernis L (2006) "Good obstetrics" revisited: too many evidence-based practices and devices are not used. Int J Gynecol Obstet 94(2):179–184

Firoz T, von Dadelszen P, Magee L et al (2013) Measuring maternal health: focus on maternal morbidity. Bull World Health Organ 91(10):794–796

Freedman LP, Ramsey K, Abuya T et al (2014) Defining disrespect and abuse of women in childbirth: a research, policy and rights agenda. Bull World Health Organ 92(12):915–917

Frøen JF, Friberg IK, Lawn JE et al (2016) Stillbirths: progress and unfinished business. Lancet 387:574–586

Graham W (2009) Criterion-based clinical audit in obstetrics: bridging the quality gap? Best Pract Res Clin Obstetr Gynaecol 23:375–388

Graham W, Woodd S, Byass P et al (2018) Diversity and divergence: the dynamic burden of poor maternal health. Lancet 388:2164–2175

Ivers N, Jamtvedt G, Flottorp S et al (2012) Audit and feedback: effects on professional practice and healthcare outcomes. Cochrane Database Syst Rev 6:CD000259

Kongnyuy EJ, Mlava G, van den Broek N (2008) Criteria-based audit to improve a district referral system in Malawi: a pilot study. BMC Health Serv Res 8:190

Kongnyuy EJ, Mlava G, van den Broek N (2009) Criteria-based audit to improve women-friendly care in maternity units in Malawi. J Obstet Gynaecol Res 35(3):483–489

Lalonde A, Herschderfer K, Pascali Bonaro D et al (2019) The international childbirth initiative: 12 steps to safe and respectful mother baby-family maternity care. Int J Gynecol Obstet 146:65–73

Lewis G (2008) Reviewing maternal deaths to make pregnancy safer. Best Pract Res Clin Obstetr Gynaecol 22(3):447–463

Liskin LS (1992) Maternal morbidity in developing countries: a review and comments. Int J Gynecol Obstet 37(2):77–87

Madaj B, Smith H, Mathai M et al (2017) Developing global indicators for quality of maternal and newborn care: a feasibility assessment. Bull World Health Organ 95(6):445–452

McCauley M, Madaj B, White SA et al (2018) Burden of physical, psychological and social ill-health during and after pregnancy among women in India, Pakistan, Kenya and Malawi. Br Med J Glob Health 3:e000625

McCauley M, Avais AR, Agrawal R et al (2020) 'Good health means being mentally, socially, emotionally and physically fit': women's understanding of health and ill health during and after pregnancy in India and Pakistan: a qualitative study. Br Med J Open 10:e028760. https://doi.org/10.1136/bmjopen-2018-028760

Miller S, Abalos E, Chamillard M et al (2016) Beyond too little, too late and too much, too soon: a pathway towards evidence-based, respectful maternity care worldwide. Lancet 388:2176–2192. https://doi.org/10.1016/S0140-6736(16)31472-6

Raven J, Hofman J, Adegoke A et al (2011) Methodology and tools for quality improvement in maternal and newborn healthcare. Int J Gynecol Obstet 114(1):4–9

Sackett DL, Rosenberg WM, Gray JA et al (1996) Evidence based medicine: what it is and what it isn't. Br Med J (Clin Res Ed) 312(7023):71–72

Say L, Souza JP, Pattinson RC (2009) Maternal near miss – towards a standard tool for monitoring quality of maternal healthcare. Best Pract Res Clin Obstetr Gynaecol 23:287–296

The Partnership for Maternal, Newborn and Child Health (PMNCH) (2011) A global review of the key interventions related to reproductive, maternal, newborn and child health (RMNCH): essential interventions, commodities and guidelines for reproductive, maternal, newborn and child health. PMNCH, Geneva

Tunçalp Ö, Hindin MJ, Adu-Bonsaffoh K et al (2013) Assessment of maternal near-miss and quality of care in a hospital-based study in Accra, Ghana. Int J Gynecol Obstet 123:58–63. https://doi.org/10.1016/j.ijgo.2013.06.003

United Nations (2015a) Sustainable development goals. Available via: http://www.un.org/sustainabledevelopment/sustainable-development-goals/

United Nations (2015b) Global strategy for women's, children's and adolescents' health, 2016–2030. United Nations, New York. Available at: http://www.who.int/life-course/partners/global-strategy/en/

van den Akker T, Beltman J, Leyten J et al (2013) The WHO maternal near miss approach: consequences at Malawian District level. PLoS One 8(1):e54805. https://doi.org/10.1371/journal.pone.0054805

WHO (2004) Beyond the numbers: reviewing maternal deaths and severe morbidity to make pregnancy safer. WHO Publications, Geneva

WHO (2009) World Health Organization, United Nations Population Fund, United Nations Children's Fund, Averting Maternal Death and Disability Program (2009) Monitoring emergency obstetric care: a handbook. http://www.unfpa.org/sites/default/files/pub-pdf/obstetric_monitoring.pdf

WHO (2012) The WHO application of ICD-10 to deaths during pregnancy, childbirth and the puerperium: ICD-MM. WHO, Geneva. http://apps.who.int/iris/bitstream/10665/70929/1/9789241548458_eng.pdf. Accessed 17 Nov 2017

WHO (2015a) WHO recommendations on health promotion interventions for maternal and newborn health. WHO, Geneva. Available via: http://www.who.int/maternal_child_adolescent/documents/health-promotion-interventions/en/

WHO (2015b) Strategies toward ending preventable maternal mortality (EPMM). WHO, Geneva. Accessed 17 Nov 2017. Available via: http://apps.who.int/iris/bitstream/10665/153540/1/WHO_RHR_15.03_eng.pdf

WHO et al (2015) Trends in maternal mortality 1990–2015: estimates developed by WHO, UNICEF, UNFPA, The World Bank, and the United Nations Population Division. WHO Publications, Geneva. Available via: https://www.who.int/reproductivehealth/publications/monitoring/maternal-mortality-2015/en/

Zafar S, Jean-Baptiste R, Rahman A et al (2015) Non-life threatening maternal morbidity: cross sectional surveys from Malawi and Pakistan. PLoS One 10(9):e0138026

Chapter 14
Sustainable Maternal and Newborn Care in India: A Case Study from Ladakh

Kim Gutschow, Padma Dolma, and Spalchen Gonbo

14.1 Excellent Maternal and Newborn Outcomes at Sonam Norboo Memorial Hospital

This chapter describes 40 years of remarkable obstetric and newborn care at Sonam Norboo Memorial Hospital (SNMH) in the Union Territory of Ladakh, which was newly established in October 2019. The Ladakh Union Territory—roughly the size of Croatia or the US state of West Virginia—is made up of Leh and Kargil districts, which each have only one public hospital that together serve a combined population of roughly 275,000 (Fig. 14.1). Its high quality of care and excellent standards are evident nation-wide. SNMH has twice won the nationwide Kayakalp Award, given to a district hospital in India in recognition of its excellence in promoting cleanliness, hygiene, and infection control and contributing to improved quality of care in India—first in 2016 and again in 2019. Given its reputation across India and the region, the SNMH maternity ward attracts women not only from Leh district, but also neighboring Kargil districts whose hospital has far lower standards than SNMH (Gutschow 2016, 2011; Gutschow and Dolma 2012).

Because of the high quality of care at the SNMH, there are no private maternity clinics in either Leh and Kargil districts, which is nearly unheard of among India's 700+ districts—most of which have multiple private maternity clinics or hospitals. By 2008, when the all-India rate of institutional delivery was only 49%, SNMH could already boast of a 90% institutional delivery rate (ICCR 2008; Gutschow and Dolma 2012). Even more notably, SNM hospital recorded an MMR of 37 over the

K. Gutschow (✉)
Department of Anthropology and Religion, Williams College, Williamstown, MA, USA
e-mail: Kim.Gutschow@williams.edu

P. Dolma · S. Gonbo
SNM Hospital, Leh, Ladakh Union Territory, India
e-mail: padmadolma29@gmail.com; spalchen@gmail.com

© Springer Nature Switzerland AG 2021
K. Gutschow et al. (eds.), *Sustainable Birth in Disruptive Times*, Global
Maternal and Child Health, https://doi.org/10.1007/978-3-030-54775-2_14

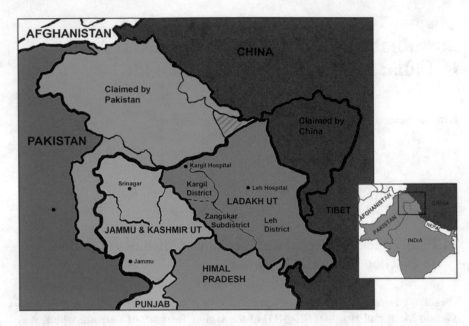

Fig. 14.1 Map showing Ladakh Union Territory (UT), Jammu & Kashmir UT, Leh hospital (SNMH), Kargil hospital, as well as both Leh District and Kargil District that together form Ladakh UT. (Published with kind permission of © Kai Gutschow 2020. All Rights Reserved)

last two decades, which is one-sixth the all-India MMR of 238 during that same period.[1] Put differently, SNMH had an MMR of 117 over the past 40 years (47 maternal deaths and 40,047 live births from 1979 to 2019) (Fig. 14.2).

In 2001, Leh district tied with the Chennai district in having the lowest total fertility rate in India (Guilmoto and Rajan 2002), while Leh and Kargil districts reported the first and second highest contraceptive prevalence rates (CPRs) across all Indian districts in 2003–2004.[2] In Ladakh, the prevalence of Himalayan socio-cultural norms that reduce fertility and promote female reproductive agency and authority, along with a culture of declining polyandry and primogeniture, has resulted in nearly universal household land ownership. The relatively egalitarian wealth distribution, lack of caste distinctions, and broad prevalence of an affirmative action category known as ST (Scheduled Tribe) status have produced a relative lack of communal violence between the Buddhist and Muslim communities, in contrast to neighboring Kashmir Valley (Van Beek 2006; Gutschow 2004, 2006; Aggarwal 2004).

---

[1] Gutschow calculated the MMR for Leh hospital between 2000 and 2020 using data from SNMH (10 maternal deaths and 27, 318 live births). She calculated the average MMR for India in a similar period using the fibe estimates for India's MMR—in 2000, 2005, 2010, 2015, and 2017—provided by the WHO (2019) and its partners.

[2] Guilmoto and Rajan (2002: 668) report Leh district's TFR as 1.3 and Kargil district's TFR as 3.4 in 2001. Contraceptive prevalence rates (CPRs) across India in 2003–2004 were reported by the Indian Institute for Population Sciences at http://www.iipsindia.org/pdf/05_b_13atab13.pdf

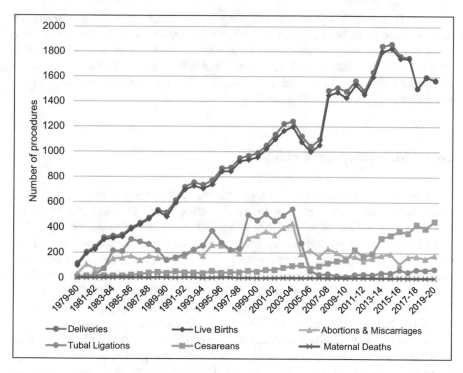

Fig. 14.2 40 years of birth outcomes from Sonam Norboo Memorial Hospital in Leh, Ladakh, annually (April–March) from opening in 1979 to 2020. (Data from SNMH records)

14.2   Methods

This chapter is based partly on Gutschow's three decades of fieldwork in Ladakh from 1989 to 2019, including participant observations and interviews with key interlocutors in the maternity unit of SNMH between 1990–1996, 2006–2007, 2011–2012, and 2019. Gutschow collected data and interviewed roughly 200 women and providers at SNM hospital during these periods, including a few dozen obstetricians, pediatricians, nurses, auxiliary nurse midwives (ANM), other doctors, and Chief Medical Officers (Gutschow 2011, 2016; Gutschow and Dolma 2012). The chapter also draws on observations and data collected by Dr. Padma Dolma and Dr. Spalchen Gonbo, conducted during their service at SNMH and summarized in their reflections below. Gutschow and Dr. Padma have worked closely together since 2006, collaborating on project design, data collection, and several international projects; the results were published and presented in Rome, Heidelberg, and India (Gutschow and Dolma 2012).

The region's high altitude, remoteness, low population density, and lack of all-weather roads create numerous obstacles to access, especially for women in labor (Gutschow 2016). The average villager needs to travel 33–42 km, often on foot, to reach a health clinic in a district where altitudes range from 3500 to 7000 m above sea level (ICCR 2008). Both Leh and Kargil districts are cut off from the rest of India by road from November to May each year due to snowfall, while roads are often blocked at other times due to landslides or road repairs (Gutschow 2011, 2016). Given this difficulty of transport, the steady rise in institutional deliveries and relative absence of maternal deaths—only 47 in the past 40 years and 6 in the last decade—is remarkable (Fig. 14.2).

14.3 Maternity Care at SNMH

The high quality of care and exceptional maternal and newborn outcomes at SNMH in the initial years were largely due to two obstetricians, Dr. Tsering Landol[3] and her niece, Dr. Padma Dolma, who have been tireless promoters of safe birth, reproductive rights, and compassionate care over the past 40 years (Gutschow 2011, 2016; Wiley 2003, 2004). After rising for nearly 25 years, the number of institutional deliveries plummeted sharply after Dr. Landol retired in 2003, but rose again from 1001 in 2005 to 1451 in 2006 after Dr. Padma joined the staff in 2005 (Fig. 14.2).[4] Deliveries under Dr. Padma's tenure dipped briefly in 2009 and 2011 when she left for more advanced training in Delhi but rose again each time she returned.

Dr. Padma and Dr. Landol and their fellow obstetricians consistently emphasized safe birth and reproductive rights for women across the region, who came to see the hospital as a place for compassionate and timely care that empowered them. Dr. Landol, who never married, was the first Ladakhi to graduate from Srinagar Medical College. The Government of India (GOI) awarded her two of the highest civilian honors in the nation, the Padma Shri in 2006 and the Padma Bhusan in 2020, for her contributions to Indian medicine, making her one of the few female recipients and the first Ladakhi ever to receive both honors. She also appears on the award's "Wall of Fame," which features those who have exhibited "excellence and glory" throughout their careers. She had been known for her consistent promotion of reproductive health and rights in Ladakh—as indicated by the rising rates of live births, tubal ligations, abortions, and IUD insertions (not shown) during her 25-year career (Fig. 14.2).

Before Dr. Landol retired in 2003, she began to face increasing backlash from religious groups against family planning, including efforts to block or prevent her mobile tubal ligation units and other reproductive health camps from operating in the villages. The final blows were the anonymous destruction of tubal ligation

---

[3] The names in this chapter have not been changed, and stories were used with permission of the interlocutors, unless otherwise specified.

[4] Dr. Lahdol once told me that her greatest influence was not her father—who was the Prime Minister or *Kalon* (*bka' blon*) and served the King of Ladakh during Partition when he organized the defense of Leh from Pakistani invaders (Gutschow 2006) but her mother—who faithfully followed the ten Buddhist virtues (*dge ba bcu*) her entire life.

machines and when she received anonymous death threats due to rising pro-natalism in Ladakh (Gutschow and Dolma 2012; Gutschow 2006).

Both total ligations and abortions sharply plummeted following Dr. Landol's retirement in 2003. Tubal ligations dropped by half in 1 year, from 545 in 2003 to 246 in 2004, and further to 56 in 2005 (Fig. 14.2). The combined number of abortions and miscarriages also dropped, from 432 in 2003 to 191 in 2004, largely driven by a precipitous decline in elective abortions. Yet miscarriages also declined slowly over the next years as prenatal care improved. Both tubal ligations and abortions/miscarriages have remained low since 2003 for a variety of reasons. Practically, the missing parts for the tubal ligation machine were never replaced, while some of the staff working in the operations theater opposed tubal ligations and voiced their concerns about the declining population of Ladakh. More importantly, the social stigma against abortions has risen during the recent trends toward pro-natalism, as both Buddhist and Muslim religious leaders have advocated against family planning and reproductive rights (Gutschow 2006; Aengst 2014; Smith 2009). The growing concern over India's sex-selective abortions also contributes to facility-based scrutiny of all abortions, although sex selection is not a pattern in Ladakh, which is known for its promotion of female rights and agency (Gutschow 2004; Aggarwal 2004). The falling demand for tubal ligations may also relate to a generation of younger women who prefer reversible methods of contraception like IUDs, condoms, and pills (Fig. 14.2).

Padma describes the difficulty of openly advocating for family planning in a close-knit community where she and other providers have been singled out for condemnation when they perform abortions. She concedes that government rules requiring a documented reason for every abortion, and consent by two providers during the second trimester, may have dampened access to and demand for abortions up until 2014. In 2012, the GOI amended the abortion laws by reducing the number of providers so that only one provider's consent was needed to perform second-trimester abortions, and in 2020 the GOI amended the bill further to extend the time limit for abortions up to 24 weeks and drop gestational limits entirely in the case of congenital abnormalities. Padma believes that these amendments may help mitigate the dampening effect of government restrictions on abortion that she has seen.

Padma and her colleagues continue to do tubal ligations via mini Lap (a small abdominal incision) or during cesarean sections and ovarian surgeries for those who request them. Yet she must often delay clients who request tubal ligations for weeks, as her schedule is already filled with obstetric and gynecological surgeries including cesareans, hysterectomies, ovarian surgeries, and myomectomies, that are privileged over elective tubal ligations. To ameliorate this situation, Padma and her colleagues have asked the hospital administrators to allow the obstetrics and gynecology department to have not one but two full days a week for elective surgeries in one of the three operating theaters at the hospital.

In their hospital, Dr. Landol, Dr. Padma, other obstetricians, as well as a team of ancillary nurse-midwives have presided over a 40-year woman-centered model of care that has facilitated the normal physiology of labor while providing skilled emergency obstetric care. This model constitutes the very essence of sustainable birth care (Introduction, this volume). The model has sustained a 40-year rise in deliveries, near absence of maternal deaths, and flexible adaptation to changing circumstances and technology using a minimum of technology and resources, given the remoteness and public status of SNMH. The lack of maternal deaths for 40 years—none at all between 2016 and 2020, and only 10 maternal deaths between 1999 and 2020—contributed to the hospital's recognition across India. Its overall outcomes and lack of corruption are far better than other public hospitals in North India (Gutschow 2016; Iyer et al. 2016; Jeffery and Jeffery 2008, 2010). The low stillbirth rate and falling neonatal mortality ratio are related to its rising cesarean rate. While the cesarean rate ranged consistently between 3% and 9% until 2009, it rose to 27% in 2019 (Fig. 14.2). Padma attributes this rise to four main factors:

- Increasing rates of ART (Artificial Reproductive Technologies) that lead women to have twin pregnancies and more high-risk pregnancies that lead to elective cesareans after 37 weeks.
- More electronic fetal monitoring (EFM) after 2009 with the arrival of three EFM machines (two in labor room and one in antenatal ward) that allow for intermittent fetal monitoring and observation of fetal distress has likely led to an increase in cesareans, even as Padma recognizes that EMF records of fetal distress are often mistaken or ambiguous.
- High rates of gestational diabetes mellitus (GDM) and intrahepatic cholestasis of pregnancy (IHCP)—now better detected due to screening and laboratory facilities—lead women to opt for cesareans, given the higher rate of sudden stillbirths after 37 weeks. The cause for the high rates of IHCP in Ladakh is not known nor well-studied. Padma wonders if there may be a causal relation to the high altitude or genetic factors and suggests more research needs to be done on metabolic diseases in pregnancy in high altitude regions.
- The hospital protocol by which each attending obstetrician takes full charge of the labor and delivery wards for a week may lead providers to opt for cesareans in the absence of shared decision making. According to Padma, the system of individual provider attendance may lead to a lower decision threshold for conducting a cesarean, compared to a team-based decision making in case of suspected fetal distress resulting from an EFM reading. Padma suspects that having an individual obstetrician be solely responsible for all labor and delivery decisions leads to provider stress, given that providers face their peers during the monthly audits on maternal and neonatal deaths and stillbirths. The pressure of decision making and concerns about the impending audit if there is a neonatal death or stillbirth may contribute to a subtle bias toward cesarean delivery.

When Dr. Padma, her colleagues in the obstetrics department, and the Medical Superintendent Dr. Tsering Samphel came together to discuss the rising cesarean rate, they identified these four primary factors and contemplated possible changes. While they have little power to lower the rates of ART or pregnancy conditions like IHCP and GDM, they were aware that EFM and the monthly clinical audits could be driving providers to opt for cesareans. Yet rather than denying or ignoring the troubling cesarean rise, they asked the Medical Superintendent to record their individual rates of cesarean, by provider, for several months. The result yielded few insights, as none of the four obstetricians was an outlier and all had months where their cesarean rates were slightly lower or higher than the average of other providers that month. The sample size is too small to tell if that was due to their patient risk profile or other factors. Yet their willingness to scrutinize each other and discussion with the Medical Superintendent shows their commitment to a sustainable model of accountability, patient-centered quality care, and the ability to adapt their obstetric practices as needed to improve care.

14.4   Dr. Padma's Story

When I was first appointed to SNMH in 2005, my main priorities were safe delivery and newborn care. I had just finished a 4-year residency and fellowship at the public Safdarjung Hospital in Delhi, where I regularly had 30–40 deliveries per day along with up to 13 cesareans on some night shifts. As such, I was hardly disturbed by a labor and delivery ward filled with women, but it was difficult to adjust to a remote district hospital whose facilities had been sorely neglected by the state government during the past 15 years of militant insurgency in the Kashmir Valley. By relying on networks with doctors I had met in Delhi and skills I had learned in my training, I was able to consult with my former colleagues in difficult cases to more accurately diagnose maternal and neonatal sepsis, for instance.

My colleague Dr. Kunzes and I implemented key changes in clinical protocols around maternal and neonatal care. By 2006, we convinced the Chief Medical Officer (CMO) in Leh to stock antenatal corticosteroids to improve fetal lung development for babies at risk for preterm delivery, 5 years before these drugs became standard protocol at hospitals across India.[5] I asked that the hospital use betamethasone rather than dexamethasone because the former only requires 24 h (rather than 48) to be effective, and so there is a greater chance that the fetus will receive the benefits when a mother arrives in an advanced state of preterm labor. Given the difficulty of road access in our high-altitude region, mothers often arrive in preterm labor and the timely delivery of antenatal steroids is critical to hasten fetal lung maturity as well as stimulate the natural production of lung surfactant in both preterm or SGA (small for gestational age) newborns with vulnerable lungs.

Across India, antenatal corticosteroids have been proven to reduce the rate of necrotizing enterocolitis (NEC) by 54%, intraventricular hemorrhage (IVH or "brain bleeds") by 46%, reduce an acute lung disorder known as respiratory distress syndrome (RDS) by 34%, and reduce overall neonatal mortality by 31% (MoHFW 2014b). They can also reduce the risk of systemic infections like meningitis and

---

[5] Padma's protocols in 2006 were far ahead of her time. Even by 2014, only 41% of eligible mothers received antenatal corticosteroids in 75 developing Countdown countries (Bhutta et al. 2014).

congenital heart disorders like PDA (patent ductus arteriosus), for which there is no surgical capacity at SNMH. Most significantly, antenatal corticosteroids are known to decrease the need for respiratory support and other neonatal interventions, reduce the length of hospital stay, and thus reduce the risk of infections and costs associated with essential newborn care (ENC).

These and other advances have no doubt improved newborn outcomes in my time at SNMH. In 2008, Dr. Laurel Spooner from the UK donated our unit's first Indian-made baby warmer, and in 2009 we began to develop our own Special Newborn Care Unit (SNCU), using funds from the Navjaat Shishu Suraksha Karyakram (NSSK) initiative that were distributed across India after 2009 to provide Essential Newborn Care (Paul et al. 2016; Mason et al. 2014). Although a district hospital was supposed to have 3000 deliveries per year to qualify for NSSK funds—and we only had half that number—we argued for an exception to be made, given the difficulties for mothers and newborns in accessing tertiary care in our region. Because there are no roads open between Ladakh and the rest of India between November and May every year, mothers and newborns can only reach tertiary level hospitals in Srinagar, Jammu, or Delhi by airplane. The closest Level III NICU (Newborn Intensive Care Unit) is in Srinagar and only accessible by one flight per week during the winter or a 2-day car journey during the summer. A plane flight carries its own risks for newborns suffering life-threatening complications, as their lungs may not adapt to the increased cabin pressure and lack of moisture on the airplane.

While a catastrophic flash flood destroyed much of our old hospital in 2010, this tragedy accelerated the construction of our new hospital with funds from the central government in Delhi. Since 2013, we have a new labor and delivery ward, with special labor rooms for women with eclampsia and infectious diseases, as well as post-op and preterm wards (Figs. 14.3, 14.4, 14.5, 14.6, 14.7 and 14.8). Our delivery room has 3 flexible tables that allow for upright or squatting delivery, with central oxygen supply for all three delivery tables (Fig. 14.3), a neonatal warmer and resuscitation equipment (Fig. 14.4), a newborn scale, and two EFM machines in the labor room for intermittent fetal and maternal monitoring (Fig. 14.5). We have equipment for vacuum and forceps deliveries, dilation and curettage (D&C) sets for abortions and post-miscarriage interventions, and an area for essential drugs such as injectable oxytocin, methergine, magnesium sulfate, carboprostone, and dinoprostone. To promote hygiene, we have a room with PPE, an autoclave for sterilizing our delivery sets, a septic labor table in a separate room for women with active infections (e.g., hepatitis) to avoid contamination, and a hand wash unit with foot pedals for improved hygiene (Fig. 14.6).

Our SNCU (Fig. 14.7) includes eight to ten incubators in two separate rooms to prevent the spread of infection and isolate the most vulnerable newborns. There are rooms for Kangaroo Mother Care (KMC) as well as breastfeeding or pumping breast milk. There are staff rooms for NICU nurses, midwives, and labor and delivery nurses to rest. We have a total of 64 patient beds, including 13 beds in our labor wards—6 for women in active labor, 6 beds for post-partum observation, 1 bed for high-risk women with eclampsia. There are 27 beds in our antenatal ward, postnatal

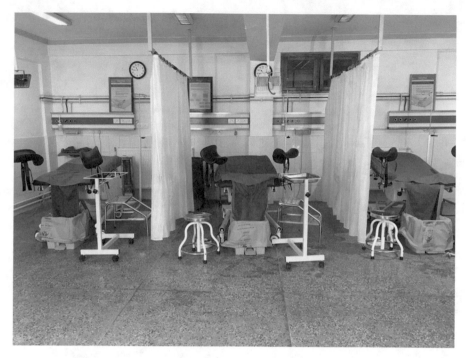

Fig. 14.3 Delivery room at SNMH. (Published with kind permission of © Kim Gutschow 2020. All Rights Reserved)

ward, and septic labor room, besides the 24 beds in our high-risk ward for women at risk of preterm labor or miscarriage and post-op women who have had cesareans, hysterectomies, and other gynecological operations. These labor and delivery wards are all connected to our operation theater (Fig. 14.8) as well as linked to our outpatient antenatal clinic, where we see over 15,000 women and children every year for antenatal care, postpartum care, newborn care, vaccinations, and infant care.

Our skill sets have increased tremendously along with our technology, such as C-reactive protein analysis that can help determine neonatal and maternal sepsis. Our current team of consultant obstetricians—myself, Dr. Ayesha, Dr. Padma Ladol, and Dr. Khatisha—have initiated key clinical protocols that WHO recommends for maternal and neonatal care, such as vitamin K injections and KMC care for all newborns, prophylactic antibiotic treatment for pregnant women who present with vaginal discharge, antenatal steroids for all women who have preterm labor, and postnatal surfactant therapy for all vulnerable newborns.

By 2011, following an all-India government initiative promoting maternal death reviews, the Departments of Obstetrics and Neonatology jointly decided to hold regular maternal and neonatal death reviews or audits to improve our quality of care and be accountable to our community (Gutschow 2016). A team consisting of the clinical staff involved in the care preceding the death and the medical superintendent now meets once a month to audit every single neonatal death, maternal death,

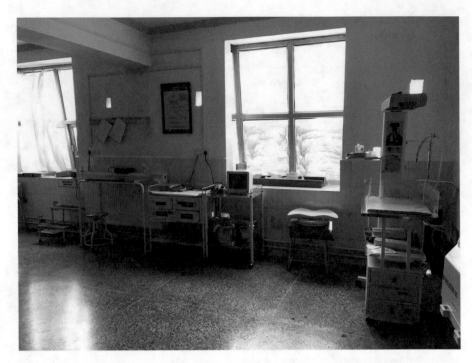

Fig. 14.4 Alternate view of delivery room. From right to left, newborn warmer, newborn delivery registers, and resuscitation table. (Published with kind permission of © Kim Gutschow 2020. All Rights Reserved)

and stillbirth. We freely discuss the care provided, what could have been done differently, and what protocols need to be changed or reviewed. These audits help avoid similar mistakes in the future and enable our hospital staff to make evidence-based recommendations around what essential skills or health commodities—drugs and equipment—are most needed to save lives at our hospital.

14.5   Dr. Spalchen's Story

Padma and her team made many improvements in maternal and newborn care between 2005 and 2009. In 2009 pediatrician Rinchen Dolma and I, as well as several nurses from SNMH spent 3 months on a neonatology fellowship at New Delhi's All-India Institute of Medical Science (AIIMS). As one of India's leading public medical colleges, AIIMS has spearheaded newborn care in India since 1990, when it hosted a national conference on medical technology for newborn care under the auspices of the NNF (National Neonatal Forum). NNF had been charged with developing the first guidelines on newborn care in India. The entire fellowship team received specialized training in essential newborn care at AIIMS, while we roomed

Fig. 14.5 Electronic fetal monitoring (EFM) machine at bedside in active labor room. (Published with kind permission of © Padma Dolma 2020. All Rights Reserved)

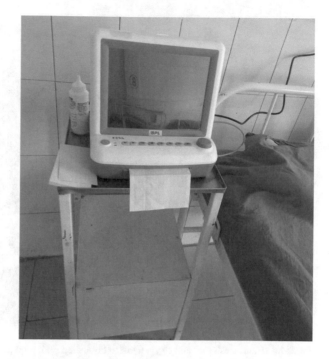

with fellow Ladakhis who lived nearby to save costs. In 2010, I received more government-funded training in facility-based newborn care for 5 days in Srinagar and for 2 weeks at Kalwani Saran Children's Hospital (KSCH) in Delhi.

My stints at AIIMS and KSCH were largely observational and did not constitute a formal residency. Like our SNMH in Leh, both AIIMS and KSCH operate with similar challenges because they have limited resources, serve a diverse demographic, have a high volume of patients, and must admit all patients who are referred there. KSCH continues to serve as a regional collaborative center that provides technical expertise, monitoring, and quality assessment for the SNCU in Ladakh and other districts across Northwest India (MoHFW 2011). After being trained in newborn fluid stabilization, resuscitation techniques, and management of newborn sepsis, Dr. Rinchen and I have moved far beyond the basic training we received while completing our MBBS (Bachelor of Medicine, Bachelor of Surgery) degrees.

By 2012, I was chosen to be a "trainer of trainers" in neonatal resuscitation and I trained over 300 doctors, nurses, and paramedics in neonatal resuscitation across Leh district. In 2013, I began collaborating with Dr. Nirupama Laroia, from the University of Rochester in New York, in order to improve neonatal resuscitation in the Leh hospital with funding from the American Association of Pediatrics (AAP) and the Helping Babies Breathe (HBB) program, which advanced basic neonatal resuscitation across India (Aneji and Little, this volume). Another pediatrician, Dr. Tsering Norbu, began to pursue a long-term study that will follow babies from birth through 5 years of age to better understand the sequelae of perinatal complications.

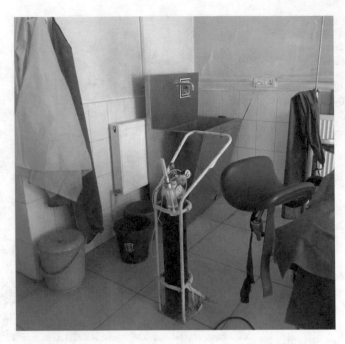

Fig. 14.6 Hand wash unit and oxygen tank. (Published with kind permission of © Padma Dolma 2020. All Rights Reserved)

By 2016, we had completed a 12-bed SNCU where all treatment to newborns is provided free of cost, including drugs and procedures. Government funding and private donations provided critical neonatal technologies including: bubble CPAP (continuous positive airway pressure)—a non-invasive method of delivering supplemental oxygen or room air into newborn lungs; a photospectrometric bilimeter to accurately measure neonatal bilirubin in order to administer appropriate phototherapy for newborn jaundice; an oxygen blender to mix oxygen and room air for compromised neonates; T-piece resuscitators that make it easier to control and deliver positive pressure ventilation; LED phototherapy units for newborns with jaundice; apnea monitors to record newborn breathing rates or cessation of breathing; and advanced warmers/monitors that can measure newborn heart rates, breathing rates, blood pressure, and oxygen levels. Future plans for the SNCU include a milk bank and the ability to provide total parenteral nutrition (TNP), a liquid nutrient via IV lines to newborns whose stomachs are too weak to handle breastmilk or formula.

Perhaps one day SNMH will venture into newborn intubation with ventilators rather than using only CPAP. Yet at this time, Padma and I believe that essential newborn care is most important and cost-effective in a remote region like Ladakh. Even during these past 9 months of Covid 19, our hospital staff used CPAP, high flow oxygen, and dexamethosone, instead of ventilation for our most critically ill patients. We have learned much about how to save newborns at this remote, district-level hospital in the last 6 years. We know that a majority of the babies born

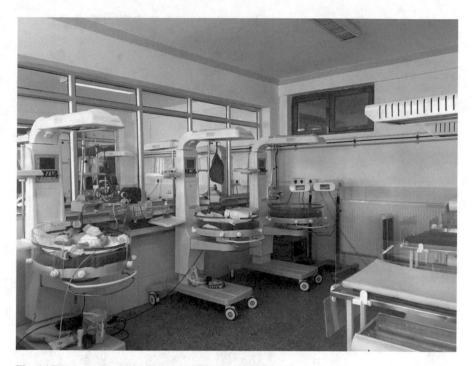

Fig. 14.7 Special Neonatal Care Unit (SNCU) room with five baby warmers, and behind glass, second room for sick or small newborns. (Published with kind permission of © Kim Gutschow 2020. All Rights Reserved)

in Leh after 32 weeks can be saved with KMC, expressed breastmilk, a high degree of cleanliness to avoid infection, and baby warmers. While the first three interventions cost almost nothing, the fourth is an expensive medical technology the government is providing across India. While some sick newborns will need this advanced care, all newborns need loving care from a trained staff who listen to the mothers and observe the minute changes in their baby's condition. As I like to say, "A smart mother is better than a poor doctor!"

14.6   Two Newborn Outcomes in the Special Newborn Care Unit (SNCU)

Dr. Spalchen recalls one of his early manual resuscitations in 2011 with a simple bag and mask device using techniques he had learned in Delhi called Helping Babies Breathe (HBB) (Aneji and Little this volume, Lawn et al. 2014). For 20 days after his birth, we gave the baby continuous ventilation with the correct air pressure of less than 40 cm/liter using a self-inflating bag and skills learned in our neonatal resuscitation training (Zodpey and Paul 2014). The baby's main complications were

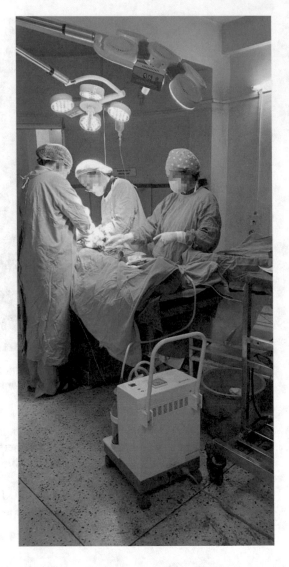

jaundice and apnea (breathing disruption), so we performed an exchange transfusion in which the baby's blood was exchanged with donor blood products to reduce excess bilirubin. Because it was the first exchange transfusion at SNMH, they had great difficulty placing the neonatal catheters to deliver the donor blood. Although the tiny baby stopped breathing twice during the procedure—causing everyone great distress—he survived, avoided infection, and the procedure cured his apnea and decreased his bilirubin levels. Given the boy's extreme prematurity, it was clear he needed an incubator, unavailable at that time in SNMH. The boy's father, an engineer, purchased an incubator in Delhi and had it flown to Leh, where it was donated to the SNCU after the boy's discharge.

In 2012, a baby boy was born weighing only 890 grams, which made him one of the smallest newborns ever to survive at SNMH. While he had no other major complications at birth, his weight declined to 850 grams after a week in the SNCU and his situation looked dire as he needed so many calories just to stay warm. But with regular kangaroo care and expressed breastmilk that his mother dripped into his mouth using a gauze and then a spoon, this newborn survived during his 2-month stay in the SNCU, where he received room air and oxygen via bubble CPAP and IV fluids for hydration. He was discharged after 2 months weighing only 1800 g, and the doctors expected he would soon be readmitted to the newborn care unit given his vulnerable size. Yet when his mother brought him for a visit after 3 months, he weighed 4.5 kg and he had no developmental delays in the first 5 years of his life!

14.7 Neonatal Care in Ladakh Versus India: Scaling Up

The National Rural Health Mission (NRHM) was launched in 2005 to improve child and maternal health across India with help from the WHO, the World Bank, and other global NGOs. In 2009, the Indian government launched the Newborn Baby Safety Program (Navjaat Shishu Suraksha Karyakram or NSSK) to help train district-level pediatricians like Dr. Spalchen in basic neonatal care, including newborn resuscitation, prevention of hypothermia and infection, Kangaroo Mother Care (KMC), and early initiation of breastfeeding (MoHFW 2009).[6] The government of India promoted access to care for mothers and newborns with the JSSK (Janani Shishu Suraksha Karyakram) initiative that provided free drugs, diagnostics, referral, and transport for mothers and newborns during the first postpartum month.

The government also committed to building a tiered set of newborn care units across all of India's districts: (1) Newborn Care Corners (NCCs) at primary health centers to provide essential newborn care and referral of sick or at-risk newborns; (2) Newborn Stabilization Units (NBSUs) to manage low birthweight or sick newborns at first referral units or Community Health Centers (CHCs); (3) Special Newborn Care Units (SNCUs) at district hospitals or medical colleges to handle all specialized newborn care except intubation and surgery; and (4) Level III Neonatal Intensive Care Units (NICUs) that provide the most advanced levels of neonatal care (MoHFW 2014a). Each SNCU was supposed to be equipped with radiant warmers, phototherapy units, oxygen concentrators, fetal pulse oximeters (which measure how much oxygen the baby's blood is carrying), IV pumps, and bag and masks for newborn resuscitation (Neogi et al. 2011).

By 2015, the Indian government had made great progress in developing newborn care facilities across most of its districts, with 565 SNCUs, 1904 NBSUs, and 14,163 NCCs completed (Paul et al. 2016). Indian companies promoted newborn

---

[6]The NSSK was first rolled out in Bihar, Rajasthan, Uttar Pradesh, Orissa, Madhya Pradesh, Uttarakhand, Jharkhand, Chhattisgarh, Assam, and Jammu & Kashmir (MoHFW 2009).

care by developing cost-effective and high-quality technology including baby warmers, phototherapy units, and resuscitation bags that met international quality standards and could be distributed across India (Kumar et al. 2016). Yet despite this success, coverage of low-tech interventions immediately before, during, and after labor and delivery remains scant in many facilities, due to poor quality of care, lack of training, and corruption in the healthcare system. Nationwide, only 45% of all newborns had three postnatal visits within 10 days of birth, roughly a third were exclusively breastfed at 6 months, and only 61% had full immunization after 1 year (Zodpey and Paul 2014; Sankar et al. 2016).

There are considerable disparities among states, between urban/rural settings, and for marginalized populations in India. The state of Kerala had the lowest NMR (7/1000) in the country, while Madhya Pradesh and Odisha's NMR of 39/1000 was six times as high in 2014 (Zodpey and Paul 2014).[7] Four northern states—Uttar Pradesh, Madhya Pradesh, Bihar, and Rajasthan—account for roughly 55% of all neonatal deaths in India (Zodpey and Paul 2014). There is a dramatic difference between rural and urban newborn death rates: India's rural NMR of 33 is double its urban NMR of 16 (MoHFW 2014a). The gender breakdown of newborn deaths and care is also a cause for concern.

There is no breakdown for male and female NMR, but India's IMR (infant mortality rate) indicates a clear preference for boys, with an IMR of 39 for male infants and 42 for females. Additionally, many district level SNCUs admit around one-third fewer female newborns than male newborns, suggesting that families are more likely to treat a sick male newborn than a sick female newborn (Sankar et al. 2016; Zodpey and Paul 2014). Death rates after discharge are also higher for female newborns (Zodpey and Paul 2014). We know that SC (Scheduled Caste), ST (Scheduled Tribe), and Dalit groups are the most disadvantaged in India, yet more research is needed to quantify the effect of discrimination on newborn mortality. A recent India-wide rural study looking at district level household surveys indicated that community-based participatory programs can help reduce NMR among SC or OBC (Other Backward Classes) communities (Houweling et al. 2013).

14.8   Neonatal Survival: India and the World

The leading causes of neonatal mortality in India today are: preterm birth complications (44%), intrapartum related events (19%), sepsis (13%), and congenital abnormalities (11%) (HNN 2020). In India, neonatal mortality still accounts for 62% of total infant deaths and more than half of the nation's under-five deaths (HNN 2020). Three-fourths of India's neonatal deaths occur in the early neonatal period, and more than a third of these deaths occur in the first 24 h of life (Zodpey and Paul 2014).

---

[7] Other states and union territories with low NMRs include Tamil Nadu (15), Delhi (16), Punjab (17), and West Bengal. There were no NMR data for India's most remote northern states (Arunachal Pradesh, Manipur, Nagaland, Mizoram, Tripura, Jammu & Kashmir, and Sikkim) in 2014.

In 2018, India was home to 17% of the world's population, 20% of its live births, 21% of under-five deaths, 15% of its maternal deaths, but 27% of its neonatal deaths—an outsized fraction of the world's newborn deaths (UNICEF 2019). With 549,000 newborn deaths in 2018, India ranks first among nations, and India's NMR of 23 is five times China's NMR (4) and is worse than Nepal's—a remote Himalayan country with far lower GDP and less infrastructure than India (UNICEF 2019). India's 7.5 million low birthweight (LBW <2500 grams) newborns are 11–13 times more likely to die than normal birthweight newborns and 10% of all LBW babies have neurodevelopmental disorders at 3 years of age (Zodpey and Paul 2014). Being low birthweight or preterm in India increases the odds of being stunted in the first 5 years of life and the risk of severe lifelong disabilities.

Globally, in 2018, there were 2.5 million neonatal deaths, 2.6 million stillbirths, and 15 million preterm births. The three leading global causes of neonatal mortality are similar to India: preterm birth complications (35%), intrapartum related complications (24%), and sepsis (15%) (UNICEF 2019). In the world, 85% of all preterm babies are born after 32 weeks and can survive with a minimum of high-quality, low-tech supportive care—yet this group contributes the majority of morbidities of preterm birth. Babies born at less than 28 weeks have a 95% chance of mortality without specialized newborn care, while babies born between 32 and 37 weeks have a seven-times increased risk of neonatal mortality than babies born at term (Lawn et al. 2014). However, due to advances in neonatal care in high-income countries, half of all newborns born at 24 weeks' gestation in those settings *survive*, while nearly half of newborns born at less than 32 weeks *die* in low resource settings (WHO 2012).

Essential Newborn Care (ENC) costs little, but requires training, motivation, and knowledge transfer to be systematically and universally applied across the developing world. Yet coverage is often lacking in the high mortality settings where ENC is needed most. In South Asia, less than 5% of all facility-based births have access to neonatal intensive care. WHO defines ENC as: immediate drying and stimulation of newborns, warming or Kangaroo Mother Care (KMC), hygienic cord and skin care (hand washing, delayed cord cutting, and chlorhexidine for cord care), immediate breastfeeding, vitamin K prophylaxis, and neonatal resuscitation for babies not breathing at birth (Lawn et al. 2014; St. Clair et al. 2014). Within ENC, cleaning the cord stump and applying chlorhexidine can reduce neonatal mortality by 23% in low resource settings and delayed cord clamping is associated with a 41% reduction in intraventricular hemorrhage (IVH), a 39% reduction in need for blood transfusions, and a 38% reduction in necrotizing enterocolitis (NEC), a life-threatening intestinal pathology (Bhutta et al. 2014).

Thermal care practices such as KMC have been estimated to reduce 20% of all neonatal deaths caused by preterm complications and 10% of deaths in full-term or slightly preterm babies caused by infection (Bhutta et al. 2014). Early breastfeeding can reduce neonatal mortality by 44%, and there are proven benefits of Vitamin K prophylaxis to prevent bleeding, and of Vitamin KMC combined with breastfeeding support, early discharge from the hospital and supportive care for stable newborns is associated with a 51% reduction in neonatal mortality, 58% reduction in sepsis, and 77% reduction in hypothermia (Bhutta et al. 2014). Finally, newborn resuscitation training has been shown to reduce intrapartum-related neonatal deaths by 30% and early neonatal deaths by 38% (Bhutta et al. 2014).

14.9 Conclusion: Sustainable Newborn and Maternal Care

The Ladakhi model suggests that the skills and equipment needed for essential neonatal and maternal care are not as costly nor as complex as once thought. Leh's experiment could become scalable across India if public hospitals in other areas have staff as dedicated as Padma and Spalchen and their team and if hospitals and communities hold providers accountable for quality of care and review of mistakes made (Gutschow 2016). Our birth model makes clear that medical staff must be open to learning new clinical protocols, to changing outmoded or mistaken practices, and to welcoming marginalized communities or women. In short, Leh's SNCU suggests that change and progress across India's district-level facilities will require willpower and commitment to equal access regardless of gender, caste, and class.

In Ladakh, Dr. Landol, Dr. Padma, and Dr. Spalchen, along with their team of dedicated obstetricians and neonatologists, worked hard to improve the levels of care long before the central government intervened. The team's commitment to transparency of care has proven itself sustainable over 40 years and sets SNMH apart from many district-level hospitals across India where corruption and staff morale are perennial problems (Gutschow 2016; Zodpey and Paul 2014; Iyer et al. 2016). Furthermore, their compassion and dedication to the people of Ladakh caused them to choose careers in Leh where they worked alongside their Ladakhi peers, instead of pursuing more lucrative medical careers elsewhere in India. The model has become sustainable because Drs. Landol, Padma, and Spalchen have collaborated with their peers in Leh to jointly develop a model of obstetric and newborn care that has received recognition in India and beyond for its excellent outcomes, dedicated staff, and compassionate care. While the revolution in newborn care in India has the potential to save millions of lives in the coming decades, it will only succeed if it includes well-trained and highly motivated staff who feel part of a functioning healthcare system that provides routine and emergency neonatal care. Hopefully and in time, more Indian hospitals will resemble the sustainable and high-quality model of care found in Ladakh.

Acknowledgments We would like to thank the wonderful women at SNMH—both patients and providers—and all the staff of SNMH including the Medical Superintendents who helped make this research possible over the past 30 years. Gutschow would like to thank Padma Dolma and Dr. Landol for help in gathering data and collegial friendship over the decades; Robin Sears for assistance in visualizing the data and reading drafts; and Kai Gutschow and Yeshe Gutschow Rai for helping create the detailed map of Ladakh UT.

References

Aengst J (2014) Silences and moral narratives: infanticide as reproductive disruption. Med Anthropol Cross-Cult Stud Health Illness 33(5):411–427. https://www.tandfonline.com/doi/abs/10.1080/01459740.2013.871281

Aggarwal R (2004) Beyond lines of control: performance and politics on the disputed Borders of Ladakh, India. Duke, Durham

Bhutta Z et al (2014) Can available interventions end preventable deaths in mothers, newborn babies, and stillbirths, and at what cost? The Lancet 384: 347-70

Guilmoto C, Rajan I (2002) District level estimates of fertility from India's 2001 census. Econ Polit Weekl 16 February:665–672

Gutschow K (2004) Being a Buddhist Nun: the struggle for enlightenment in the Indian Himalaya. Harvard University Press, Cambridge, MA

Gutschow K (2006) The politics of being Buddhist in Zangskar. India Rev 4(6):470–498

Gutschow K (2011) From home to hospital: the extension of obstetrics in Ladakh. In: Adams V, Schrempf M, Craig S (eds) Medicine between science and religion: Explorations on Tibetan grounds. Berghahn Books, London, pp 185–214

Gutschow K (2016) Going 'beyond the numbers': maternal death reviews in India. Med Anthropol: Cross-Cult Stud Health Illness 35(4):322–337. https://doi.org/10.1080/01459740.2015.110146 0

Gutschow K, Dolma P (2012) Global policies and local implementation: maternal mortality in rural India. In: Kappas M, Gross U, Kelleher D (eds) Global health: a challenge for interdisciplinary research. Universitaetsverlag Goettingen, Goettingen, pp 215–238

Healthy Newborn Network (HNN) (2020) Leading Causes of Neonatal Deaths in India. https://www.healthynewbornnetwork.org/country/india/

Houweling TAJ et al (2013) The equity impact of participatory women's group to reduce neonatal mortality in India: secondary analysis of a cluster-randomised trial. Int J Epidemiol 42(2):520–532. https://doi.org/10.1093/ije/dyt012

Indian Council of Social Science Research (ICCR) (2008) Baseline Survey of Minority Concentration Districts of India. Leh (Jammu & Kashmir). Institute for Human Development Publications, New Delhi

Iyer V, Sidney K, Mehta R, Mavlankar D (2016) Availability and provision of emergency obstetric care under a public– private partnership in three districts of Gujarat, India: lessons for Universal Health Coverage. BMJ Glob Health 1(1):e000019. https://doi.org/10.1136/bmjgh-2015-000019

Jeffery P, Jeffery R (2008) Money Itself Discriminates': obstetric emergencies in the time of liberalisation. Contribut Indian Sociol 42(1):59–91

Jeffery P, Jeffery R (2010) Only when the boat has started sinking: a maternal death in rural North India. Soc Sci Med 71(10):1711–1718

Kumar VS, Paul VK, Sathasivam K (2016) Innovating affordable neonatal care for equipment for use at scale. J Perinatol 36:S32–S36

Lawn JE et al (2014) Every newborn 2: Progress, priorities, and potential beyond survival. Lancet 384:189. https://doi.org/10.1016/S0140-6736(14)60496-7

Mason et al (2014) From evidence to action to deliver a healthy start for the next generation. Lancet 384:455–467

MoHFW (Ministry of Health and Family Welfare) (2009) Navjaat Shishu Suraksha Karyakram: basic newborn care and resuscitation training manual. Government of India Publications, New Delhi

MoHFW (Ministry of Health and Family Welfare) (2011) Facility based newborn care operational guidelines. Government of India Publications, New Delhi

MoHFW (Ministry of Health and Family Welfare) (2014a) India newborn action plan. Government of India Publications, New Delhi

MoHFW (Ministry of Health and Family Welfare) (2014b) Use of antenatal corticosteroids in preterm labor: operational guidelines. Government of India Publications, New Delhi

Neogi SB, Malhotra S, Zodpey S, Mohan P (2011) Assessment of special care newborn units in India. J Health, Popul Nutr 29(5):500–509

Paul VK, Kumar R, Zodpey S (2016) Towards single digit neonatal mortality rate in India. J Perinatol 36:A1–S2

Sankar MJ et al (2016) State of newborn health in India. J Perinatol 36:S3–S8

Smith S (2009) The domestication of geopolitics: Buddhist-Muslim conflict and policing of marriage and the body in Ladakh, India. Geopolitics 14:197–218

UNICEF (2019) Levels and Trends in Child Mortality, Report 2019: Estimates by the United Nations Inter-agency Group for Child Mortality Estimates. UNICEF Publications, New York

Van Beek M (2006) 'Sons and daughter of India': Ladakh's reluctant tribes. In: Karlsson BG, Subba TB (eds) Indigeneity in India. Kegan Paul, New York, pp 118–141

WHO (2012) Born Too Soon: The Global Action Report on Preterm Birth. WHO Publications, Geneva. Available via: https://www.who.int/maternal_child_adolescent/documents/born_too_soon/en/

WHO (2019) Trends In Maternal Mortality 2000-2017: Estimates Developed by WHO, UNICEF, UNFPA, The World Bank, and the United Nations Population Division. WHO Publications, Geneva. Available via: https://apps.who.int/iris/handle/10665/327596

Wiley A (2003) Increasing the use of prenatal care in Ladakh (India): the roles of ecological and cultural factors. Soc Sci Med 55(7):1089–1102

Wiley A (2004) Neonatal size and infant mortality at high altitude in the Western Himalaya. Am J Phys Anthropol 94:289–305

Zodpey S, Paul VK (eds) (2014) State of India's newborns 2014: a report. Public Health Foundation of India, AIIMS, and Save the Children, New Delhi

Chapter 15
Giving Birth at Home in Resource-Scarce Regions of India: An Argument for Making the Women-Centric Approach of the Traditional Dais Sustainable

Bijoya Roy, Imrana Qadeer, Mira Sadgopal, Janet Chawla, and Sandhya Gautam

15.1 Introduction[1]

Globally, India ranks first in the number of births and until recently ranked first in total maternal and neonatal deaths as well (WHO 2015). Institutional births increased across the country after the implementation of Janani Suraksha Yojana (JSY), an Indian government cash transfer scheme that began in 2005. It provides

---

[1]This paper is based on a project titled The JEEVA Study, "Establishing the Scope and Pattern of Care by Dais during and after Childbirth in Four Cultural and Geographic Settings in India." This study was carried out between 2011–2015 with a focus on the multiple roles of dais in childbirth and their working linkages with Health Providers (PI, Dr. Mira Sadgopal; co-researchers, Prof. Imrana Qadeer, Dr. Janet Chawla, Dr. Leila V Caleb, Dr. Anuradha Singh, Sandhya Gautam and Dr. Bijoya Roy).

B. Roy (✉)
Centre for Women's Development Studies, New Delhi, India
e-mail: bijoyaroy@gmail.com

I. Qadeer
Centre for Social Medicine and Community Health, Jawaharlal Nehru University, New Delhi
& Currently the Visiting Professor, Council for Social Development, New Delhi, India
e-mail: imranaqadeer@gmail.com

M. Sadgopal
Principal Investigator, JEEVA Project & Managing Trustee, Tathapi Trust, Pune, India
e-mail: miradakin@gmail.com

J. Chawla
Janet Chawla, Director, MATRIKA, New Delhi, India
e-mail: janchawla@gmail.com

S. Gautam
Project Coordinator, JEEVA Project & Consultant, Centre for Health and Social Justice, New Delhi, India
e-mail: sandhyagautam570@gmail.com

© Springer Nature Switzerland AG 2021
K. Gutschow et al. (eds.), *Sustainable Birth in Disruptive Times*, Global Maternal and Child Health, https://doi.org/10.1007/978-3-030-54775-2_15

pregnant women with cash in exchange for documented antenatal care visits and delivery at accredited health facilities. The policy focus on increased institutional births did not truly address the quality of care at these health facilities, their ability to provide emergency obstetric and essential medicines or technologies for that care, the increased workload for the providers at the facilities, and the treatment marginalized women face at these facilities. By policy fiat, the Indian government projected institutional births as safer than homebirths, despite the evidence that facility-based care was often of very poor quality (Jefferey and Jefferey 2008, 2010; George 2007; Iyer et al. 2016). In recent decades, traditional birth attendants or *dais*[2] have been marginalized in maternity care policy, and the value of the maternal and neonatal care that dais provide during labor, delivery, and the postpartum period has been underappreciated (Qadeer et al. 2015; Sadgopal 2009).

Despite their marginalization, dais continue to assist in homebirths in large tracts of the low-resource areas of the country, such as the rural areas and urban slums. Studies of dais' knowledges or skills have tended to focus on either rural or urban low-income and marginalized communities (Bhattacharya et al. 2016; Devasenapathy et al. 2014; Iyengar et al. 2008; Pinto 2008; Chawla 2006). These studies examine why poor women prefer homebirths as well how dais embody familiarity, respect, and rapport with marginalized women who are often subjected to disrespect or discrimination at facilities (Chawla 2006; Pinto 2006). Georges and Daellenbach (2019) refer to the cultural rapport between dais and mothers as "cultural safety" and see it as a source of strength for poor women. Other scholars have argued that dais bring women comfort, a sense of empowerment over their bodies, and agency during the labor process (Qadeer et al. 2015; Sadgopal 2009). This chapter examines how dais' traditional knowledges and practices can manage low-risk births while empowering low-income women during labor and delivery. We show why many Indian women still choose dais in rural areas with poor infrastructure and low quality of facility-based care.

15.2   Methods and Study Areas

Our study was conducted in marginalized communities of Himachal Pradesh (HP), Jharkhand (JH), Maharashtra (MH), and Karnataka (KR). In each region where our partner NGO was already working, we chose 5–35 relatively contiguous villages.

---

[2] We use the term "traditional dai" and argue that they "represent thousands of years of experience in attending to birthing women and newborn babies in India and south Asia. Surprising to many, the term *dai* arises from British colonial usage, perhaps of Arabic origin" (Van Hollen 2003:39). Dais are not the only "traditional birth attendants" in India, as there is a larger category of women and rarely men, who perform tasks during childbirth and afterwards, in rural and urban settlements. Birth work may be divided between attendance during labor and birth, immediate care of mother and baby, and the ritually polluting postpartum tasks of cord-cutting, cleaning up, and disposing of the placenta (Pinto 2006; Sadgopal 2009).

Ultimately, our study encompassed 56 villages and 6990 households, with a total population of 41,621. We conducted a survey by randomly sampling roughly one-third of the households from each of our four regions. Our retrospective survey (completed in 2013) included 2309 households and 498 live births in the past 2 years. We initially found a total of 261 dais: 108 from MH, 62 from HP, 38 from JK, and 23 from KR. The low numbers in KR and JK may be due to the earlier shift to institutional delivery in KR as well as the remoteness of Adivasi (tribal) villages in those regions. We interviewed 498 women with children under the age of two and a total of 60 dais (the 15 most popular or experienced dais in each of our four regions). Our team of researchers[3] conducted participant observation of the dais and collected retrospective survey data in the local languages (MH: Mainly Pawra, Bhili and Marathi; HP: Hindi and Pahari; JH: Hindi and Bengali; KR: Kannada). We asked informants for informed consent and explained that they were not required to participate nor answer all questions.

Most of the families in our survey performed agricultural work, although lack of land, seasonal weather challenges, and inadequate income led to annual out-migration for farm or construction work within or outside the state. Women worked hard in the fields and at home, fetching water, fuel, and fodder, cooking, cleaning, and caring for children or the ill. One woman in Maharashtra voiced women's everyday hardships, echoing many of our interviews:

> I wake up early morning near about 5, then clean the house, the cattle-house, give the previous night's food to my children, and prepare hot water for my husband's bath. Thereafter I drink black tea and go to our farmland. I come back around 1:00 PM from there and then I prepare food for everybody in our home…..at the end I will eat. In November, my husband will migrate and I will stay here to look after land- and farm-related work …..Women during pregnancy also go with their husbands for labor work. This is the question of our survival.

In all four regions, the public healthcare systems had inadequate maternity services. We found deserted Community Health Centres (CHCs) and first referral units (FRU), nonfunctional clinics, as well as vacant paramedical staff and absent physicians. In Jharkhand, ANMs (Auxiliary Nurse-Midwives) and ASHAs (Accredited Social Health Activists) did not reach out to the most marginalized Dalit or Dom[4] communities. Discrimination against and neglect of marginalized communities within the public healthcare system are also reported in other states like Gujrat and Uttar Pradesh (Iyer et al. 2016; Jeffery and Jeffery 2008).

---

[3] Research teams in HP: Asha Bharti and Sangeeta Maurya, Kusum and Shanta and (Late) Khajana Ram and Kokila. JH: Neha Srivastava, Anita and Chandana and Yamuna and Tumpa Mudi. KR: Annapoorna and Savitri, Sunanda and Yashoda, and Mrusiddamma and Suprita. MH: Sneha Makkad, Munni, and Ismal and Roop Singh Pavra. Regional partners: (1) Jan Chetna Manch, Bokaro in Bokaro District of Jharkhand, (2) Janarth Adivasi Vikas Sanstha in Nandurbar district of Maharashtra, (3) Society for Rural Development and Action in Kangra/Mandi district of Himachal Pradesh, and (4) Mahila Samakhya Karnataka in Bellary district of that State.

[4] Dalits include several castes and Dom is one among them.

In all four regions, roads to referral centers were often in poor condition and providers in remote Primary Health Centres (PHC) or Community Health Centres (CHC) were not equipped to address complications or even to arrange for immediate safe transport of women to better institutions. Many remote PHCs had only two to three providers, and many lacked the required medicines such as antibiotics, anticonvulsants, uterotonic drugs, or the necessary skills to conduct manual removal of the placenta, vacuum or manual removal of retained products of conception, assisted delivery (forceps or vacuum extraction), and neonatal resuscitation. The CHCs that were expected to provide Comprehensive EmOc (emergency obstetric care) rarely had facilities for cesarean sections or blood transfusions and often could barely provide basic EmOC. Even the secondary level maternity services at the district hospitals in our study regions lacked healthcare providers such as obstetricians and anesthesiologists and essential medicines for EmOC, as well as transfusion technologies, adequate laboratory facilities, or instruments needed for routine or emergency obstetric care such as neonatal laryngoscopes, vacuum extractors, and ultrasound machines (WHO 2009).

15.3 Mother's Attitudes Towards Homebirths

Within our survey population, 66% of births took place at home. We will show why women chose to give birth at home and how the dais have been accepted and respected within these low-resource settings. We will show how dais handle low risk or "normal" deliveries by providing a set of supportive services that are low-cost, appreciated, and flexibly appropriate for the context.

Many of our interlocutors explained that they preferred to deliver at home because of *apana pan* (familiarity and belonging) by which they meant the supportive environment of caring home helpers. Unfamiliar and distant hospitals lack this important emotional, social, and physical support. Women feared the hospital environment, as well as the *chid-phad* (surgical procedures) routinely performed on birthing women such as painful episiotomies, cesarean sections, and tubal ligations. In contrast, dais were trusted, regardless of whether or not they were close relatives or familiar faces.

Women described how dais considered labor pain as a natural process and waited patiently for babies to be born, rather than seeking to intervene or hasten labor as is common at facilities. They felt the dais helped women to gain strength and prepare them for birthing, while guiding them in breathing to help them to relax or feel less fear. All of the women we interviewed were given instructions by their dai about abdominal breathing during labor, and many were told that short breaths and forceful exhalations will help the baby move down the birth canal. Women repeatedly mentioned that the assistance they received from dais and family members made them feel both safe and secure. This warmth and safety acted as a source of power, while facility-based births made them feel lonely, alienated, and isolated. The dai's reassuring touch, confidence-building conversation, and the constant presence of family helped them do their best during labor and delivery. Their husbands called the dais and helped out by heating water and if required called other knowledgeable women and arranged transport if necessary.

Women appreciated that dais supported both mother and newborn after birth. The postpartum continuity in care helps to restore woman's psychological, emotional, physical, and social well-being. After the placenta (*sui/aawal*) is expelled, dais help cut the umbilical cord (*naal*) and clean up both baby and mother. They advise post-birthing women to eat light foods and also to drink *jhol*—a yoghurt drink—and rice water) for the next few months. They advise women not to carry heavy goods after birth to prevent uterine prolapse and to protect the mother's pelvic floor.

Many women and dais reported regular visits by the dais on the first, third, and seventh days after birth and further visits up to 2–3 weeks depending upon region and tradition. In Himachal Pradesh and Maharashtra, dais would visit on the third day after birth, while in Jharkhand dais came almost twice a day; in Karnataka the dais visited less often. They checked both mother and newborn and inquired if there was any problem with either. Women with less breast milk are advised to take a drink called *peuva* made with one handful of rice and one glass of milk with a pinch of salt. Dai also provide *sek* (dry fomentation) and *tel-maalish* (oil massage) to both the child and the mother. Dais in Karnataka prepared dry packs with dry *neem* leaves, *lassan* (garlic) peels, *ajowan* (carom seeds), and *raagi* (finger millet) and applied these around the woman's belly to give strength to the body, for cleansing and to prevent women from getting sepsis. Dais also provided vaginal fumigation to help speed the healing of minor tears or infections. One of the dai describes this process:

> To give *dhuna sek* (dry smoke from burning incense*)*, first I ask the *puvaati* to hold her *sari* up and sit on the cot. I take a piece of cloth and put some burning coals on that and put some *dhuna* (incense) on this fire, I put this just below her cot. This *dhuna* directly goes to the puvaati's *asthaan/yoni* (perineum) and she gets cured.

Dais believe that *dhuna sek* helps to heal minor tears or infections, and they also help mothers by washing clothes, cleaning the birth room, and offering incense to purify both mother and newborn. These processes restore the mother and integrate the newborn into everyday mundane life and social relations.

15.4 Dais' Skills in Normal Births

Dais' narratives reiterate and amplify the mother's reasons for wanting homebirths. Nearly all the dais expressed explicit support for homebirths and saw their work as far more than a source of livelihood. For the dais we interviewed, work is a social responsibility, a spiritual act, and *dharam ka kaam* (righteous work). As a dai from Himachal Pradesh explained, this work allows them to do "good deeds for others' well-being." They are keen to attend birthing women when called and stay until the entire birthing process is completed. The dais do not fear traveling long distances alone or at night, even if the road conditions are bad and flooding or landslides are common during the monsoon season. As one dai explained, "Sometimes I have to go in the night also, there is no cause for fear. This is our own area and our own people, our relatives, all ours, and then, there are other people along with us, so what is there to be afraid of?"

All dais interviewed expressed their familiarity with their community, and many spoke of how this comforts and empowers them during the birth process. They have the trust of local people, unlike the providers at government facilities who are often from outside the region and may be responsible for abusive or disrespectful behavior. The dais do not discriminate nor target cases based on their existing relationship with the families. According to one dai, they visit houses "whether it is a relative or enemy." Birth is a sacred time when mundane relationships are suspended.

A dai's knowledge is shaped by her material and social context. She is trained by a mentor who can be a mother, mother-in-law, or a senior dai, and her experience of helping women generates a relationship of interdependence with the community. Unlike the practices of "skilled birth attendants," as defined by the WHO, dais' practices cannot be defined as a set of technical skills acquired through training. Our interviews with dais indicate that most learned their skills as apprentices from a very young age, by accompanying and closely observing their mentors. They were slowly introduced to small tasks such as heating water and cleaning the birth space, but over time their mentors began to ask them to give oil massage or offer physical support to mothers to help with labor pain. Most of the dais started practicing independently only after getting married and having babies themselves, slowly gaining community recognition as they demonstrated their abilities. Their training derives largely from oral tradition and experiential learning (Jordan 1993; Davis-Floyd and Davis 1996), in which emphasis is laid on how to use their senses and hands to understand what is happening in a birthing woman's body.

Dais are called as soon as labor pains start and will provide or arrange for basic materials (hot water, clean cloths, razor blade, thread, etc.) and help the woman in labor by talking encouragingly, telling jokes and giving her back and abdominal massages in order to assess the position and descent of the baby. They also encourage mothers to walk in early labor and help them conserve energy by showing them how to breathe; these services resemble doula work in high-resource settings. Light food and fluids are given to the laboring woman to keep up her strength, including herbal decoctions, hot tea, rice starch, or gruel. It is not uncommon for dais to open up or loosen threads, buttons, clothes, and jewelry or to untie a woman's *guth* (hair braid)—believed to help her relax. By performing these actions, dais monitor the progress of labor, help the mothers gain confidence in their bodies and labor, and facilitate their mental and physical preparation for birth.

In response, women tolerate pain, loosen and warm up, and ease into the final stages of labor and delivery. Some of the Maharashtra dais were inclined to normalize labor pain by seeing births and labor pain as unremarkable events within mundane life. In contrast, the dais in Himachal Pradesh and Karnataka verbally guide women on how to endure pain, by explaining how labor pain differs from other kinds of bodily pain. They explain that early labor pains are mild with longer intervals between contractions and that the body can be looser at this time. They see progress when the birthing woman's face becomes red, she sweats, and her body becomes tighter. Only late in labor do dais urge women to push; they understand the danger of pushing before full cervical dilation that can lead to a swollen cervix (Jordan 1993). Several dais explained that the degree of pain a woman feels helps coordinate her labor and helps them know when to signal a woman or push (or "give pain"). As one dai explained:

> Labor pain comes on its own. When baby pushes, at that time we say, "give pain." We say when there is slight pain, do not give pain. We tell woman to give pain when there is heavy/strong pain. When there is *prasoota* pain [pushing contractions], the woman starts to sweat. But even then we do not ask to give pain continuously. We should not ask her to give pain forcefully as the woman herself is suffering and then giving pains forcefully causes difficulty. If some women get strong pains then there is no time even to look at the *raasta* [vaginal opening], she should just be made to sit for *prasoota* [delivery] to happen. In some women, if there is time for *prasoota* to happen then we do check the raasta also.

All dais described the bodily changes that accompany the process of labor. An elderly dai explained the shift that happens just before delivery:

> According to dais, when woman is about to become *prasoota* [give birth] then the baby comes down to the lower abdomen and the space on the upper side becomes empty. During the time of *prasoota*, the abdomen becomes tight as a rock. If a woman does not give pain in a timely fashion, the baby stays inside and then the woman has more difficulty. We keep telling the woman to give pain when it is strong. As the woman gives pain, the baby keeps coming out.

The dais' physical assessments of labor progress, their observational skills, and their detection of early signs of fetal distress are individualized to the mother at hand. They allow time to flow as needed. Several dais confirmed that the lithotomy position was rarely used. As one dai stated:

> We do not do deliveries like a doctor...we make the woman kneel down on the floor, place the palms on the floor and apply all the weight on the hands and knees (*mundi*) and do birthing....The way doctor do *prasoota*, the woman does not get pain properly. The way we follow for prasoota, the woman pushes properly.

This hand-and-knee position for birth is well-known across many midwifery traditions, including Guatemala, where Ina May Gaskin first encountered it before making it central to her teaching and writing. It has been proven to expand the pelvic outlet by 2–3 cm, thereby greatly facilitating women's ability to give birth. Thus, it is widely recommended across the globe for breech births, shoulder dystocia, and other complications (Daviss and Bisits 2021). The dais' use of this hand-and- knee position indicates their deep awareness of the normal physiology of labor. In contrast, the lithotomy position used in most Indian facilities (as elsewhere in the globe) has been proven to be one of the worst possible birth positions, as it narrows the pelvic outlet, works against gravity, and inhibits the mother's ability to push effectively. Because many Indian medical staff who work in first referral units do not guide labor using the WHO recommended partograph, their ability to detect symptoms of distress is somewhat arbitrary and depends on staff experience, quality of care, patient load, and regularity of monitoring. The dai's monitoring of labor is more woman-centered, more pelvic friendly, more experience-based, and thus more sustainable than the poor quality of obstetric care that is delivered in many first referral units in our regions of study.

15.5 Birth Patterns and Complications

In all four regions, most rural households depended largely on dais for childbirth. Roughly two-thirds of all births took place at home, and between 70% and 90% of homebirths were conducted by dais. Government-employed midwives and other "skilled" providers with officially recognized training assisted at less than 10% of the births. In Karnataka and Jharkhand, there is a sharp shift towards institutional births, especially among women under the age of 25 (Table 15.1).[5]

Of the 329 homebirths in our survey, 69% of births were reported as normal, while the remaining third had some complications. Women from the Maharashtra site reported the most complications. We explored these difficult births to better understand how dais resolve complications and how they advise women on when to transfer to a facility.

According to our survey (Table 15.2), prolonged labor, delayed placental delivery, and premature labor were the three most common complications that dais handled. Even when dais recommended transfer, mothers were often reluctant to go to facilities, especially if they were at an advanced stage of labor or had delivered but

Table 15.1 Place of birth in retrospective survey

| | Place of birth | | | | | | |
| | At home | | In hospital | | On way | | |
Study site[a]	No.	%	No.	%	No.	%	Total births
HP	77	74	24	23	3	2.9	104
Jh	75	66.3	38	33.6	0	0	113
Kr	20	20.4	77	78.5	1	1	98
Mh	157	86.2	21	11.5	4	2.2	182
Total	329	66.2	160	32.2	8	1.6	497

Source: Singh et al. (2016)
[a]Himachal Pradesh (IIP), District and Block, Kangra (Baijnath) and Mandi (Darang); Jharkhand (Jh), District and Block, Bokaro (Chandan Kiyari); Karnataka (Kr), District and Block, Bellary (Kudligi); Maharashtra (Mh), District and Block, Nandurbar (Dhadgaon)

---

[5] Sharp shift towards institutional births in KR and Jharkhand: one of the main focuses of the National (Rural) Health Mission (2005) was to increase institutional births, since it was a key indicator to assess the performance of the health workers and of the health institution in Jharkhand. Karnataka's aggressive approach against traditional birth attendants and private informal practitioners/Rural Medical Practitioners stopped them from attending childbirth. Also homebirths made it difficult to get a birth certificate and the entitlements under various government sponsored schemes.

Table 15.2 Classification of birth complications in retrospective survey. Source: Survey data, Prepared by Imrana Qadeer and Bijoya Roy. Adapted from Singh et al. (forthcoming) The Role of Indigenous Midwives (DAIS) in the Health and Wellbeing of Birthing Women and Newborns in Four Diverse and Remote Locations in India, The Jeeva Project Study Report

Homebirths	Births (4) at study sites				Total births
	HP	JH	Kr	MH	
Total homebirths	77	75	20	157	329
Normal births	59 (77)	57 (76)	17 (85)	94 (60)	197 (69)
Complicated births	18 (23)	18 (24)	3 (15)	63 (40)	102 (31)
Excessive delays in labor	2	10	–	9	21
Delayed placental delivery	1	2	1	16	20
Footling or frank breech	–	–	–	2	2
Nuchal cord or cord prolapse	–	–	1	–	1
Frank, footling breech	1	–	–	–	1
Delayed placental delivery and cord issues	1	–	–	–	1
Premature labor	–	2		3	5

not yet expelled the placenta. According to the dais, the most likely reasons for labor delay are poor nutrition and the hard physical work that women continue to perform all through pregnancy. There is no system of formal help for homebirths nor transport in case of complications. Dais were not supported by providers at referral units or by the government health systems. They were only expected to bring women to facilities, regardless of the quality of service, and largely ignored after arrival.

Although dais base their assessments on experience of both normal and complicated deliveries, mothers may ignore their recommendations to go to a facility. In such cases, dais have little choice but to handle complications at home, even as they tend not to intervene without good reason. As such, dais have the ability to stretch beyond strict obstetric norms and thereby "normalize uniqueness" in individual labor situations (Davis-Floyd and Davis 2018). All of the 60 dais interviewed could monitor and assess the baby's position in labor and 80% of them could assess cervical dilation manually (Table 15.3).

Most of the dais we interviewed checked the amount of bleeding postpartum and had an ability to recognize "too much bleeding." They counted and looked at the cloths mothers used as pads to assess the rate of bleeding. We only heard of two very experienced dais who knew how to manually remove the placenta (one was interviewed). Most dais used a combination of putting their hands into the vagina to pull out the placenta, using massage, external manual manipulation, healing herbs, and rituals to help expel the placenta and ensure that all placental clots or fragments were removed. If all else failed, they referred women to institutions.

Dais cut the umbilical cord only after the placenta was expelled and the baby was observed to be doing well. They understood the critical connection between placenta, umbilical cord, and newborn and knew how to "milk the cord" or massage the placenta to revive the baby if needed, using heated bricks or stones. Many of these midwives understood that the baby's life force or breath (*jeeva*) resided in the placenta and spoke of treating a weak or severely compromised newborn by milking the cord to draw upon this life force and transfer its energy to "awaken" the newborn.

Table 15.3 Manual techniques dais knew in retrospective survey. Source: survey data prepared by Mira Sadgopal

Sl. No.	Manual techniques	HP	Jh	Kr	Mh	Total of 60 (%)
1	Assessment of baby's position in the womb	15	15	15	15	60 (100)
2	Assessment of dilation (PV)	15	15	13	5	48 (80)
3	Releasing nuchal cord	11	5	8	1	25 (41.6)
4	Post-birth massage and binding the belly	10	15	13	1	39 (65)
5	Placental stimulation	1	10	10	10	31 (51.6)
6	Perineum support and massage	15	7	8	5	35 (58.3)
7	Supporting breech delivery	12	4	3	5	24 (40)
8	External manipulation to correct breech	5	6	1	8	20 (33.3)

In all four regions combined, roughly half of the dais we interviewed spoke of cord stimulation to revive a struggling newborn that was blue, limp, or unresponsive. Other methods used to revive newborns included blowing in the baby's ear or mouth; splashing the baby with water; beating a plate or drum with a stick to produce sound and vibration; gentle slaps, especially on the newborn's feet; massage; turning the baby upside down; and checking to see that that the airways and mouth were clear. The dais understood that manual resuscitation might be necessary if the newborn had experienced a difficult labor or delivery, cord pressure or prolapse, nuchal cord (around the neck), or placental placement (such as placenta previa) that kept "breath" from reaching the newborn. Many of our mothers spoke of dais who could stimulate and revive unresponsive newborns.

In all four regions, dais explained that they would manually assess fetal position after the start of labor. Roughly 40% of the dais we interviewed had handled breech births, and 41% could remove a nuchal cord (wrapped around a baby's neck). They reported successful breech deliveries during which they had to remove a nuchal cord while the head was in the birth canal. The procedure was described as a delicate one requiring patience, first slowly loosening the cord with a finger if the dai felt it was hindering the delivery. Birma,[6] a dai from JH, describes a breech birth as follows:

> Difficulty happens when baby is *ulta* (breech) because water gets filled in baby's nose and mouth. I insert my fingers and then search for baby's face and lips. When I find it then I press it towards the body and then take out the baby holding it with the other hand.

Like the hand-and-knee position, this kind of head flexion is an evidence-based practice, as is delayed cord-cutting. The following quotation from a mother illustrates how a dai helped in removing a nuchal cord *after* the head was delivered:

> The naal was stuck around my baby's neck. The dai gently put in her fingers and loosened it before she took out the naal from around her neck. The baby cried immediately after the cord came out. My placenta was also not coming out. Then the dai massaged my abdomen. She gently shook the placenta and thereafter she took it out by putting her hand inside.

---

[6] Names and identifying details of dais have been changed.

15.6 Newborn Care and Birth Rituals

Dais cared for newborns as much as for birthing women. They explained their newborn care in order of priority and need:

> After birth the baby is wrapped in a cloth....The cord is cut only after the *sui* (placenta) comes out and baby is carried in the arms. It is important to put the babies to breast after cutting the cord, otherwise baby forgets to suckle. The first milk is important as it has a lot of advantages for the baby.

Dais were conscious of the nutritious value of colostrum and other aspects of newborn care. They taught mothers how to hold newborns while bathing them and how to massage them with oil twice a day so that their newborns would get proper sleep. They also told the mothers to feed the baby while sitting down, not while lying down, so that newborns don't suffocate. Dais also asked mothers to check the baby's breathing after the baby falls asleep.

Rituals are integral parts of labor and delivery, and there are common features across the four regions despite great diversity in cultures and environments. The common rituals that dais perform include unbraiding hair, removing jewelry, and opening of doors and locks. These rituals serve the symbolic purpose of moving women from the identity of a bound and obedient daughter-in-law—the space of "culture"—into unbound, open, fertile, and strong birth givers, the space of "nature" (Chawla 2014).

Mothers are considered ritually polluted during labor, delivery, and the postpartum period until they are ritually initiated back into mundane life (Pinto 2008; Chawla 2006). The dais, who themselves are considered polluted in this period, help clean the lower body parts of the woman after delivery, cut the umbilical cord,[7] clean away the blood and other bodily effluents from birth, bury the placenta, help the woman and newborn to have their first bath after a few days, and give them both an oil massage. Postpartum rites conducted by the dais mark the end of the "pollution" period and ritually transfer women from pollution to purity. Until the postpartum rites, the mother and the newborn are isolated from outsiders in order to protect them from the "evil eye" or malevolent spirits and harmful energies that could provoke illness or misfortune. The rituals protect the mother/newborn dyad and produce ritual purity that allows them to re-enter sociality.

The ritual burial of the placenta indicates a deep respect for the placenta and its role in the newborn's development. Care is taken to protect the buried placenta from being eaten by animals or taken by another person for black magic. The following quotes express some traditional beliefs:

---

[7] In the KR site, dais and women reported the use of a new blade for cord-cutting; in JH dais reported using a blade and heating/burning it in fire before cutting the cord; Ii KR, coconut oil and/ or turmeric powder were used on the cord stump; in JH they used mustard oil or a white powder they get from hospital) on the cord stump.

Sui [placenta] is inside the *bachchedaani* [uterus] and baby is inside the placenta. While cutting the cord if it is not tied, baby can die. Baby's saans [breath/life] is in that placenta. Baby gets strength and is nurtured through the placenta. (HP)

In the *naadu* [cord] and placenta is the space for life/breathing. . . the placenta and cord work to give breath/life to the baby. The baby takes food from the placenta. That's why it is *jeev* [life force]. (HP)

Baby's life is in the *phool* [placenta] only. That's why after being born if the baby does not cry then I milk the *naal* [cord] and bring it towards the baby and then baby starts crying. (JH)

Rituals surrounding the birth contribute to improving well-being and releasing anxiety for the mother, her family, and the wider community. The rituals comfort and support the birthing woman, and collectively they bind families to their communities and emphasize the sacredness of a new human life. Paradoxically, birth is considered both auspicious and polluting for the family and the community. It is the dai who orchestrates the ritual practices while also serving as skilled midwife in her community. If dais were to be formally recognized for their services to women and their communities, their status elevation could serve as a critical social intervention to tackle the pervasive caste and gender bias that undermines their livelihoods and social roles.

15.7   Conclusion

We argue that the skills of dais should be recognized and that they should be treated as the *traditionally skilled birth care providers that they are.* Such recognition would include them as official partners in India's formal maternity care system, dramatically increase the numbers of birth providers in rural India, and help facilitate the connection between homebirths and transport to government hospitals or private facilities. This would also allow them to stay in the hospital with women they have transported, provide continuity of care, and alleviate women's fears of birthing in these unfamiliar facilities. Integration of dais into government facilities might help increase women's willingness to use facilities for birth in emergency situations and erode the pervasive bias against marginalized groups such as Adivasi (tribal), Dalit, and low-income women.

Apart from their skills, dais are effective because they share the culture, language, and social background of their clients, thereby providing a network of "cultural safety." Our narratives show that dais do not rush women through labor; nor do they push women into an artificial time frame set by obstetric standards that may bear little relation to local cultural practices (Davis-Floyd and Cheyney 2019; Buffington et al. 2021). Our data on birth patterns and complications provides evidence of key skills that dais use to manage minor intrapartum and postpartum complications at home. They continuously assess the progress of labor and know when to recommend transfer, even if that recommendation is not always followed. Many of their practices challenge and contradict the norms of the obstetric model of birth that are followed in most Indian hospitals and clinics.

Our interlocutors noted that while dais are not equipped to handle severe emergencies at home, they do accompany women to hospitals or clinics. If they could be able to continue providing labor and delivery care for their clients and postpartum care for mother and newborn at these referral units, there would be better continuity of care between home and hospital (Davis Floyd and Davis 2018, Dunham and Hall this volume).

A global movement for humanized births respects local knowledges, local cultures, and the quality of women's birthing experiences. In this process, the voices and roles of traditional birth attendants and midwives in other parts of the world where they are not government-recognized are needed to underscore how home-births can be seen within their broader social and cultural context. The most critical lesson the fractured formal healthcare system of India—and other nations—needs to draw from homebirths is the need to develop a women-centric approach towards birthing.

The humanization of birth care has shown that collaboration between midwives and doctors can produce an environment supportive of the normal physiology of labor and improved maternal satisfaction (Buffington et al. 2021; Fujita et al. 2012). Yet traditional midwives will require a formal set of skills in order to be recognized as trained traditional birth attendants. According to WHO, such skills include being able to handle basic emergency obstetric situations including preeclampsia, eclampsia, intra- or postpartum hemorrhage, dysfunctional progress in labor, and manual removal of the placenta or its fragments, but not cesarean section or high-risk neonatal care (WHO 2002). They should have both skills and social competence.

The current debate in India is about who qualifies to become an official skilled birth attendant (SBA). Auxiliary Nurse-Midwives (ANMs) and general nurses who work in labor wards receive some midwifery training, and a proposal to develop full-scale midwifery training programs is being considered. Today in India, the ANMs, who originally were community level workers doing home visits, now work only in FRUs (first referral units) and hospitals, as will this new group of professional midwives if the proposal is adopted. Reid (2012) shows how by the beginning of the twentieth century in Britain the bias against community or lay midwives who had served the poor with very good outcomes produced a push for middle-class government-trained midwives, who soon replaced community midwives. In India today, there is a similar push for training middle-class midwives more formally, although the proposal is still under consideration.

Women depend on dais in rural or marginalized urban areas of India with low-quality facility-based maternity care, little access to transport, and little prenatal care. The sheer number of dais across rural India where they attend many home-births is testament to their critical roles in their communities. It has long been clear that *women want care in their communities* (Davis-Floyd et al. 2009). Maternity facilities are distant, under-resourced, and overcrowded, while medical staff are overburdened and often underskilled. They need relief to even offer basic services, not to mention the practice of humanized birth care. An awareness of the poor quality of public healthcare and of the valuable roles of dais in imparting maternity care is necessary to avoid eliminating or side-lining them—thereby leaving no option of community level care. Reports from urban areas show that middle-class Indian women are increasingly employing doulas to provide the kind, compassionate care that dais also provide (Sood 2017). In remote rural areas, government-trained midwives could learn from dais and begin to create partnerships with dais by encouraging low-risk homebirths and thereby eliminating unnecessary hospitalizations. These partnerships could increase the skills of dais, improve maternal and newborn outcomes for homebirths, facilitate referrals to facilities when needed, and prevent unnecessary transport. Almost all dais in our study welcomed additional training and knowledge but were not keen on being treated as inferior and polluted.

Pushing low-risk births to poorly managed first referral units increases the burden on both institutions and on families who cannot afford costly transport or the risks of poor maternity care. This situation is complicated by well-documented disrespectful, even abusive, attitudes towards women during facility-based maternity care in India (Vishvanathan and Walia 2015; Iyengar et al. 2009). The challenges include (1) improving maternity care at the existing first referral units of primary care for primigravidas, high-risk, and/or medically complicated pregnancies and assuring the availability of transportation from home to first level referral units and/or to hospitals and (2) acknowledging the persistence of the present system of homebirths with the support of skilled dais in low-resource areas, where families frequently choose dais' skills and humanized approach over undependable existing facilities. There is a need to accept homebirths attended by dais as part of primary level maternity care, to recognize dais' knowledge and skills as essential resources, and to encourage and include them in providing antenatal and postpartum care—through need-based, well-conceived participatory trainings if necessary. With health budgets dropping in India, we argue that the formal incorporation of dais into the Indian maternity care system is the best path to strengthen Comprehensive EmOC in resource-scarce areas and to create a viable and sustainable maternity care system in that country.

Acknowledgments We thank all the field researchers who helped us in the collection of data from different research sites. We are grateful to Kim Gutschow and Robbie Davis-Floyd for their comments and editorial work on the chapter.

References

Bhattacharyya S, Srivastava A, Roy R et al (2016) Factors influencing women's preference for health facility deliveries in Jharkhand state, India: a cross sectional analysis. BMC Pregnancy Childbirth 16:50:1–50:9
Buffington ST, Lynn S, Armbruster D et al (2021) Home based life saving skills: working with local leaders and families to prevent maternal and perinatal mortality. In: Daviss BA, Davis-Floyd R (eds) Birthing models on the human rights frontier: speaking truth to power. Routledge, New York/London. in press

Chawla J (ed) (2006) Birth and birthgivers: the power behind the shame. Har-Anand Publication, New Delhi

Chawla J (2014) How will the children be born? Shakti and satta in the context of childbirth. Samyukta: J Women's Stud XIV 2

Davis-Floyd R, Cheyney M (2019) Birth as a culturally marked and shaped. In: Davis-Floyd R, Cheyney M (eds) Birth in eight cultures. Waveland Press, Long Grove, IL, pp 1–16

Davis-Floyd R, Davis E (1996) Intuition as authoritative knowledge in midwifery and homebirth. Med Anthropol Q 10(2):237–269. https://doi.org/10.1525/maq.1996.10.2.02a00080

Davis-Floyd R, Davis E (2018) Intuition as authoritative knowledge in midwifery and homebirth. In Davis-Floyd R and Colleagues, Ways of knowing about birth: mothers, midwives, medicine, and birth activism Waveland Press, Long Grove, pp 189–220

Daviss B-A, Bisits A (2021) Bringing back breech: dismantling hierarchies and re-skilling practitioners. In: Daviss B-A, Davis-Floyd R (eds) Birthing models on the human rights frontier: speaking truth to power. Routledge, New York

Devasenapathy N, George MS, al GSJ (2014) Why women choose to give birth at home: a situational analysis from urban slums of Delhi. BMJ Open 4:e004401. https://doi.org/10.1136/bmjopen-2013-004401

Fujita N, Perrin XR, Vodounon JA et al (2012) Humanised care and a change in practice in a hospital in Benin. Midwifery 28(4):481–488

George A (2007) Persistence of high maternal mortality in Koppal district, Karnataka, India: observed service delivery constraints. Reprod Health Matters 15(30):91–102

Georges E, Daellenbach R (2019) Divergent meanings and practices of childbirth in Greece and New Zealand. In: Davis-Floyd R, Cheyney M (eds) Birth in eight cultures. Waveland Press, Long Grove, pp 129–164

Iyengar SD, Iyengar K, Martines JC et al (2008) Childbirth practices in rural Rajasthan, India: implications for neonatal health and survival. J Perinatol 28(2):23–30. https://doi.org/10.1038/jp.2008.174

Iyengar K, Iyengar SD, al SV (2009) Pregnancy-related deaths in rural Rajasthan, India: exploring causes, context, and care-seeking through verbal autopsy. J Health Population Nutr 27(2):293–302

Iyer V, Sidney K, Mehta R, Mavlankar D (2016) Availability and provision of emergency obstetric care under a public–private partnership in three districts of Gujarat, India: lessons for universal health coverage. British Med J Glob Health 1(1). https://doi.org/10.1136/bmjgh-2015-000019. Accessed 25 May 2018

Jeffery P, Jeffery R (2008) 'Money itself discriminates': obstetric emergencies in the time of liberalisation. Contr Indian Sociol 42(1):59–91

Jeffery P, Jeffery R (2010) Only when the boat has started sinking: a maternal death in rural North India. Soc Sci Med 71(10):1711–1718

Jordan B (1993) Birth in four cultures: a cross-cultural investigation of childbirth in Yucatan, Holland, Sweden and the United States, 4th ed,revised and updated by Robbie Davis-Floyd. Waveland Press, Prospect Heights IL

Pinto S (2006) More than a dai: birth, work and rural Dalit women's perspectives. Seminar, Special issue Dalit Perspectives No. 558. Available via http://www.india-seminar.com/2006/558/588%20sarah%20pinto.htm

Pinto S (2008) Where there is no midwife: birth and loss in rural India. Berghahn, New York

Qadeer I, Roy B, Gautam S (2015) Must history repeat itself? The role of dais in maternity care in backward districts of Himachal Pradesh. In: Qadeer I (ed) India: social development report 2014: challenges of public health. Oxford University Press, New Delhi

Reid A (2012) Birth attendants and midwifery practice in early twentieth-century Derbyshire. Soc Hist Med 25(2):380–399. https://doi.org/10.1093/shm/hkr138

Sadgopal M (2009) Can maternity services open up to the indigenous traditions of midwifery? Econ Pol Weekly XLIV 16

Singh A, Roy B, Qadeer I et al (2016) Establishing the scope and pattern of care by dais during and after childbirth in four cultural and geographic settings in India, the Jeeva project study report. CWDS, New Delhi

Singh A, Roy B, Qadeer I et al. (forthcoming) The Role of Indigenous Midwives (DAIS) in the health and wellbeing of birthing women and newborns in four diverse and remote locations in India, The Jeeva Project Study Report

Sood V (2017) Home births: why are more women choosing it over c-section? https://fit.thequint.com/health-news/advantages-of-home-birth-over-cesarean-3

Van Hollen C (2003) Birth on the threshold: childbirth and modernity in South India, University of California Press, Berkeley; Los Angeles; London

Vishvanathan N, Walia M (2015) Birthing experiences of marginalised women in a peri-urban public health system: a qualitative study of maternity care. In: Qadeer I (ed) India: social development report 2014: challenges of public Health. Oxford University Press, New Delhi

WHO (2002) Essential antenatal, perinatal and postpartum care: training module. www.euro.who.int/__data/assets/pdf_file/0013/131521/E79235.pdf

WHO, UNFPA, UNICEF. and Mailman School of Public Health (2009) Monitoring emergency obstetric care: a handbook. www.who.int/reproductivehealth/publications/monitoring/9789241547734/en/

Chapter 16
It Takes More Than a Village: Building a Network of Safety in Nepal's Mountain Communities

Vincanne Adams, Sienna R. Craig, Arlene Samen, and Surya Bhatta

16.1 Introduction: Sustainable Maternal Health in Mountain Communities

Remote mountain communities can be particularly difficult places for birthing women. In high-altitude environments (over 3000 m), physiologic risks for child-bearing women increase, especially for individuals who are not native to such environments (Beall 2001; Wiley 2004; Beall et al. 2010). Such risks include pregnancy-induced hypertension, preeclampsia, and low birth weight/small-for-gestational-age infants.[1] Emergency evacuations to well-equipped facilities are often challenging if not treacherous, especially where physical infrastructure such as motorable roads or airstrips are unreliable or nonexistent. Fundamental infrastructural supports, including clean water and electricity, are often absent in remote

This chapter was originally published, in a slightly different version, as a "Report from the Field" in a special issue of Maternal and Child Health Journal dedicated to mountain communities. Reprinted by permission from Springer Nature: Springer, Maternal and Child Health Journal, It Takes More than a Village: Building a Network of Safety in Nepal's Mountain Communities, Adams V., Craig S., Samen A., et al. Copyright © Springer Science+Business Media New York 2016. Some modifications to the text were made. https://doi.org/10.1007/s10995-016-1993-1

V. Adams (✉)
Department of Anthropology, History, and Social Medicine, UCSF, San Francisco, CA, USA
e-mail: Vincanne.Adams@ucsf.edu

S. R. Craig
Department of Anthropology, Dartmouth College, Hanover, NH, USA
e-mail: Sienna.R.Craig@dartmouth.edu

A. Samen
One Heart Worldwide, San Francisco, CA, USA

S. Bhatta
One Heart Worldwide – Nepal, Kathmandu, Nepal
e-mail: surya@oneheartworldwide.org

[1] http://www.summitpost.org/pregnancy-and-altitude/286351

© Springer Nature Switzerland AG 2021
K. Gutschow et al. (eds.), *Sustainable Birth in Disruptive Times*, Global Maternal and Child Health, https://doi.org/10.1007/978-3-030-54775-2_16

mountain regions of poor countries. Mountain environments can limit the provision of basic healthcare in situ as well as compromise communication efforts between periphery and center when it comes to meeting healthcare needs. Sometimes these dynamics manifest in shortages of essential medicines and other supplies, in the difficulty of transporting medical equipment to build a birth center, or in retaining qualified staff. Cultural differences and linguistic divides between mountain communities and urban centers can also hinder the provision of care for women and children, especially when centralized policies are designed for urban lowland settings rather than high-altitude mountainous environments. Cultural hierarchies can also play out within ethnic or caste groups, as well as between genders and generations. These dynamics, too, can manifest differently between lowland and mountain communities.

In this chapter, we discuss some of the links among infrastructure, cultural, and geographic challenges in the social ecologies of risk and care[2] in relation to maternal and neonatal outcomes. Our case materials come from the experience of one NGO that has focused solely on birthing women in mountain environments, specifically in the Nepal and the Tibetan plateau. In what follows, we will map this NGO's approach, called a *Network of Safety*, to overcoming some of these obstacles and improving care for mothers and newborns.

Sustainable and successful networks of care should involve local initiatives and social organizations. Such networks are not only about building roads and clinics but also are about helping communities to navigate the sometimes treacherous risks created by socioeconomic inequality, miscommunication, bureaucratic barriers, and points of cultural conflict over the course of a pregnancy, labor, and delivery.[3] Sustainability also means reliable access to essential medicines and basic medical technologies, such as misoprostol and intrauterine balloon tamponades, which can be lifesavers in rural settings when hospital care for postpartum hemorrhage remains out of reach. This NGO's Network of Safety begins with women and their families but extends far beyond the village, reaching up to tertiary care facilities and government ministries. The network model considers navigation of *social* infrastructures to be an essential ingredient of effective material infrastructural support–especially in remote mountain areas where supporting a network helps to overcome obstacles imposed by a history of marginalization by the state in terms of the provision of basic services. What follows is a brief overview of how this strategy works.

---

[2] See Janes (2004) on the social ecologies concept as related to maternal health and death in Mongolia and Craig, Chase and Lama (2010) on impacts of mountain environments in Nepal on patterns of resort for health seeking behavior, and Black (2018) for a review of the ethics and aesthetics of care.

[3] See Justice (1986) and Subedi (2018) for general discussions of the relationships between state policies, socioeconomic dynamics, infrastructures of development, and healthcare in Nepal.

16.2   The NGO: One Heart Worldwide

One Heart Worldwide (OHW) began its program in Nepal in 2010, after having successfully developed similar programs in the Tibet Autonomous Region, China (3500–4000 m), starting in the late 1990s. Over the past two decades, OHW has developed their Network of Safety approach to address the particular challenges of serving women and infants in mountain communities. Many of the regions where OHW works are both geographically remote and socioeconomically disadvantaged. As we describe here and in other works (Adams et al. 2015; Adams et al. 2015; Adams et al. 2005; Craig 2011a), such regions are often marked by a lack of paved roads, little-to-no transport for emergencies, and minimal functioning government-supported healthcare resources, including lack of essential drugs. Some communities where OHW works practice agropastoralism, such that members of households, including pregnant women, are on the move, for trading or in high-altitude pastures during the summer months. In other communities, particularly in Nepal, the relative absence of married and younger men, due to the pervasive practice of labor migration abroad, has created further challenges in meeting the needs of pregnant and laboring women (Lewis et al. 2015; Craig 2011b).[4] Extreme weather conditions add to the on-the-ground complexities of serving mountain communities, which are also marked, even in more proximal hill regions of Nepal, by a great deal of cultural and sociolinguistic diversity: communities of belonging distinguished by a deep valley or a high mountain pass.

Addressing maternal and child health issues in Nepal has a long history, some of which replicates MCH international health history elsewhere in the world (World Health Organization 2015). Institutions such as the United States Agency for International Development (USAID) have been partnering with the Nepali government and nongovernmental actors for more than four decades in the area of MCH to implement a wide range of interventions: support for Female Community Health Volunteers (FCHVs), vitamin A supplementation, immunization and family planning support, integrated management of childhood illnesses, and safe motherhood programs. With respect to Millennium Development Goals 4 and 5, Nepal has been lauded as a country that has had remarkable success. Between 1990 and 2015, the MMR (maternal mortality ratio or maternal deaths/100,000 live births) declined from 901 to 258, while the under-5 mortality rate (deaths in children under age 5 /1000 live births) declined from 140 to 32, and the IMR (infant deaths/1000 live births) declined from 97 to 27 (WHO 2015; UN IGME 2019). These steep decreases were the result of combined efforts by multilateral agencies, private donors, Nepal's government, and multiple players on the ground at the village and regional levels.

---

[4] Nepal is experiencing some of the highest rates of labor-driven outmigration in the world, with more than four million of Nepal's 30 million people working outside of the country, and remittances accounting for more than a third of GDP. Migration dynamics have been exacerbated by political instability and natural disasters.

Nepali programs such as the AAMA Initiative, begun in 2007, have helped to subsidize and perhaps incentivize the cost of deliveries in known healthcare institutions by eliminating obstacles based on finance–at least theoretically. Between 2006 and 2011, the proportion of deliveries assisted by a skilled birth attendant (SBA)[5] rose from 19% to 36%.[6] The proportion of births assisted by SBAs is a key indicator for assessing progress toward maternal mortality reduction, according to both the UN Sustainable Development Goals (SDG) and Nepal's Health Sector Strategy (2016–2020). In line with the SDGs, Nepal's target reduction of MMR is 125/100,000 live births, while the target for NMR is 17.5/1000 live births by 2020, with further goals to lower these ratios to MMR 70/100,000 live births and NMR 12/1000 live births as per the SDG 2030 agenda. Intensive human resources for health (HRH) including the increase in SBAs, are necessary to achieve these ambitious targets.

Nepal envisions these targets, in part, because the country has seen successes, as illustrated above. These results are deeply connected to increasing female literacy and education, as well as to efforts at poverty alleviation (LeVine et al. 2012). And yet these positive effects have been uneven: women in mountain environments that have been politically and geographically marginalized as well as the poorest and socially disadvantaged women from *dalit* (or "untouchable") backgrounds continue to bear the greatest structural and embodied burdens, including more deaths and poorer birth outcomes overall (Pandey et al. 2013).

Despite many areas of improvement in maternal and infant health, as well as the right to free primary healthcare mandated in the new 2015 constitution, the gap between government policy and actual services delivered in remote mountain regions of Nepal remains wide. Likewise, despite subsequent decentralization of government according to new federalist parameters, privatization of the healthcare sector in Nepal remains significant, and public-private partnerships in healthcare remain highly variable (Citrin et al. 2018, Maru and Uprety 2015; Harper 2014). Often, resources are channeled to districts where there is greater population density and easier infrastructural accessibility. Some might also argue that, although the government of Nepal goes to great lengths to provide services, it is simply too expensive and resources are too sparse to reach remote areas. OHW is committed to working with governmental partners at all levels, recognizing that reproducing parallel health systems on a solely NGO model does not produce durable and sustainable health systems (cf. Farmer et al. 2013). Likewise, the Network is attentive to–and builds on–lessons learned about "continuum of care" models in the country (Bhandari et al. 2011).

---

[5] The World Health Organization defines an SBA as "an accredited health professional – such as a midwife, doctor or nurse – who has been educated and trained to proficiency in the skills needed to manage normal (uncomplicated) pregnancies, childbirth, and the immediate postnatal period and in the identification, management, and referral of complications in women and newborns." OHW follows this definition of the term.

[6] http://blogs.worldbank.org/health/maternal-and-child-health-nepal

16.3   The Network of Safety Model in Nepal

In the rural locations where OHW works, the Network of Safety (see Fig. 16.1) approach provides a model for intervention that is flexible and that focuses on being responsive to the particular needs of each community. The Network emphasizes cultural respect, local ownership, education, and both physical and social infrastructures. Education includes community and provider trainings that are aimed at mothers, husbands, health workers, and other stakeholders, all the way to policy makers in the government. The aim here is to *scale across* rather than simply "scale up" (Adams et al. 2015). "Scaling across" means prioritizing bonds of knowledge, trust, and infrastructure that move in specific and unique ways from households to referral hospitals and halls of government–and back again–as opposed to exporting and imposing the same specific tactics across diverse regions and communities. The Network of Safety (Fig. 16.1) attempts to surround a mother and her child with the resources and skills needed for health and safety as illustrated below:

Similarly, the Network pays attention to the quality of experience. The organization places an emphasis on the idea that every individual served by the Network "counts." In an era in which global health success has become dominated by quantitative metrics and the push to "go to scale," OHW maintains that an "n of one" is still a crucial index of success (Adams et al. 2015; Fisher 2012). The organization also emphasizes a "high-touch" rather than exclusively "high-tech" local approach to project management and impact evaluation (Adams et al. 2015). By this we mean not simply privileging high-tech solutions or approaches to community intervention that require large-scale data production but an approach that values particular and individualistic cases, in which women are quite literally within range of members in

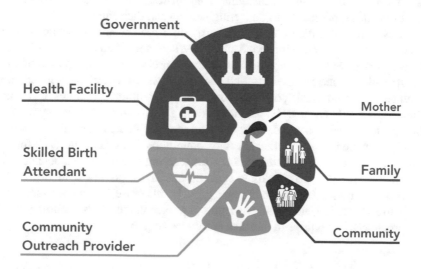

Fig. 16.1 The Network of Safety Model as described in One Heart Worldwide's Manual of Operations. Used with permission of © One Heart Worldwide 2020. All rights reserved

the Network and are taken as a singularly important data point regardless of their ability to generate usable data points for larger-scale program building. Thus, rather than relying more exclusively on large-scale statistical or experimental platforms for survey data collection, the Network of Safety takes each woman as an "n-of-one" (Adams et al. 2015).

OHW began its Nepal programs in Baglung (650 to 4300 m elevation) and Dolpa (1525–7625 m) districts; it has now expanded programs to 15 of Nepal's 35 under-served districts. In collaboration with the Ministry of Health, OHW envisions implementing programs in all 35 districts, representing about 7.5 million people and 200,000 pregnancies annually (Nepal Census Report 2011). However, the success of OHW's work in Nepal over the past 10 years has also led to difficult questions about monitoring and evaluation as well as organizational structure and leadership, highlighting the benefits and challenges of being successful enough to now contemplate "going to scale" by expanding the Network of Safety model to more communities.

What makes the Network of Safety work is collaboration with village- and district-level partners on MCH strategic plans that pave the way for systemic change, from supporting village-based Female Community Health Volunteers (FCVHs) to working with the Ministry of Health and Population (MOHP) to consider national MCH policies such as the inclusion of misoprostol on Nepal's "essential medicine" list or the use of intrauterine balloon tamponades to manage postpartum hemorrhage. OHW also addresses infrastructural gaps and obstacles to safe delivery by investing in improvements in health facilities; again, this usually involves partnering with government institutions even if they are at some distance from the intervention site. Sometimes the organization finds itself in the position of being a "culture broker," navigating between government policies and Kathmandu-based expectations and local lived realities, including what matters most to, and what remains most difficult for, pregnant and delivering women and their families.

The Network of Safety attempts to surround a mother and her child with the resources and skills needed for health and safety, depicted schematically in Fig. 16.1. The Network of Safety is capable of addressing problems mountain communities face in relation to access, diversity, and geography. As a practice, the Network aims to attune to the physical, political-economic, and cultural structures that shape people's lives. Whenever OHW begins work in a new place, the organization uses ethnographic research methods to understand the specific histories, diverse experiences, and challenges within that specific community. The OHW approach focuses on one community or catchment area at a time, trying to build a complete network in a small area, rather than trying to scale up quickly or provide a single, vertical intervention across a vast region or population. In this sense, the organization's aim is akin to Partners in Health's human rights approach that devotes attention to multiple problem-solving tasks in one area before moving to another.[7]

---

[7] Partners in Health Human Rights Approach https://donate.pih.org/page/s/declaration

The Network of Safety model is nimble and can be flexibly adapted to different regions within one country. For example, it is currently undergoing feasibility studies to determine how the Network of Safety would need to change for interventions in Nepal's Tarai region, on the southern border with India. Needs will be different, even in neighboring communities–in terms of infrastructure, culture, or accessibility–and the Network adapts (Acharya and Cleland 2000). This flexibility becomes especially important in mountain communities, where cultural, religious, and economic conditions can vary dramatically from one valley to the next. For instance, in Dolpa, as one moves up in altitude, communities change from middle hill villages consisting largely of Hindu sedentary farmers to higher elevation villages, home to largely culturally Tibetan Buddhist pastoralists, farmers, and traders. Within one Nepali administrative unit, there is immense diversity.

Attitudes toward delivery in these areas include some common ideas about the physical and spiritual "pollution" brought on by childbirth, but "pollution" is conceived of differently across geographic and cultural terrains. Hindu women must often abide by extended rules of seclusion associated with pollution based on pregnancy status and associated fears of contamination, including by bodily fluids; these practices can be further inflected by caste (Pinto 2008).[8] Buddhist understandings of pollution are not tied to caste but rather associated with the blood of childbirth and protecting specific household spaces from "defilement" (Gutschow 2011). Likewise, while it is more common that only women attend births in Hindu communities, men may assist women with birth in Buddhist households, yet the containment and subsequent purification of birth-related pollution remains a central concern.

Using the Network's adaptive tactics can mean recruiting and training different key players in caregiving in each community and working *with* rather than against non-biomedical understandings of what makes a birth "safe" (Adams et al. 2005). As a result of cultural diversity, OHW developed two different curricular approaches for the communities it has worked with in one district, Dolpa, where the population can be broadly categorized into Hindu and Buddhist communities. Specifically, the Network of Safety training curricula harnessed vernacular ideas about "containing" pollution. In primarily Hindu communities, the emphasis was placed on arguing for more guided or assisted seclusion and using birth kits to limit physical contact with polluting substances. Refurbished birth centers offered separation yet safety, where women could deliver without the presence of male relatives but with skilled help. In the culturally Tibetan Buddhist communities, the OHW team encouraged monks and householder priests (*ngakpa*) as well as and traditional medical practitioners (*amchi*) to participate in birth attendant training, a tactic that also enabled them to be at the ready for postpartum purification rituals and infant naming ceremonies and that also created opportunities to share knowledge in both directions. This gave these local authority figures space to articulate their knowledge and practices surrounding pregnancy and birth and to listen and learn from OHW staff who imparted

---

[8] Such cultural concepts are also reflected in practices of menstrual seclusion, or *chaupadi,* which can result in serious injury or death for women. See Atreya and Nepal (2018).

basic information in both local Tibetan and Nepali languages about basic biomedical danger signs in infants and new mothers as well as good practices during pregnancy. OHW's goal with this approach was to validate the community authority of local experts, rather than undermine them. In most cases, this effort has created opportunities to talk about "purification" also in a biomedical sense, namely, cleanliness of instruments and supplies, with people that women and their families are most likely to trust.

Similarly, villages in OHW catchment areas may have radically different profiles when it comes to existing healthcare infrastructure. These differences can be seen in the comparisons between OHW programs in places like Baglung or Sindhupalchok districts in Nepal's mid-hills, which are actually mountains themselves by any standard–to the higher-altitude extremes of villages and hamlets in upper Dolpa, on the Tibet (China) border. In some areas, OHW programs are often the only interventions and resources the villages have had, despite the fact that government health services should, theoretically, be available. Initially the Network approach focuses on setting up personnel and facilities. This often means obtaining commitments from the local, regional, or national governments to provision clinics and pay skilled birth attendants who are initially trained by OHW. Often, however, the kinds of resources each village has, or has access to, vary, requiring distinct approaches to training and infrastructural support. Villages that have skilled birth attendants already, for instance, may need refresher training and support, whereas villages with no such healthcare workers will need recruitment, more training, and ongoing support. OHW works hard to recruit, train, retain, and support local women as SBAs wherever possible, as having SBAs on the ground increases community trust and facilitates communication.

Given the centrality of SBAs to the organization's model, it is worth describing in detail how OHW recruits and trains these individuals. SBA trainings are facilitated by the National Health Training Center (NHTC) which falls under the purview of the Ministry of Health and Population (MoHP). All SBA trainers are nationally certified by this body. Individuals are selected from among the cadres of nursing staff at the district as well as municipal level; this can include someone trained as a staff nurse or an auxiliary nurse midwife (ANM) who has graduated from this program and is registered with the Nepal Nursing Council. Permanent nursing staff who have completed their probationary periods and who have not received SBA training in the past are given first priority. OHW also looks to recruit from existing and well-functioning government birthing centers, with priority given to those with high caseloads. OHW also prioritizes sites where no other trained service provider is available to assist with pregnancy, labor, and delivery. Likewise, staff who are working in marginalized, remote, communities and/or among those of lower socioeconomic status are also priorities. Although SBA training can be provided to contract staff (e.g., nonlocal healthcare providers), again the priority is on identifying individuals who are local wherever possible, who have a record of providing good services within their capacities in previous years, and who are willing to commit to work for 2 years after completion of SBA training.

Prior to recruiting a cohort of new SBA trainees, OHW works with government partners to assess the number of nursing staff or other potentially eligible trainees, collect MNH data from all birthing centers in each district as well as from these centers' catchment areas, and gather demographic information about expected numbers of pregnancies, percentages of institutional deliveries, and, as available, information about ANC visits and BCG vaccines given in the last fiscal year. OHW staff then conduct meetings with local rural municipality health coordinators and other relevant local authorities so that they can prepare a district-level plan in coordination with the rural municipality leadership. Together OHW and local government leaders prioritize the health facility within a given district that is in greatest need of SBA training. OHW's Training Coordinator then works with the NHTC and specific training sites to finalize schedules and sites for a specific SBA training and to invite participants to join the training. OHW provides financial support for the trainings in line with norms established by the NHTC–including cost of the training site, trainer expenses, and NTHC certification. All participants receive travel allowances as per government norms so that this is not a barrier to participation. In relation to sustainability, it is worth noting that OHW is working to encourage local government to support part of the costs of SBA training from municipal budgets, including costs incurred by SBA trainees for travel. These are ongoing points of negotiation as part of this public-private partnership.

OHW's SBA course is designed to deliver competency-based training covering knowledge and skills as defined by the National Policy on SBAs–itself reflective of goals and guidelines set by the WHO. The duration of this training is 60 days; however, due to the nature of competency-based training, the trainers may release any participants (in coordination with NHTC) up to 1 week prior to the course duration if the trainee fulfills all evaluation criteria. Alternatively, the trainers may add an additional week for any participant who is unable to achieve competency by week 10. The competency-based curriculum focuses on the development of 27 core skills of healthcare providers such that they are able to deliver high-quality maternal and neonatal services. The overall objectives of these trainings are also to ensure that there are not only high-quality SBAs but a sufficient number of trained individuals deployed at different levels of health facilities in the districts where OHW works. Furthermore, the objectives of this training are to strengthen referral services for safe motherhood and newborn care, particularly at the first referral level, which is usually the government district hospital. These trainings also aim to equip SBAs with the skills to support and participate in well-managed birthing centers. Alongside the training provided to SBAs, OHW also provides facilities upgrades to government birthing centers. OHW's model for SBA training also includes mechanisms for follow-up supervision and support for these trainees to help ensure that MNH services are being performed to national standards and protocols. This includes, but is not limited to, evaluation of local MNH service utilization before and after SBA training as well as tracking of the data that SBAs collect on-site about birth outcomes.

OHW works in a similar way for supporting and sustaining the infrastructure in clinics, medicines, technologies, and the financing for such resources. Each community may have distinct starting points, necessitating a flexible approach to investments in each place. Over time, OHW efforts can lead to further growth in primary care services. In upper Dolpa, for instance, government health workers were virtually nonexistent prior to the work of OHW; now there are equipped health posts and health workers who provide a range of support, from family planning and childhood immunizations to general medical support and referral. In this way, the Network and OHW's approach also reflects forms of public-private partnership to build and implement working healthcare systems, with care for women and children at their core. Tailoring the Network to local circumstances creates a sense of community ownership, which is vital to sustainability. This too helps people to gradually trust biomedical care in areas where it has either not existed or has been ephemeral and unreliable in the past.

Problems of healthcare accessibility and the provision of emergency evacuations in mountain regions are daunting at best for OHW teams. They can also be absolutely terrifying for the skilled birth attendants and, in some cases, Female Community Health Volunteers (FCHVs) who are tasked with ensuring that women deliver safely in the Himalayan communities of Nepal. Often there is no option for emergency evacuation. Approaching these problems from the perspective of a Network of Safety means determining contingency plans for different cultural, geographic, and socioeconomic terrains and for various medical emergencies. To this end, one of OHW's education goals is to create channels of communication that allow birth attendants to reach out to other community members to learn who has animals or vehicles that can be used for transport or teams of men who can carry women to facilities.[9] OHW stresses the importance of sharing information about deliveries when they are in progress so that such resources can be mobilized. An important focus here is also on helping people recognize problems in delivery earlier, so that it is possible to get women to a skilled and equipped clinic in time.

Even with efforts to get women to clinics if needed for delivery, timing can be a challenge. An OHW-trained skilled birth attendant in a high-altitude village in Dolpa recalled a frightening incident in which she was called to help a mother who was partway through her delivery of a stillborn. Faced with one of the most dreadful and difficult scenarios of her life, the birth attendant had to find a way to extract the dead baby with rudimentary instruments and without anesthesia. She saved the mother's life but wondered if she could have done more. And she carries the ongoing stress and anxiety over the thought of a similar situation happening again. Having to make such decisions about how to save lives is often radically different than being a healthcare worker in one of Nepal's urban areas, let alone in a fully industrialized and well-resourced context. And yet, this birth attendant was able to act in ways that saved a mother's life. She was then given training for and use of a handheld ultrasound device so that she could recognize complications sooner and

---

[9] Such structural and geographic contingencies are dramatically illustrated in the opening scene of Kesang Tseten's film "Hospital," which focuses on the district hospital in Kalikot, western Nepal (http://www.shunyatafilm.com/?p=947).

refer or evacuate a woman before this sort of event occurred. This tactic also helped bolster her sense of confidence and, crucially, local trust in her abilities.

The Network of Safety model often takes the OHW team in unexpected directions that pose new challenges that are often unique to a given village or moment in time. We see this quality as resonating with the reality of the communities where OHW works. That is, in mountain communities, people have learned to adapt to demanding environments, to survive and even thrive in some of Earth's most challenging locales. People who are used to facing these challenges are often quite receptive toward working with an organization whose approach embraces a sense of adaptability that rewards local resilience. These qualities as well as ethics of mutual aid and social support are valuable and instructive models for OHW and for the kind of work that is involved in keeping women alive and improving their chances for survival in mountain regions. In turn, people with whom OHW partners often value an organization that acknowledges the gaps–geographic, economic, cultural, and political–between remote places and urban centers, even as it works to close these gaps.

In summary, we have endeavored to offer some key insights about the challenges and achievements of working in mountain communities. These dynamics not only include those of geography but also of social and cultural, political, and economic conditions that shape pregnancy and birth in high country. Although OHW offers only one among many possible approaches to improving maternal and infant outcomes in underserved mountain communities, the results of these efforts have so far been quite good. For more details on project impact, we refer readers to the organization's website.[10] There, interested readers can find annual reports, stories, and links to research papers that emerge from the organization's data. Here we offer a few key results.

In upper Dolpa, the highest altitude and most remote region in which the organization has worked; in the first 2 years of program implementation, maternal deaths decreased from an average of 15 per year (out of 1000 deliveries) to 12 and then 9. In the subsequent 2 years, the region experienced only one maternal death out of roughly the same number of deliveries. These results are based on verbal autopsy and reporting by the district health officer; they were confirmed by either FCHVs or SBAs. In Baglung District, a more densely populated region with greater capacity for addressing obstetric emergencies in the district hospital, results have been equally promising. Maternal deaths appear to have dropped from an average of 30 per year out of approximately 8000 deliveries to 0 deaths in this same 2-year reporting period (2013–2015), with roughly the same number of live births.[11] Although not the focus of this chapter, OHW also responded nimbly and with direct positive impact on pregnant and laboring women and infants to the spring 2015 earthquakes

---

[10] https://www.oneheartworldwide.org/

[11] Similar results are seen in reduction of infant deaths: in Dolpa from 85–90 deaths out of 1000 births to 75, then to 35, and in the last 2 years between 3 and 5 deaths; in Baglung from 300 newborn deaths (again out of 8000 deliveries) to 150, to less than 50, and now to 0 newborn deaths in 2015.

in Nepal, not only in Baglung but also in two heavily impacted districts (Sindhupalchok and Dhading) where the organization had been poised to expand its programs in collaboration with the Ministry of Health.

16.4 Building Trust and Local Knowledges

OHW relies on local knowledge and resources to build from the ground up. This focus helps ensure that programs resonate with community needs and desires; such an approach helps to mitigate points of conflict, contradiction, or confusion over program activities. Take the community health worker described in the vignette below, for instance, who became interested in working with OHW after OHW's founder introduced the project to a group of male health post directors. She queried the men about their involvement in safe deliveries by first asking them to imagine how their lives would be different if their own mothers had died in childbirth. They then began to talk in new ways about how they have contributed to the problems that women face in not having safe deliveries. Some of the men at this meeting expressed their desire to be part of the solution as follows, as illustrated by these field notes from Samen, OHW's founder, taken during this time:

> On our last visit to Baglung District, we had to drive six hours from Kathmandu over a bumpy, winding dirt road, across rivers … you know, remote. When we finally got up to one particular village in the mountains, the senior auxiliary health worker came out to meet us. He began to tell us about how our program was working. He knew all the statistics about who delivered and how many delivered, and all the progress they had made. He said that as a leader in the community he established a no-home births policy. "No women should deliver at home, and no one should deliver alone," he said. He went around to every household in the community and collected money and with that money he built a birthing center. This was probably also related to the fact that our organization had promised to supply the equipment for the center.

> Another man in the village donated his land for the building site. He was not wealthy. Together the community built this space. It was one of the best I have ever seen: well-constructed, clean, organized, attached bathroom, a separate room for intake and prenatal care, a room for labor and delivery, and a room for postpartum care. All of the decisions and effort that created this facility were initiated by the men in this community. Not just the raising of the money and setting the policy, but the community outreach as well. The District Health Officer was a man. The head of the hospital was a man. Most health post supervisors were men. The person who donated the land was a man. In many ways it is always men who are decision-makers about healthcare for women. So, of course, men will need to be key driving forces for change.

We note that Network of Safety interventions often produced unpredictable windfalls as side effects of our focus on birthing women. When OHW began its work in Baglung, the team anticipated meeting resistance from local men, given the practices of female seclusion and cultural suspicion of and fear of the blood of menstruation and childbirth that has prevented women from receiving biomedical care during delivery.[12] In fact, the opposite occurred. Not only did the men end up taking part in decision-making about safe motherhood, but they also became active contributors to the programs that OHW helped to launch. While such interventions have not fundamentally altered aspects of Nepali culture that remain patriarchal when it comes to decision-making and control over women's reproductive lives, the heightened awareness and sense of responsibility, as illustrated in this example, can still be an important force for better birth outcomes.

We acknowledge that the push out of the home and into the clinic offered by the male health worker in the vignette above is a directive that some view as "best practice" and that others–including laboring women themselves–may hope to avoid, often for good reason, as other chapters in this volume have shown and has been illustrated elsewhere in Nepal (Vidnes 2015). Yet we also understand that some of the reticence about institution-based births can be mitigated by community-led efforts to create inviting, warm, safe, and connected local birthing centers–spaces that may be endorsed and supported by male community leaders but that are still primarily female domains. This narrative highlights the politics of donor-NGO-community dynamics, even as it indicates an empowered citizenry holding its government accountable for meeting local healthcare needs, in collaboration with an organization whose fingers rest on the pulse of national and international MCH policy, as well as local values and concerns.

16.5   Conclusion: The Sustainability of OHW's Network of Safety

With specific reference to questions of sustainability, OHW was fortunate to have come to an understanding about what it takes to create durable programs in challenging conditions during the organization's tenure in Tibet. Some of this learning was conscious and strategic; other lessons were learned inadvertently (Craig 2011a, b). After OHW set up the skilled birth attendant program in Lhasa Prefecture over a 9-year period, the training and outreach approach became fully integrated with the Lhasa Municipal Health Bureau and Tibetan physicians were teaching most of the curriculum. This development reflected overt choices and program management. But after political riots broke out in 2008 and the Chinese government mandated that all foreign NGO personnel leave the country, OHW was under threat of closure, and the few foreigners regularly involved in teaching did not have their visas renewed. However, because OHW supported a strong team of local collaborators who were already running the programs, they continued working without foreigners involved, eventually applying for government permits to operate as a local NGO, which, in turn, enabled them to receive both state funding and resources from

---

[12] See Nepal Safer Motherhood Project: http://www.nsmp.org/pregnancy_childbirth_nepal/index. html

Chinese and Tibetan philanthropists. The Tibet programs continue today and have been used as the model for safe motherhood throughout the Tibetan Autonomous Region, China.

It is unrealistic to assume that in all places, governments will be able to absorb the costs that come with managing and supporting a Network of Safety or that there will always be health infrastructure within which to integrate, but it is reasonable to assume that what funding is available can be leveraged across scales. Thus, while sustainability is often a desired outcome (and an implicit goal) of global health programs, few actually count this outcome in ways that see it as a type of evidence of success in global health work. *Attentiveness to local ownership should be a priority* from the initial planning phases all the way to the time when the implementing agency leaves, and this outcome should count as much, if not more than, making sure such interventions are being done in statistically robust ways.

OHW learned from its formative Tibet experience that local ownership should be a priority and considered primary evidence of success and sustainability. The Network of Safety approach also foregrounds, from the beginning, what a viable, ethical, and sustainable exit plan will look like. OHW found that at least a 3- to 4-year period was needed for initial assessment and ethnographic work, implementation, and building multiple stages of transition, including training programs and upgrading existing facilities. And yet sustainability also means sustaining *relationships*. This, in turn, means a commitment to refresher training courses and ongoing sources of advice, support, and respect for people working across the Network. It also means working to maintain supply chains of needed equipment and medicines, all the while pushing the state to live up to its stated fiscal and political commitments in this regard. Again, these are not unfamiliar goals for any global health program, but we stress *the importance of building in the exit plan from the start* and monitoring its progress at every step of the way. As OHW continues to work in Nepal, indicating which stage of implementation it is in, in each district where the organization is working, has also become a transparent part of its planning and reporting process.

Strategic investment in local health personnel and advocacy for living wages, rewards, and incentive structures and recognition of practitioners for their work as government health workers are all part of what the organization calls "success" and also why it relies on tactics of *scaling across*, not just up. These issues of support, recognition, and remuneration for the demanding physical, technical, and emotional labor involved in attending to pregnancy and birth are now reaching a tipping point in Nepal with respect to the "foot soldiers" of care, namely, FCHVs. As educational and employment opportunities for rural Nepali women continue to change, in part driven by labor migration abroad (particularly of men), the idea that the government or organizations such as OHW can continue to expect these women to *volunteer* their time and labor is being called into question and requires reevaluation.

The needs of delivering women in remote regions of the world are often overlooked simply because the challenges they face are so much more extreme than those in easily accessible places. Even though these challenges are daunting, and even though many organizations are unwilling to face these challenges, we argue that with the right approach, the provision of high-quality maternal and child health-care in mountain communities can be sustainably accomplished.

Acknowledgments The authors thank the Nepal- and US-based staff of One Heart Worldwide, including Dr. Sibylle Kristensen and Michaela Hayes, as well as the many local healthcare workers without whom the Network of Safety would be impossible to implement. The authors also acknowledge partners at Nepal's Ministry of Health and Population, as well as its funders and partner organizations.

References

Acharya LB, Cleland J (2000) Maternal and child health services in Nepal: does access or quality matter more? Health Policy Plan 15(2):223–229

Adams V, Miller S, Chertow J et al (2005) Having a 'safe delivery': conflicting views from Tibet. Health Care Wellness Infor 26(9):821–851

Adams V, Craig S, Samen A (2015) Alternative accounting in maternal and infant health. Glob Public Health https://www.tandfonline.com/doi/abs/10.1080/17441692.2015.1021364?journalCode=rgph20

Atryea A, Nepal S (2018) Menstrual exile – a cultural punishment for Nepalese women. Med Leg J:1–2. https://doi.org/10.1177/0025817218789600

Beall CM (2001) Adaptations to altitude: a current assessment. Annu Rev Anthropol 30:423–456

Beall CM, Cavalleri G, Deng L et al (2010) Natural selection on EPAS1 (HIF2alpha) associated with low hemoglobin concentration in Tibetan highlanders. Proc Natl Acad Sci 107(11):459–464

Bhandari KC, Pradhan YV, Upreti SB et al (2011) State of maternal, newborn, and child health programmes in Nepal: what may a continuum of care model mean for more effective and efficient service delivery? Nepal Health Res Council 19:92–100

Citrin D, Mahat A, Bista H (2018) Partnerships and public-private discontent in Nepal's health care sector. Med Anthropol Theory 5:2. https://doi.org/10.17157/mat.5.2.529

Craig S (2011a) Not found in Tibetan society? Culture, childbirth, and a politics of life on the roof of the world. Himalaya 32(1–2):101–114

Craig S (2011b) Migration, social change, health, and the realm of the possible: women's stories from Mustang, Nepal to New York. Anthropol Humanism 36(2):193–214

Craig S, Chase L, Lama TN (2010) Taking the MINI to Mustang: methodological and epistemological translations of an illness narrative interview tool. Anthropol Med 17(1):1–26

Farmer P, Kim JY, al KA (2013) Reimaginging global health: an introduction. University of California Press, Berkeley

Fisher M (2012) Conclusion. In: Beihl J, Petryna A (eds) When people come first. Princeton University Press, Princeton NJ, pp 347–373

Gutschow K (2011) From home to hospital: the extension of obstetrics in Ladakh. In: Adams V, Schremph M, Craig S (eds) Medicine between science and religion: explorations on Tibetan grounds. Berghahn Press, London, pp 185–214

Harper I (2014) Development and public health in the Himalayas: reflections on healing in contemporary Nepal. Routledge, London

Janes C (2004) Free markets and dead mothers: the social ecology of maternal mortality in post-socialist Mongolia. Med Anthropol Q 18(2):230–257

Justice J (1986) Policies, plans, and people. University of California Press, Berkeley

LeVine R, LeVine S, Schnell-Anzola R et al (2012) Literacy and mothering: how women's schooling changes the lives of the world's children. Oxford University Press, Oxford

Lewis S, Lee A, Simkhada P (2015) The role of husbands in maternal health and childbirth in rural Nepal: a qualitative study. BMC Pregnancy Childbirth 15:162. https://doi.org/10.1186/s12884-015-0599-8

Maru D, Uprety S (2015) The high costs of Nepal's fee-for-service approach to health care. Health Affairs Blog, 20 July. https://www.healthaffairs.org/do/10.1377/hblog20150720.049382/full/

Ministry of Health and Population (MOHP) [Nepal], New ERA, and ICF International Inc (2012) Nepal demographic and health survey 2011. Ministry of Health and Population, Kathmandu, Nepal, New ERA, and ICF International, Calverton

Pandey JP, Dhakal MR, Karki S et al (2013) Maternal and child health in Nepal: the effects of caste, ethnicity and regional identity - Further analysis of the 2011 Nepal Demographic and Health Survey. Nepal Ministry of Health and Population, New ERA, and ICF International, Calverton

Pinto S (2008) Where there is no midwife: birth and loss in rural India. Berghahn, New York

Subedi M (2018) State, society, and health in Nepal. Routledge India, Delhi

Suwal JV (2008) Maternal mortality in Nepal: unraveling the complexity. Can Stud Popul 35(1):1–26

United Nations Inter-agency Group for Child Mortality Estimation (2019) Levels and trends in child mortality, report 2019. UNICEF Publications, New York

Vidnes T (2015) Challenging global advocacy of biomedical institution-based birth: a review with reference to Nepal and South Asia. Himalaya 35(1):103–116

WHO (2015) Trends in maternal mortality: 1990 to 2015. Estimates by the WHO, UNICEF, World Bank Group, and the United Nations Population Division. WHO Publications, New York

Wiley A (2004) An ecology of high-altitude infancy: a biocultural perspective. Cambridge University Press, New York/Cambridge

World Health Organization (2015) Success factors for women's and children's health: Nepal country report. World Health Organization Library, Geneva

Chapter 17
Tranquil Birth: Revising Risk to Sustain Spontaneous Vaginal Birth

Kathleen Lorne McDougall

Elma's second labor was very different from her first, an unnecessary "emergency" cesarean section (CS) in an expensive private clinic in Cape Town in 2013.[1] Elma was not unusual in having an unnecessary cesarean (CMS 2020). In 2015 in South Africa, private hospitals had CS rates of almost 70% and public hospitals had rates of around 30%, much higher than the WHO's (2015) suggested national rate of 10–15%. Elma was unusual in perceiving that hospital birth was too risky, in terms of its likelihood of resulting in subsequent cesareans with their risks of, for instance, placenta accreta, placenta perccreta, and ill effects on her psychological well-being. She was also unusual finding a midwifery practice experienced in vaginal births after cesareans long before she conceived again, and so had plenty of time to let go of her fears about birth before her vaginal birth at home in 2015.

For her second labor in 2015, Elma chose an independent midwife whose hospital transfer rate was only 9%, and who was very experienced with vaginal births after cesareans (VBACs) and twin births (both considered extremely high risk in hospitals). Elma's second delivery took place under tranquil conditions at home, accompanied only by her husband, doula, and midwife. Her labor took roughly 40 h, most of which were peaceful, quiet, and almost uneventful. While in early labor, Elma cleaned her home and slept; later she used the warm water of a shower to ease the pain of her contractions. A midwife checked Elma's blood pressure and the fetal heart rate regularly with unobtrusive hand-held devices and found no reasons for concern. After 38 h, when she was dilated to 6 cm and tiring, the midwife, with Elma's permission, briefly manually stretched her cervix. Elma had prepared for the birth by exercising, researching, and attending intensive antenatal classes.

---

[1] Names and identifying details of people described in this chapter have been changed to protect their privacy.

K. Lorne McDougall (✉)
University of Cape Town, Cape Town, South Africa

© Springer Nature Switzerland AG 2021
K. Gutschow et al. (eds.), *Sustainable Birth in Disruptive Times*, Global
Maternal and Child Health, https://doi.org/10.1007/978-3-030-54775-2_17

Elma had decided to give birth at home mainly to avoid the culture of fear that was so pervasive in institutional health settings across South Africa.

The attitude and ideology of providers can have a profound influence on the outcome of a birth (Hodnett et al. 2013; Byrom and Downes 2015). This chapter describes "tranquil birth"—a term I use to describe what my interlocutors would term a "peaceful," "positive" or "compassionate" or even "traditional African" birth. Since COVID-19 emerged, societies worldwide have become ever more highly medicalized, and South Africa is no exception. In this context, where people are fearful of infection, it is possible that birth will be further institutionalized and, in the early days of the first South African lockdown in March 2020, non-hospital midwives and doulas were excluded from institutional births and further delegitimized as non-medical workers (even if for their own safety). However, along with reducing pressure on hospitals, tranquil birth methods may enable birthing mothers to avoid hospitals, as which are epicenters of infection.

My ethnographic fieldwork in Cape Town from 2014 to 2017 focused on observing one midwifery practice that was very effective in producing extraordinarily low cesarean and transfer rates. Fieldwork included interviewing parents and attending about 150 prenatal appointments and classes, where some parents invited me to attend their births. I also interviewed health professionals and prominent clinicians, attended professional meetings for obstetricians, and visited birthing facilities across Cape Town, including public and private hospitals. Independent midwives were, for the most part, registered nurses who were regulated by the South African nursing association, while others were traditional healers regulated by the Traditional Health Practitioners Council in South Africa. Some few independent midwives were direct-entry midwives (midwives who do not pass through nursing training first) who had taken international courses and then interned with midwives in South Africa. As such, these direct-entry midwives had less hospital time than registered nurses, although they were also allowed to register with the nursing association, even if it took years to complete this registration. I also spent time with a traditional midwife who ran a practice from her shack home in a very poor neighborhood. As was typical of traditional midwives, she did not charge a fee, though she would accept gifts. She had a day job as a housekeeper, with an employer who was understanding about her needing to leave sometimes for births.

South Africa's maternity care system can be characterized as providing care that is both "too much too soon" (TMTS) *and* "too little too late" (TLTL) (Miller et al. 2016). Neither poorly resourced public hospitals nor well-resourced private hospitals consistently offer tranquil birthing. Despite great concern for maternal and infant mortality rates, public health policy tends toward centralized TMTS overmedicalization that cannot be consistently implemented in public hospitals, where TLTL care prevails as Freedman (2016) notes. This situation strips midwives of decision-making authority in both public and private sectors. Given the vast divide between South African haves and have-nots—in 2015 the widest gap in the world (according to the GINI coefficient)—public and private health sectors are usually considered as having nothing in common, and there are very few studies of private South African healthcare. My study is unusual for including higher income families and for considering birthing practices across income. The women in my study differed greatly in terms of their financial resources, yet were drawn together by their desire to avoid (1) cesareans and (2) birth humiliation.

17.1 Fearfulness and Institutional Apartheid

The midwives, families, and doulas I interviewed reiterated that caregivers and parents need to let go of their fears about a woman's physical capacity to give birth without instrumental or pharmaceutical assistance. Yet what I observed in Cape Town was more than letting go of fears about pain or rupture. To support tranquil birth, South African midwives, families, and doulas also needed to let go of their beliefs about apartheid social divisions and birth as an imminent emergency. Effectively, they needed to let go of their belief in the modernist order that apartheid doctrine had enforced.

"Emergency talk" has long been a dominant feature of South African sociality. Afrikaner Nationalist stalwarts motivated their apartheid policies by convincing a White electorate that they were constantly under threat from their Black compatriots (Lorne McDougall 2013). While it could be argued that there is considerable urgency to reduce the national maternal death rate, framing this effort as a social-clinical emergency pushes a lot of buttons locally. A predilection to crisis thinking is a feature of our times, and not limited to South Africa (Roitman 2013), and the conflation of social and clinical emergency is at the heart of many humanitarian health interventions. According to Peter Redfield (2013), the focus on short-term geopolitical clinical emergencies allows for evading the political inequities that make such emergencies chronic.

In South Africa, there was nearly a decade of political emergency before the end of Apartheid. White South Africans were taught in state schools to fear violent Black uprisings, though the anti-apartheid movements eschewed non-strategic (civilian) targets and worked actively for 40 years to find peaceful resolution (Lorne McDougall 2013). Considering forms of birth, and even birth itself, as an emergency in this historical context of political fearfulness brings into play all kinds of residual fears. As a doctor told me about ordering an emergency cesarean in a public hospital in the middle of the night: "I am the one to marshal the troops." The metaphors of war and conflict pervade maternity care discourse and practices in ways that are unhealthy and traumatic for families and birth practitioners.

Apartheid doctrine enforced and insisted upon obedience to false racial distinctions as well as different standards of education, housing, and healthcare (Coovadia et al. 2009) for different racial groups as well as totalitarian control and other forms of violence to uphold those distinctions. To help tranquil births emerge, the caregivers I met traveled across racialized boundaries in the city and accepted learning from traditional African midwives who were mistakenly viewed in mainstream medicine as medically "less evolved." Well-off families left what they had considered the safety of plush hospitals to visit shabby midwives' offices in edgy neighborhoods, and registered for births at public hospitals they had previously characterized as chaotic, because CS rates in private hospitals stand at around 70% while those in public hospitals stand at around 26% (Gonzalez and Grant 2019). Less well-off families believed that they deserved better care than that provided at public hospitals and mobilized financial resources for their daughters to birth in less rushed settings such as homes and private birth centers. The resulting antenatal care and births could require many hours of labor support, but far fewer resources in terms of technology and post-birth interventions. According to my interlocutors, when mothers felt empowered during birth, they were able to heal psychologically from previous humiliations experienced during birth.

Elma persevered through a long labor in order to birth vaginally because she was convinced that this would be *safer* than a repeat cesarean. For her first birth, as soon as labor started, Elma and her husband had called an ambulance to rush her to the private hospital, a very uncomfortable (and expensive) ride. Although neither Elma nor her infant were in any distress, the obstetrician on call advised a cesarean since Elma's cervix was dilating at a rate of less than 1 cm per hour. When Elma resisted this suggestion, he said with some annoyance that he was in danger of missing the start of his rugby match. The second time he advised a cesarean, Elma relented but then changed her mind. She was physically restrained while receiving an epidural and screaming at the anesthetist to stop, to no avail. Unsurprisingly, Elma suffered severe post-natal depression, and decided she could not endure another cesarean. I found that many women, like Elma, experienced some degree of coercion during their labor or delivery at either private or state hospitals. Coercion took the form of rushing consent, specifically through not advising about reasonable alternatives, not advising of the risks incurred with physician-preferred treatment, by threatening to withdraw emergency care or threatening to exclude preferred birth partners.

Most of the women who chose this midwifery practice had experienced births in both private and public hospitals. Only 17% of South African women could afford private medical care in 2015 (CMS 2016). Private hospital care emerged in the last years of apartheid, as a way of replacing Whites-only public hospitals, but now cater to all upper income earners. However, low income and impoverished South Africans tend overwhelmingly to be people of color, so public healthcare is effectively racially distinct. In South Africa, once having had one cesarean, subsequent vaginal birth (whether in a private or public hospital) is unlikely. Support for vaginal birth after cesarean (VBAC) has been declining dramatically over the last 5 years, and what works (as in Elma's birth) is so far contrary to hospital protocols as to make VBACS almost impossible to achieve in hospital settings.

Studies have shown that birthing in South Africa's predominantly Black public hospitals can be a humiliating experience (Honikman et al. 2015). However, I found that women who birthed in predominantly White private hospitals *also* routinely found their birth experiences to be humiliating, albeit sometimes in different ways. Women in both public and private hospitals were regularly subjected to invasive protocols they found unnecessary—in the name of "reducing risks" of maternal and newborn death. This unfortunate situation suggests a broader problem than the actions of individual providers and extends to a fearful institutional obstetric culture in both public and private sectors. For South African women whose families were subjected to apartheid-era humiliations, the continuation of institution-based humiliation during birth is devastating. The consequences of humiliation during birth extended far beyond the mother's psychology to include long-term negative health impacts for mothers and families. It appears that the experience of humiliation may lengthen labor in subsequent deliveries, leading to a higher likelihood of surgeries overall (Hodnett et al. 2013).

17.2   Risky Definitions of Risk

The families and health professionals I spoke with felt that pervasive risk-thinking led to unnecessary surgeries and trauma. Alternative providers and their clients judged it less risky to: (1) allow labor to start spontaneously; (2) avoid epidurals; and (3) promote deliveries without vacuum suction or cesareans. Elma and many others like her chose to move away from a TMTS obsession with risk, intervention, and duration of labor in order to reduce the likelihood of creating a situation that requires further interventions.

In addition to the medical risks associated with repeat cesareans, increasing cesarean rates are unsustainable for lower income countries whose maternity care systems are already stressed with poor outcomes and provider shortages. There are ongoing national efforts in China, Brazil, and other countries to reduce the numbers of cesareans in order to create more sustainable healthcare and improve outcomes for mothers and newborns (Van Lerberghe et al. 2014). Inefficient medical interventions do not only waste money and time, but are also likely to result in more extreme medical interventions, which further contradict sustainability (Renfrew et al. 2014, 1134).

The reason for high cesarean rates even among homebirth midwives is what midwives termed a "culture of fear." Midwives told me repeatedly that doctors supporting homebirth or birthing center vaginal deliveries were haunted by a very few cases with adverse outcomes. Doctors spoke of the fear of malpractice suits that could end their careers. If homebirth midwives wanted the support of clinicians, they needed to adhere to the stringent protocols the clinicians set, including cutting labor short. Toward the end of my fieldwork, hospital groups asked midwives to sign liability documents that forced them to follow protocols the doctors alone had set and over which the midwives had no influence. For doctors, childbirth risk could be controlled through risk stratification, strict labor protocols, and the always available cesarean.

High cesarean rates in South African public and private hospitals were produced by extending the category of "high risk" women, as well as by obscuring the risks of repeat cesareans. Women over 35 years of age, pregnant with multiples or breech babies, are automatically classified as high risk, as are prior cesareans. In the private sector, when pregnancies are classified as high risk, cesareans are routinely scheduled for one week prior to the due date. In addition, most private sector pregnancies seem mysteriously to become high risk in weeks 38–40. During my three years of fieldwork, women would repeat the same refrain about why they had cesareans: "The doctor said the baby was too big for my hips." Many private sector cesareans were scheduled following diagnoses of cephalopelvic disproportion (CPD), insufficient amniotic fluid, and placenta calcification. These diagnoses can be highly subjective prior to delivery and many are not confirmed after delivery.

No woman I spoke with was ever informed by her doctor about the risks of repeat cesareans, nor the risks associated with babies not carried to term. If "high-risk" women insisted on a trial of labor by not scheduling a cesarean before their due date, they were allowed a maximum of ten hours of labor before cesareans were advised. The possibility that labor can proceed safely far beyond ten hours in these cases was not considered (Simpson 2014, Littlejohn 2011), and women were not advised that they could continue to labor beyond ten hours. Doctors and many independent midwives did not acknowledge that latent labor (up to 6 cm dilation) may take days in a woman's first pregnancy. Women who had not had prior cesareans routinely received synthetic prostaglandins to speed up or induce labor, which is known to be a factor related to higher cesarean rates. The same women who might need longer labor times due to the use of prostaglandins would then receive cesareans if they were not fully dilated within ten hours of hospital admission.

In both Cape Town's public and private sectors, unless a woman and her family were very, very determined, and had support from a select handful of experienced birth practitioners, a first cesarean led inexorably to subsequent ones, and with each subsequent cesarean the possibility of vaginal birth became ever more remote. High private sector cesarean rates as well as the racially structured division of wealth in Cape Town meant that cesareans came to be associated with privilege, and many poor women longed for the special attention of an obstetrician during surgery. While cesareans in private hospitals were relatively safe in the short-term and mostly performed under optimal conditions, public sector cesareans incurred far greater risk (Gebhardt et al. 2015). Further, women who had a first cesarean with medical insurance at a private facility were destined for public sector cesareans if they lost their jobs and/or their medical insurance.

Sustaining spontaneous vaginal birth has considerable health and economic benefits (Simpson 2014, Renfrew et al. 2014). In the first place, pharmaceutical, instrumental, and surgical interventions require expensive infrastructure that is limited in most South African public hospitals. In South African hospitals, a cesarean typically means three nights in a facility, during which time breastfeeding and maternal bonding can easily be undermined. Physical recovery from cesareans is costly to individuals, families, and society, in terms of the extended recovery time during which a woman might lose her job or be unable to perform necessary tasks at work or home. As previously noted, even in well-resourced private hospital settings, repeat cesareans pose considerable risks to future pregnancies due to the increased likelihood of placenta previa, placenta accreta and perccreta, as well as uterine rupture after cesarean (Spong et al. 2012). Further, increased bleeding in labor and instrumental delivery lead to higher rates of HIV transmission to the infant. Roughly 30%

of mothers were HIV-positive in South Africa in 2012 and some four million women lived with HIV in 2017.

There is growing concern that pre-labor cesareans (typical in South Africa for high-risk pregnancies) deprive infants of beneficial developmental effects of labor stress and the microbiome of the vaginal canal (Odent 2015). Other significant health benefits to infants and mothers from spontaneous vaginal birth include: less chance of childhood diabetes, allergies and obesity; increased likelihood of successful breastfeeding and its benefits (neonatal immunity and nutrition), and breast cancer reduction benefits for mothers (Childbirth Connection 2012). In a country with very high rates of diabetes, extreme food insecurity for many households and high child mortality due to malnutrition, successful breastfeeding can literally save lives, as well as help reduce the cost of public health care.

While childbirth risk is managed through cesareans in the private sector, this form of risk management is too expensive for the public sector. Yet the two arenas of birth are connected, as ideas about how to define and manage childbirth risks circulate between private and public sectors. All South African medical staff complete training in state hospitals before they move to the private sector. In efforts to meet UN Millennium and Sustainable Development Goals, public sector maternity care has seen increased standardization of labor management and increased medicalization of childbirth.

About ten years ago, state facilities started programs to reduce mother to child HIV transmission, including HIV tests during pregnancy and administering ARVs in antenatal care; such programs increased medicalization at public facilities. Now, although public maternity facilities are severely under-staffed and under-equipped, and although public transport is unreliable and/or requires expensive travel through dangerous areas (Ferreira 2016), women are increasingly encouraged to birth at hospitals. Public sector midwives told me that one consequence of a more standardized regulation in public sector settings is a rise in transfers from midwife-run obstetric units, and a rise in cesarean rates. As I noted above, cesareans are more risky in public hospital settings than in private ones, especially in rural areas where there may not be enough staff to check for hemorrhages during the night, or where surgeons or operating theaters may be poorly equipped (Moodley 2010). Although money does not move between private and public sectors, staff and ideas do, including the idea that childbirth is an emergency that needs to be controlled with interventions such as cesareans.

17.3   Sustainable Birth

In the context of historical anxiety around birth, decisions to trust in the natural physiology of labor and delivery are radical innovations. As a counterpoint to the fearful imaginary of emergencies, both clinical and political, a midwife's birthing space in an informal settlement can be viewed as a sanctuary from overly medicalized maternity care in both private and public facilities. "Informal settlements" are low-status neighborhoods, precarious in standing with the Cape Town City Council, characterized by shack dwellings and inadequate infrastructure such as a lack of plumbing. Patience was a midwife whose home in an informal settlement was sometimes a birthing center. Patience's clients were typically treated more harshly in public maternity care because of their African immigrant status, religious beliefs, and language. In some cases they knew of women experiencing harsh treatment in hospital and aimed to avoid hospitals if at all possible. Patience's clients were very poor, and, as was typical of traditional midwives, she did not ask any fee, though she accepted gifts. Her home was small and dark, without windows, yet the effect was not at all claustrophobic, but rather cozy, like a ship's cabin. Patience's space was clean and efficiently organized, and, while noises from the street and neighboring shacks could be heard clearly, it felt more private than the hospital laboring rooms I visited, because no one went in and out. For a time, the shack was a bounded space, a sanctuary within which it is easier to birth (Stenglin and Foureur 2013). Women coming here typically delivered without pharmaceutical or instrumental intervention within a few hours of arrival, and the last labor had lasted only an hour. I learned that short labor times were typical of second and subsequent spontaneous vaginal births. In her ten-year practice, Patience said she had never needed to transfer a client for a cesarean.

One of the midwives I met told her clients, "All you need to birth is the space between your legs." Margaret could always get a laugh with that slightly risqué comment, but her main aim was to reassure them that they merely needed the relaxation to allow their bodies to take over and to stop the production of adrenaline that would slow labor. Michel Odent (2004), among others, has argued that the clinical management of labor and delivery causes stress, cortisol, and adrenaline to rise, while blocking oxytocin and other hormones that promote physiologic labor, maternal well-being, and maternal-infant bonding. In conditions where a clinical risk model is easily triggered, it is difficult for women to fully relax and labor to proceed as easily in a tranquil, bounded space that the female body needs. A tranquil labor requires physical privacy, with the support of trusted birth companions who know how to step back and let natural labor proceed without excessive restrictions, interventions, or humiliations, all of which can bring labor (and cervical dilation) to an abrupt halt (Littlejohn 2011; Hodnett et al. 2013; Erhardt 2011; Scamell and Stewart 2013). Sometimes home is the most tranquil setting, but if the home setting is too crowded or busy with relatives, then Margaret would offer her home as a setting, reserving her bedroom and ensuite bathroom for birthing clients. She also had a room with emergency equipment, should the mother or newborn need assistance.

Tranquil birth providers have experienced how a calm setting reduces clinical risk. Rachel, a registered traditional healer, told me of a case of shoulder dystocia—a dangerous situation in which the baby's shoulder is stuck behind the mother's pelvis. Rachel used the McRoberts technique for manipulating the mother's body and was able to free the shoulder within a short time. When I asked her what caused the dystocia, I expected an answer I had heard from hospital-based providers, who describe shoulder dystocia as resulting from cephalopelvic disproportion, which would generally be an indication for an emergency cesarean. Rachel surprised me by stating that the cause was a lack of privacy that prevented the mother's pelvic muscles from opening up as wide as they should have, given how many people attended this birth. She blamed herself for failing to make the birthing environment more private by asking some family members to leave.

Midwives like Rachel, Patience, and Margaret actively create a tranquil birth space in order to reduce and manage perinatal risk. Keeping the lights low, using massage and warm water to relax the laboring woman, keeping vaginal exams to a minimum, and monitoring the mother's contractions and fetal heart rate unobtrusively and intermittently using a hand-held fetoscope all facilitate a woman to move into an optimal laboring state. Midwives try to help women connect with their bodies, rather than overthinking, which actually slows or halts their labor progress (Odent 2004). For a mother to labor comfortably, she needs to lose her own sense of time, which the midwife protects as sacred from outside interventions. Above all, the providers tried to maintain their own emotional awareness and calm, which allowed them to access their deepest intuition (Davis-Floyd and Davis 2018).

There is more to tranquil birth than what happens during labor. Tranquil birth providers work hard at establishing trust by *preparing* families for labor. Antenatal consultations I attended with Margaret and a doula were at least an hour in length, and most of the time was spent chatting with clients about labor and birth. These sessions could be intense when mothers revealed previous traumatic experiences, but such sessions were also quite raucous as Margaret made jokes that encouraged her clients to overcome bodily taboos. The sessions created invaluable trust and bonds between the midwife/doula duo and their clients. Margaret believed that the baby becomes familiar with her voice and her touch as she palpates the uterus and that this familiarity contributes to birth tranquility and easier labor. Margaret also spends a lot of time during antenatal sessions informing clients about how to prepare for birth physically, by encouraging them to exercise and control their diets. She began offering antenatal classes in which where she and her doula team taught their clients and families about physiologic labor and worked through potential psychological stumbling blocks such as past physical or sexual trauma that could prevent a mother from fully opening up and letting go during the various phases of labor.

Lastly, the midwives and doulas I interviewed built confidence in their methods by keeping themselves informed about techniques, ideas, and clinical experience, and by building a community. Margaret and her team of doulas/midwives draw on their own experiences as well as on the international literature they read in support of natural birth, and they travel within Africa and internationally at times to learn about traditional methods and midwifery practices that have withstood the test of time. Keeping in touch with other midwives who practice tranquil birth methods— even by WhatsApp during labor—and sharing their empirical experiences and birthing skills with each other helps them build a knowledge community to empower midwives to make births safer and more tranquil.

17.4   Conclusion

The tranquil birth attendants I studied sustain the skills necessary for spontaneous vaginal birth by creating a peaceful and safe space in which labor and delivery are not emergencies waiting to happen. There have been significant innovations in scaling up this effort across facilities in Cape Town. For instance, one public sector midwifery unit has partnered with an NGO to provide a doula for local clients when possible. The doulas donate their time to complete their training and clients receive the much-needed birth support that helps advance their labor and ward off some interventions. Two midwives from Margaret's practice formed a partnership with a public maternity care training branch in Cape Town, where midwives learn the midwifery model of care, or what I call "tranquil birth" methods.

Neither South African public nor private maternity care is sustainable in terms of improving birth outcomes for mothers or newborns: the cesarean rate in private hospitals is far too high to be necessary or affordable (as recently pointed out in a Medical Schemes Council Report), and consistent claims of coercion are worrying. Public hospitals are currently simply too over-crowded and under-staffed to be consistently safe places to birth, despite the best intentions. In Cape Town as elsewhere in South Africa, travel to and from public institutions is often unaffordable and also unsafe for low income or impoverished women, so safely localizing birthing at home or non-medical birth centers would help poorer families to have better access to midwifery care and make birth in South Africa more sustainable and lower cost. The tranquil birth model outlined in this chapter is flexible and builds on traditional bodies of knowledge. Its de-centered approach that shifts births away from private and public hospitals makes better use of existing human and financial resources. If widely implemented, this approach would reduce the fears and risks so prevalent in hospital birth and generate a much more sustainable future for birth in all of South Africa.

South Africa is on the verge of a (slow) public health revolution, as proposed in the 2015 draft National Health Insurance Bill, intended to even out resources between the public and private sectors. The COVID-19 State of Disaster Regulations may kick-start health resource sharing—time will tell. Certainly, everyday life has become dramatically more medicalized since COVID-19 was defined as a public threat in South Africa in March 2020; it is not yet clear whether birth will be further medicalized—especially since avoiding medical institutions for birth makes even more sense now. However, I have heard of obstetricians suggesting early cesareans in order to avoid pressuring hospitals later, when more coronavirus patients are expected, and, since the advent of COVID-19, even more severe restrictions have been placed on birth companions in South African private and public institutions, just as they have been in many other countries. Hospitals and clinics have come to be considered epicenters of contagion, and so birth partners are considered both to be at risk and to carry risk. For midwives and doulas working in institutions and already feeling delegitimized, and for clients hoping for birth support, the new regulations provoke anxiety. Midwives and doulas express concern at the trauma for birthing mothers of unassisted and highly medicalized births in South African private and public hospitals under COVID-19 conditions. Given the higher chance of in-hospital infections, and the pressure on such institutions to prioritize virus patients, it seems clearer than ever that tranquil and sustainable birthing must rely on homes and non-medical birthing centers to decentralize care.

References

Byrom S, Downes S (eds) (2015) The roar behind the silence: why kindness, compassion and respect matter in maternity care. Pinter and Martin, London

Childbirth Connection (2012) Vaginal or cesarean birth: what is at stake for women and babies? Childbirth Connection, New York

Council for Medical Schemes (CMS) (2020) Epidemiology and trends of caesarian section births in the medical scheme population, 2015–2018. Council for Medical Schemes, Cape Town

Council for Medical Schemes (CMS) (2016) Annual report 2015/2016. Pretoria, South Africa

Coovadia H, Jewkes R, Barron P, Sanders D, McIntyre D (2009) The health and health system of South Africa: historical roots of current public health challenges. Lancet 374(9692):817–834

Davis-Floyd R, Davis E (2018) Intuition as authoritative knowledge in midwifery and homebirth. In: Davis-Floyd R, Colleagues (eds) Ways of knowing: mothers, midwives, medicine, and birth activism. Waveland Press, Long Grove, pp 189–220

Erhardt R (2011) The basic needs of a woman in labor. True Midwifery, Capetown

Ferreira N (2016) Enduring "lateness": biomedicalisation and the unfolding reproductive life, sociality, and antenatal care. Dissertation, University of Cape Town

Freedman L (2016) Implementation and aspiration gaps: whose view counts? Lancet 388:2068. https://doi.org/10.1016/S0140-6736(16)31530-6

Gebhardt GS, Fawcus S, Moodley J et al (2015) Maternal death and caesarean section in South Africa: results from the 2011–2013 saving mothers report of the National Committee for confidential enquiries in maternal deaths. S Afr Med J 105:287. https://doi.org/10.7196/SAMJ.9351

Gonzalez LL, Grant L (2019) A changing birth: what's behind SA's skyrocketing c-section rates? BHEKISISA Center for Health Journalism. https://bhekisisa.org/article/2019-01-09-00-a-changing-birth-whats-behind-sas-skyrocketing-c-section-rates-map-district-rates/

Hodnett ED, Gates S, Hofmeyr GJ et al (2013) Continuous support for women during childbirth. Cochrane Database Syst Rev 7:CD003766. https://doi.org/10.1002/14651858.CD003766.pub5

Honikman S, Fawcus S, Meintjes I (2015) Abuse in South African maternity settings is a disgrace: potential solutions to the problem. S Afr Med J 105(4):284–285

Littlejohn M (2011) Protecting mother and baby during the second stage of labor. http://www.spiritualbirth.net/protecting-mother-and-baby-during-second-stage-of-labor. Accessed 24 May 2017

Lorne McDougall K (2013) The threat of history: post-apartheid genea-logic and apartheid life chronicles. Dissertation, University of Chicago

Miller S, Abalos E, Chamillard M, Ciapponi A, Comande A, Diaz V, Geller S et al (2016) Beyond too little, too late and too much, too soon: a pathway towards evidence-based, respectful maternity care worldwide. Lancet 388:2176. https://doi.org/10.1016/S0140-6736(16)31472-6

Moodley J (ed) (2010) Saving mothers: a monograph on caesarean section 2013. Department of Health, Pretoria

Odent M (2004) The caesarean. Free Association Books, London

Odent M (2015) Stress deprivation in the perinatal period. Midwifery Today 116. https://midwiferytoday.com/mt-articles/stress-deprivation-perinatal-period/

Redfield P (2013) Life in crisis: the ethical journey of doctors without borders. University of California Press, Berkeley

Renfrew MM, Bastos M, Campbell J et al (2014) Midwifery and quality care: findings from a new evidence-informed framework for maternal and newborn care. Lancet 384(9948):1129–1145

Roitman J (2013) Anti-crisis. Duke University Press, Durham

Scamell M, Stewart M (2013) Time, risk and midwife practice: the vaginal examination. Health Risk Soc 16(1):84–100

Simpson K (2014) Labor management evidence update: potential to minimize risk of cesarean birth in healthy women. J Perinat Neonat Nurs 28(2):108–116

Spong CY, Berghella V, Wenstrom KD et al (2012) Preventing the first cesarean delivery. Obstet Gynecol 120(5):1181–1193

Stenglin M, Foureur M (2013) Designing out the fear cascade to increase the likelihood of normal birth. Midwifery 29:819. https://doi.org/10.1016/j.midw.2013.04.005

Van Lerberghe W, Matthews Z, Achabe E et al (2014) Country experience with strengthening of health systems and deployment of midwives in countries with high maternal mortality. Lancet 384:1215–1225

Western Cape Department of Health (WCDH) (2016) First 1000 days rapid situational analysis for the Western Cape December 2016: Survive, thrive, transform. Cape Town, WCDH

World Health Organization (2015) WHO statement on caesarian section rates: executive summary. WHO, Geneva. Available via http://who.int/reproductivehealth/publications/maternal.perinatal_health/cesarean-statement/en/

Chapter 18
Sustainable Birth Care in Disaster Zones and During Pandemics: Low-Tech, Skilled Touch

Robbie Davis-Floyd, Robin Lim, Vicki Penwell, and Tsipy Ivry

18.1 Introduction: Effective Disaster Care as a Critique of Technocratic Birth

Many chapters in this book and others heavily critique what Davis-Floyd (2001, 2003) has long called "the technocratic model of birth." Following Ivry et al.'s (2019) suggestion that disasters may provide a differing and powerful perspective for such critiques, this chapter examines effective care in the immediate aftermaths of disasters that render the technocratic model, with its reliance on high technologies, inapplicable in the absence of those technologies. Midwife Robin Lim (2021) brings into geopolitical focus the issues this chapter is designed to address:

> Climate change, geological events and socio-political struggles are contributing to disasters devastating communities worldwide. Pandemics, superstorms, ocean surges, tsunamis, rising tides, landslides, floods, blizzards, droughts, bitterly cold and scorching hot weather, earthquakes, volcanic eruptions and wars fought over resources, territories, food security, dogma, and precious water, all destabilize our planet Earth. When the hospitals are reduced

R. Davis-Floyd
Department of Anthropology, University of Texas Austin, Austin, TX, USA
e-mail: davis-floyd@outlook.com

R. Lim
Bumi Sehat Foundation, Ubud, Bali, Indonesia
e-mail: iburobin@bumisehat.org

V. Penwell (✉)
Department of Anthropology, Rice University, Houston, TX, USA
e-mail: vickipenwell@mercyinaction.com

T. Ivry
Department of Anthropology, University of Haifa, Haifa, Israel
e-mail: tsipy.ivry@gmail.com

© Springer Nature Switzerland AG 2021
K. Gutschow et al. (eds.), *Sustainable Birth in Disruptive Times*, Global
Maternal and Child Health, https://doi.org/10.1007/978-3-030-54775-2_18

to rubble, electricity is gone, water is not flowing, and people are left homeless, hungry and thirsty, who will receive the babies? Where will the mothers birth? What childbirth protocols will best support life as communities heal in the aftermath?

In this chapter, in response to Robin's questions, we examine effective care in the immediate aftermaths of disasters that render the technocratic model of birth both unsustainable and ineffective at providing optimal maternal and perinatal care. Many assume that maternity care in disaster settings requires high-tech equipment. Yet as Lim asks above, when the normative spaces usually assigned to birth, such as clinics or hospitals, lie in ruins or are in danger of collapse, how might we create safe and sustainable models of birthing care? When the clock on the wall that indicated time for another cervical check lies shattered and the electricity for monitoring mother and fetus is down, what tools will sustain us? When epidemics and pandemics add to the preexisting risks of hospitals as sites of contagion, where indeed should the mothers give birth?

The accounts presented in this chapter will demonstrate that what is most needed for sustainable care in disaster settings are dedicated and skilled midwives, low-tech equipment, referral to sites with emergency obstetric care or on-site obstetricians, and courageous flexibility of all involved–including administrators, providers, mothers, and their families. We will illustrate how a midwifery model of care that is both "low-tech" and "high-touch" and is based on the 12 Steps of the *International Childbirth Initiative* (ICI) (Lalonde et al. 2019) can provide nimble and high-quality care for MotherBaby dyads and their communities in times of enormous upheaval and destruction and can produce maternal and perinatal outcomes that match or even improve upon nationwide statistics collected in the absence of disasters and other climate-related shocks. And, as a result of the 2020 global COVID-19 pandemic, we must also ask, what spaces for care and which practitioners will best serve mothers and babies and avoid ongoing disease transmission?

Herein we will focus on the highly sustainable disaster zone maternity care provided by Bumi Sehat under the direction of Robin Lim in Indonesia and the Philippines (see Lim and Leggett 2021; Lim and Davis-Floyd 2021), by Mercy In Action in the Philippines as directed by Vicki Penwell (2020), and in Japan as described by Tsipy Ivry and colleagues (Ivry et al. 2019). While Lim's and Penwell's accounts focus on the experiences of the providers, Ivry's account from Japan offers first-hand descriptions of how mothers successfully delivered their babies in extreme conditions with the help of midwives and nurses. Davis-Floyd describes some of the rapid changes in global maternity care as a result of the coronavirus pandemic and their effects on both practitioners and childbearers. Thus, our chapter seeks to understand optimal maternity care in disaster settings from the perspectives of both providers and mothers.

18.1.1 Obstetric Disaster Responses: A Brief Note

A team of international relief doctors deployed by the Israeli Defense Forces reported that they saw 44 pregnant and 24 nonpregnant patients as early responders covering the earthquake disasters in Haiti in 2010 and Japan in 2011. They handled 16 births, 3 by cesarean section. One-half of the births were complicated by preeclampsia, and 31% were preterm (30 to 32 weeks gestation), leading them to believe that obstetrical specialists plus technological equipment, including fetal heart monitors, gynecologic chairs (birth tables), and an ample supply of blood for transfusions were necessary in order to effectively attend births in disaster zones (Pinkert et al. 2013). Yet the accounts presented in this chapter will demonstrate otherwise. Collectively, we will show that what is really needed in disaster birth care is dedicated and skilled midwives–both traditional and professional, low-tech equipment, courageous mothers and families, some available obstetricians, and flexibility on the part of all involved.

18.1.2 The International Childbirth Initiative as a Template for Optimal Care

The basic elements of maternity care that are required in disaster or any other settings are laid out in the *International Childbirth Initiative* (ICI)*: 12 Steps to Safe and Respectful MotherBaby Family Maternity Care* (Lalonde et al. 2019; see also www.internationalchildbirth.com and the Appendix to this book). The two nongovernmental organizations (NGOs) we focus on here–Bumi Sehat and Mercy in Action–have created flexible, adaptive models of maternity care that implement all 12 Steps of the ICI and exemplify the MotherBaby-Family Model of Care chartered in the ICI. As their statistics show, this model of care is cost-effective,

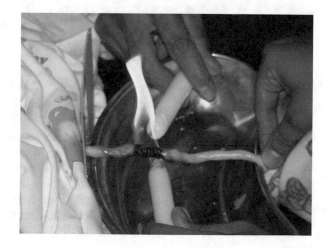

Fig. 18.1 A Bumi Sehat midwife and an Acehnese traditional midwife burn a baby's umbilical cord to prevent tetanus in the absence of other sterile tools in a disaster setting, 2004. Published with kind permission of © The Bumi Sehat Foundation. All Rights Reserved

life-saving, and sustainable, even in the context of utter devastation. In this era of the climate crisis and the global COVID-19 pandemic, where destruction, damage, and tragedy will only increase, birth can and should be gentle, respectful, and holistic. When disaster and tragedy strike, our Birthkeepers must be ready (see Fig. 18.1).

18.2   Bumi Sehat's Disaster Relief Efforts as Recounted by Founder Ibu Robin Lim

Yayasan Bumi Sehat (http://bumisehat.org/) was founded in 1995 in Bali, Indonesia. "Yayasan" means not-for-profit, "bumi" means "earth-mother," and "sehat" translates as "healthy," so our name translates to Healthy Mother Earth Foundation. We operate four Community Health and Education and Childbirth Centers within Indonesia (in Bali, Aceh, Lombok, and Papua) and two childbirth centers in the Philippines (Leyte and Palawan). Additionally, we helped organize and operate post-disaster birth units in Jacmel, Haiti; Dhading, Nepal; and Palu, Sulawesi. At our clinics, we offer a comprehensive range of allopathic and holistic medicine, as well as pre- and postnatal care, breastfeeding support, infant, child and family health services, nutritional education, prenatal yoga, childbirth education, and safe, gentle loving natural birth services. Funding for Bumi Sehat's work comes from many generous donors including Direct Relief International, Earth Company, WADAH Foundation, Every Mother Counts, Dining for Women, IDEP Foundation, Kopernik, We Care Solar, Rotary Clubs International, and the anonymous generosity of friends.

After providing disaster relief in Aceh, Sumatra, Indonesia, we became early responders after the earthquakes that wreaked havoc in Yogyakarta, Padang, Lombok, Sumatra, Haiti, and Nepal, during the 2017–2018 eruption phase of Mount Agung in Bali and following the super typhoon Haiyan/Yolanda in the Philippines. We still support one of the birth centers there, which is run by Filipino midwives. Bumi Sehat Foundation International and Bumi Wadah Foundation (a partnership between Bumi Sehat and the Wadah Foundation–an Indonesian charity) have taken teams of practitioners into the lowest-resource, highest-risk settings possible. Upon arrival in each disaster area, we liaison and work with surviving medical professionals and traditional/cultural healers in the devastated communities; this collaboration greatly facilitates the recovery process.

Based in Bali yet highly mobile during disasters, we distribute food, tools, shelter tarps, solar lanterns, and precious water filters. We treat illnesses and wounds, both physical and psychological. We carry water in buckets. And we receive babies in tents, by the light of solar lanterns and with rudimentary supplies. Our outcomes in all these settings were and remain far better than the national statistics for these countries. In most of these sites where possible, Bumi Sehat has stayed on following its disaster relief, because we work without an explicit exit strategy; instead, we build sustainable healthcare in cooperation with local midwives or medical staff until they can take over the clinics we establish.

18.2.1   The Aceh Tsunami 2004

Bumi Sehat's abrupt initiation into disaster relief began with the tremendous tsunami and earthquake (measuring 9.3 on the Richter scale) that hit Aceh, Sumatra, in Indonesia on December 26, 2004. The official death toll was estimated at over 200,000, although the military admitted it may have buried as many as 400,000 victims. Within days of the earthquake, Bumi Sehat collaborated with the Wadah Foundation to provide volunteer midwives, nurses, doulas, emergency responders, and doctors of allopathic medicine, naturopathy, and Chinese medicine, into a very lowest-resource but highest-risk setting. Upon arrival in Aceh, as elsewhere, Bumi Sehat first liaisoned with the surviving medical professionals and traditional/cultural healers to see what was most needed by the devastated communities. Over the next 3 years, Bumi Sehat helped over 1000 mothers give birth, with basic traveling birth kits, no fetal monitors, gynecologic chairs, or whole blood supplies. We originally camped close to the heart of the disaster, where almost 100% of the population was homeless, with no electricity, little food, and not enough drinking water. According to our estimates, most Acehnese survivors had lost an average of 12 relatives.

To forge liaisons with local Acehnese midwives, we called a meeting of Birthkeepers, including both professionally trained midwives (*dukun bayi*) and traditional midwives (*bidan kampong*), as the latter are often the most trusted in disaster settings. Thirty-two midwives showed up; all had experienced severe loss of family and property. One midwife had walked an entire day to attend; another midwife–who was 7 months pregnant–had walked through fallen trees and mud flats after losing her husband, two children, parents, and home. Although everyone had experienced deep trauma themselves, all were there to support mothers in childbirth in this tragic time. Each midwife received mother-baby kits for their estimated number of surviving clients, as well as supplies of high-energy bars, water filters, and midwifery equipment. Our day-long seminar knit the women closer to each other and ended in a moment of silence for those who had not survived the quake/tsunami. We later learned that while the Meulaboh area had 156 midwives before the tsunami, the 32 midwives who attended were the only surviving midwives in the region.

Over the next days, weeks, and months, we found that many women could manage to safely birth with little risk, even in the absence of clinics, hospitals, obstetricians, and extensive medical technology or equipment. We learned that midwives, nurses, and doulas were critical, even as obstetricians and other physicians were lacking. Those obstetricians/gynecologists who did join our team worked closely with the midwives, providing a natural, simple model of supportive and respectful care for mothers in labor, delivery, and postpartum. We found that sound midwifery skills, essential medicines, and simple tools plus a transport vehicle for emergency complications when possible constituted the most effective and sustainable model of maternity care in disaster settings. In the case of complications that required a cesarean section or blood transfusion, transport to clinics or sites in more densely populated areas made more sense than trying to keep obstetricians on hand in widely dispersed rural areas. Home visits to the shacks or tents where survivors lived offered important support to breastfeeding mothers.

Our outcomes were surprising to others in the Indonesian healthcare system, who had underappreciated how effective a midwifery model of care can be. Out of 1000 births that were attended and followed by the Bumi Sehat Aceh midwives after the tsunami, there were 14 intrapartum and neonatal deaths:

- Four stillbirths, including an intrapartum death at the clinic, an intrapartum death at home, and two stillbirths after transport for fetal distress.
- Six neonatal deaths after preterm delivery of babies between 20 and 32 weeks gestation and birth weights between 500–800 grams.
- Two deaths due to congenital abnormalities.
- One intrapartum death due to shoulder dystocia.
- One early newborn death at one week to a mother suffering from "smallpox".

Not counting the 4 stillbirths, the 10 neonatal deaths among the 1000 births were better outcomes than Indonesia's nationwide neonatal mortality rate of 14/1000 in 2017 (UNICEF 2017). There were no maternal deaths during the 3 years that we attended over 1000 births in Aceh.

The traditional midwives–*bidan kampong*–within the catchment area of over 11 villages that were close to epicenter of the disaster organized and worked closely with Bumi Sehat. The *bidan kampong* have lifelong skills that they have learned from apprenticeship as well as from their own experiences of supporting mothers during childbirth, but no professional medical training. Each *bidan kampong* was given a hand phone and a paid phone plan from Bumi Sehat, as well as hand crank chargers and electric chargers, as much of Aceh province had no electricity for up to 4 years following the tsunami, and even now electricity is not always dependable. Training the *bidan kampong* how to use a phone took time, but the Bumi Sehat team was determined to help these community leaders have a means to communicate with health centers and each other. Furthermore, we conducted monthly trainings for these elderly Keepers of Birth, as the *bidan kampong* are known within the community.

Once they had cellphones and knew how to use them, the *bidan kampong* could and would call the professionally trained midwives of Bumi Sehat to attend births with them when mothers preferred home births. The *bidan kampong* also bring their clients to the Bumi Sehat Aceh clinic for prenatal care and delivery, where they attend their laboring clients side-by-side with the professional midwives. This system of collaboration helps build the skills of the *bidan kampong*, while also fostering trust in and increasing awareness of the quality of Bumi Sehat's maternity care. The resulting partnerships help us stay connected to the community, earn the trust of the families we serve, and foster long-term growth and sustainability. Fifteen years after the 2004 tsunami, the Bumi Sehat Aceh Community Health and Childbirth Clinic, which we built with grant-funding, continues to sustainably thrive. We at Bumi Sehat feel that it is critical to enter a disaster area without planning an exit strategy because trust in care and continuity of care are critical for devastated communities.

18.2.2   Volcanic Eruptions in Bali 2017–2018

Between 2017 and 2018, Bali's volcano Gunung Agung erupted multiple times, causing more than 140,000 people to be evacuated from their homes. Bumi Sehat's medical team was responsible for bringing healthcare and supplies to the displaced people (*pengungsi*) in the evacuation camps. The government had planned to evacuate pregnant women among the *pengungsi* who were near full-term to tents in a parking lot outside a government hospital, where these women were supposed to wait alone until their babies were born. This isolation went completely against Balinese culture, where no one, especially a pregnant woman, wishes to be separated from their families. So we arranged for the expectant mothers plus their immediate families to be housed at the Bumi Sehat clinic.

We provided all services including a kitchen for the displaced, and truckloads of vegetables were donated twice weekly by the Ubud community. After we had attended births for 7 weeks, the families were permitted to return home, but 3 weeks later when the volcano erupted again more violently and lava and lahar (destructive mud flow) filled the rivers, the evacuees returned to Bumi Sehat for another 13 weeks. By December of 2019, the volcano had quieted, and the evacuees had returned home, but the volcano is still off-gassing and disaster could strike again.

18.2.3   Disasters on Lombok and Sulawesi 2018

In 2018, Bali's nearest neighbor island, Lombok, suffered a devastating earthquake. Aftershocks and landslides continued to plague the survivors living in makeshift shelters for months, and more violent earthquakes are expected. Across Lombok, many government health centers (*Puskesmas*) were destroyed, and the main hospital in Mataram was so damaged that all patients had to be evacuated to the parking lot, where they were exposed to blistering sun and torrential rains. Bumi Sehat, led by a professional midwife and Lombok native, provided medical relief in tents; there are plans to build a permanent clinic and childbirth center in Lombok with funding from Direct Relief International. Also in 2018, Bumi Sehat responded to the widespread destruction by earthquake, tsunami, flooding, landslides, and liquefaction on the island of Sulawesi. In 2018 alone, Bumi Sehat's relief efforts reached 52,121 homeless patients in the aftermath of these disasters. Violent flooding in Papua in March of 2019 led evacuees to flee to the Angel Hiromi-Bumi Sehat Childbirth Clinic in Sentani after their homes were destroyed. When violence broke out across the nearby region of Wamena later that year in August and September, 30 families fled the violence and sheltered at the clinic in Sentani. The increasing rate of natural disasters in Indonesia has only intensified Bumi Sehat's efforts to tend to communities and families across the region.

18.3 Mercy In Action's Disaster Relief Efforts as Recounted by Founder Vicki Penwell

Mercy In Action (www.mercyinaction.com) was established in 1991 to build birth centers for impoverished families across the Philippines. By 2019, Mercy In Action staff had attended 15,000 births, while tens of thousands of lives have been helped and healed in medical outreaches. At present, Mercy In Action still runs several birth centers and outreach clinics across the Philippines, while many others that it founded have been turned over to local Filipino professional midwives who continue to sustainably practice our model of care, which is based on the ICI. All medical services are provided at no cost, and funding comes from private donors, grants, and the Philippines health insurance system for qualifying individuals.

18.3.1 Mercy in Action's Disaster Response after Hurricane Haiyan/Yolanda

Super typhoon Haiyan (locally called Yolanda) was the largest storm to ever make landfall in human history, on November 8, 2013. Although our medical staff in the Philippines had lived through and learned from many smaller disasters in the past 25 years, we were struck by the force of this storm, which gave us ample opportunity to put into practice the Disaster Preparedness course we had painstakingly prepared for our midwives.

Within a few days after the hurricane had passed, we loaded up our ambulance, arrived at Ground Zero of the disaster, set up canvas birthing tents, and began to provide free medical care (see Fig. 18.2). Over the next 65 days, we treated 3616 patients, despite having limited food, no running water, no electricity, with area clinics damaged or destroyed, and most of our patients homeless and traumatized.

When we had patients with complications that needed cesareans we could not provide, we transported them to tent hospitals staffed by our partners Doctors Without Borders. We also partnered with UNICEF to create a Mother/Child-Friendly Space for breastfeeding and other services. These were our statistical outcomes:

- Total primary health and wound care: 1532.
- Total deliveries: 116.
- Cesarean section rate: 2%.
- Stillbirths: 1.
- Neonatal deaths: 1 (tetanus at 8 days).
- Maternal mortalities: 0.
- Total breastfeeding women: 648.

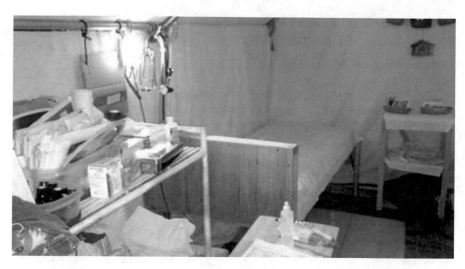

Fig. 18.2 Mercy In Action's small but clean and well-stocked birth tent at Ground Zero. Mercy In Action public domain staff photo collection, 2014. Published with kind permission of © Mercy in Action. All Rights Reserved

- Rate of breastfeeding by mothers when we left: 100%.
- Total women given prenatal care and food: 367.
- Total survivors who attended our healing trauma seminars: 196.

In the months after the typhoon, we raised donations and grants to completely rebuild and restock two clinics/birthing centers in the disaster area and conducted 40 hours of capacity-building training for local midwives. We equipped all midwives who graduated from that training with basic birth kits and emergency equipment so that they could continue to serve as community midwives. The continuity of care by trusted local professional midwives has been critical for women and their families after such traumatic loss and destruction of family and kin networks. Mercy in Action remains involved with rebuilding efforts in 2020, including midwifery training and ongoing partnership with a local midwife and the rebuilt Cumpio clinic. The Center for Disaster Philanthropy provided donations to rebuild the Cumpio birth center, while GlobalGiving was a valuable partner during the typhoon rebuilding stage and for subsequent disasters, including the 2019 earthquake in the Philippines. In addition, Mercy In Action's nonprofit board members were incredibly generous with general funds during the typhoon disaster and now keep a savings account ready for future disaster responses.

18.4   The Great Japanese Earthquake of March 11, 2011: Mothers' Perspectives as Recounted by Tsipy Ivry and Robbie Davis-Floyd

It is a pity that we've lost practicing independent midwives who could deliver babies close to home. We wouldn't have been in such trouble if there had been enough midwives in the community. –Japanese midwife as quoted by Etsuko Matsuoka (2019)

Ivry et al.'s (2019) description of births outside a badly shaken hospital in the aftermath of the March 11, 2011 earthquake in Japan shows the power of women. These authors describe how, with the elevators inoperable, mothers protectively cradling their newborn babies, as well as those who were in all stages of labor, including the pushing stage, were able to descend several flights of stairs and walk into the hospital parking lot, where they delivered their babies in cars or on furniture dragged by staff from the hospital. (Fortunately, none of them had epidurals, which Japanese women choose far less often than women in other high resource countries (Williamson and Matsuoka 2018)). Midwives and nurses were able to provide effective care in that parking lot with only the most minimal equipment that was grabbed hastily on the way out–or that they bravely ran back for.

For example, when the shaking ceased, one of the pregnant women took advantage of the intervals between contractions to walk down the stairs, pressing her contracting belly and resting during the contractions. She was told to take refuge in the parking lot, though it was about to start snowing. The nurses grabbed a sofa from the hospital waiting room and laid her down on it, wrapped in thick blankets, but, given that she was wearing a thin hospital gown, the blankets were not enough. So her husband brought their car, and folded the rear seat down. She did lie down there for a bit but soon was up and walking at the height of the contractions. She said that she believed the walking helped to push her baby down. When he was about to be born, she got back into the car, thinking "Let's get him out!" The car was crowded with the doctor, nurse, and midwife, who had all climbed in to catch the baby. With powerful aftershocks going on, the nurses ran in and out of the hospital building, finding and bringing necessary items "such as water and bath towels and other things" (Namikawa and Kawaguchi 2012: 88–89, cited in Ivry et al. 2019: 174).

In their analysis of this story, Ivry et al. (2019: 179) note that this woman acknowledged her own perseverance in the face of danger, "yet attributed the safe conclusion of her birth to the nurses' and midwives' efforts to secure a closed, safe and private place for the birth and low-tech necessities rather than high-tech interventions." These authors point out the evidence-based nature of her certainty that walking during the contractions accelerated her birthing process–which is in line with the evidence about the benefits of mobility during labor (Lawrence et al. 2013).

A common thread among the narratives of these Japanese birthing mothers was these women saying to themselves, "Let's get this baby out quickly!" They acknowledged the roles played by their own strong wills, which enabled them to birth safely in spite of the disruption of the technological surveillance they had previously thought necessary. Yet they also emphasized that they were able to give birth under such extreme circumstances in large part due to the calm and flexible support provided by their providers, mostly nurses and midwives. In other words, as Ivry et al. (2019: 179) state, "the midwifery model of care provided an example of fluid adaptation to mothers' needs within an urgent and unpredictable situation."

Tellingly, after the earthquake, the Japanese Nursing Association (JNA) produced a formal recommendation that "all birth professionals providing care in any setting learn how to attend 'freestyle' childbirth" (quoted in Ivry et al. 2019: 181)–just as the Bumi Sehat and Mercy in Action midwives do. The JNA statement (2013) echoed one made in 2006 by the White Ribbon Alliance for Safe Motherhood in the aftermath of Hurricane Katrina, which recognized the critical importance of "homebirth skills" in times of disaster, when hospitals may be unavailable, inaccessible, or overwhelmed with casualties. Had this statement been acted upon at the time, it is likely that the United States would have been better prepared for the maternity care challenges presented in 2020 by the COVID-19 pandemic.

18.5   Global Impacts of COVID-19 on Maternity Care

In 2020, the rapid spread of the novel coronavirus SARS-CoV-2 and the disease it produces, COVID-19, caused a large increase in demand for midwife-attended homebirths and births in freestanding birth centers across high-income countries (HIC). This demand was due in part to families' fears of contagion in hospitals and in other part to hospitals' sudden refusals to admit partners or doulas into birthing rooms or to force the laboring woman to choose only one support person, who might have to leave immediately after the birth (Davis-Floyd et al. 2020). During this pandemic, many hospitals in HIC were often overwhelmed, while home birth midwives and freestanding birth centers were also overwhelmed by childbearers' requests for transfers from hospital-based care. Unfortunately, in the United States and in European countries where the numbers of midwives who attend out of hospital births are few, there were not enough community midwives to cover the demand. As a result, many women who sought out-of-hospital births were turned away. Thousands of hospital practitioners faced shortages of personal protective equipment (PPE) for weeks or even months, while many providers and patients contracted COVID-19. Some families resorted to unattended "freebirths," for which outcomes are difficult to track (Davis-Floyd, Gutschow, and Schwartz 2020). And no statistics for mortality and morbidity in that time period are available as of yet. Clearly, much new research is needed on the global impacts of COVID-19 on maternity care and will soon be forthcoming (Davis-Floyd and Gutschow 2021).

18.6   Conclusion: Lessons Learned from Disaster Zone Maternity Care

Ironically, disasters provide valuable opportunities to examine what happens when high technologies cannot be used during labor and birth (Fortun and Frickel 2012; Hofman 2005). Maternity care in the aftermath of natural disasters that ends with healthy mothers and babies stands in stark contrast to the iatrogenic outcomes of the technocratic model of birth, in which births are seen as potential disasters-in-the making, and interventions that cause harm are routinely employed. *In the face of natural disaster, childbirth risk emerges as secondary, and the lack of need for high-tech intervention in most births is revealed* (Ivry et al. 2019: 181). In short, disasters, including pandemics, provide a mirror through which to see birth anew and reevaluate the shrill narrative of risk promoted by the technocratic model (Ivry et al. 2019: 165, 180).

As Lim shows, collaborations and partnerships between traditional and professional midwives work to generate an emergent "human resources model" that "promotes a non-bureaucratic system of flexible emergency response" (Monteblanco and Leyser-Whalen 2019:146). This model of flexible response can highlight the need for adapting maternity care to be less institutionalized and lower tech, both during and after disasters. These authors continue:

> This model rejects the argument that disasters cause human panic, instead encouraging and challenging scholars and practitioners to view local community members (trained healthcare providers or not) as emergency response resources. . . In [so doing], the emergent human resources model also indicates the necessity for identifying and using non-mainstream and non-institutionalized medical care providers during and post-disasters.

How can we apply the insights from sustainable disaster care provided in this chapter to revolutionize maternity care in non-disaster settings? Can low-tech, high-quality disaster care proceed to unsettle the seeming inevitability of the technocratic management of childbirth? How might analysis of both providers' and women's experiences of childbirth in disaster settings contribute to more sustainable model of birth?

More research is needed on the impact of using evidence-based midwifery care in disaster zones and the outcomes produced by midwifery care. Yet already, these accounts of birth experiences in disaster settings help us recognize the value of skilled community midwives who are more flexible and mobile, less tied to hospital or clinic settings, and less reliant on technology than obstetricians and facility-based midwives (Monteblanco and Leyser-Whalen 2019). And their value also extends to local epidemics and global pandemics like the one caused by the coronavirus.

Ultimately, several clear lessons emerge from our study of maternity care in disaster zones:

- Birthing women can be resilient and powerful. Their greatest need is for emotional and physical support from their caregivers and families.

- Skilled community midwives and facility-based midwives collaborating with one another provide invaluable resources in disaster and pandemic settings as well as in all settings during times of normalcy.
- Sustainable midwifery care that is decentralized and locally available is the most appropriate care in disaster settings, during epidemics or pandemics, and in low resource settings, especially when midwives have basic birth kits, cellphones, and the possibility of transport to referral units.
- Obstetricians should be reserved for complicated births, in both disaster zones and in normal circumstances, and they should be concentrated in cities as well as in referral units where women and newborns experiencing complications can be transported.
- Maternity care providers in disaster zones should not enter with an exit strategy but rather with strategies for building trust and providing long-term models of care that continue after the disaster ends.
- Breastfeeding and non-separation of the mother/baby dyad are essential, as are providing potable food and water for breastfeeding mothers; infant formula should be avoided due to contamination risks.
- Maternity care should be decentralized, everywhere.
- All birthing facilities should fully implement the 12 Steps of the *International Childbirth Initiative* (ICI), which work under all circumstances to improve quality of care and support normal physiologic birth.

Given our ongoing climate crisis, which contributes to global and regional pandemics like COVID-19 and vector-borne illnesses such as dengue, chikungunya, and Zika virus, as well as to natural and human-made disasters and conflicts, the rate of internal and external migrations will inevitably increase and birth care will need to adapt. All these processes will require ongoing, decentralizing shifts in maternity care. We stress that *decentralizing birth care in favor of localized systems of support for normal physiologic birth will better prepare low-and-middle-income countries (LMIC) and high-resource nations alike for effective disaster and pandemic responses.* Large tertiary care facilities are:

- Extremely costly and thus often economically unsustainable, especially in LMIC.
- In LMIC, plagued by lack of essential supplies and poor quality of care, in part due to their economic unsustainability,
- Highly vulnerable to earthquake, superstorm, and epidemic-caused damage. Hospitals are especially dangerous places to be during large-scale epidemics, due to the large numbers and proximity of staff, patients, and visitors, all of whom can acquire and/or transmit infections. Even in high-resource nations, as the coronavirus pandemic has revealed, hospitals may lack essential supplies such as personal protective equipment (PPE) and thereby become even more unsafe as sites of contagion (Davis-Floyd et al. 2020).
- Sometimes completely unavailable. For example, thousands of women across Latin America have to go while in labor to multiple hospitals trying to find one that will accept them–a terrible situation occurring so frequently that it has been given a name, "peregrination" (Menezes et al. 2006), and was exacerbated during

the 2020 COVID-19 pandemic. Many women, especially in Venezuela, ended up giving birth alone on a sidewalk, sometimes with disastrous results (Turkewitz and Herrera 2020).

Using the human resources model, *the push for facility-based birth across LMIC should be turned around 180 degrees and transformed into a push for the support and empowerment of local community midwives, homebirths, and births in smaller clinics or first-referral units* rather than tertiary care centers. In smaller birth facilities staffed primarily by midwives, or at home (or in tents), there is less risk of infection and the midwifery model of care can prevail, resulting in vast improvements in the quality of maternity care in general (Johnson and Daviss 2005; Cheyney et al. 2014; Alliman et al. 2019) and enormous cost savings. For instance, Anderson et al. (2021) showed that the United States would save $9.1 billion each year if only 10% more US births took place in homes and freestanding birth centers. Professional midwives should be allowed and encouraged to practice autonomously in varied settings; and instead of being phased out, traditional midwives, wherever they still exist, should be fully incorporated into their country's maternity care system and supported to continue their community-based care.

We must reiterate that, as Davis-Floyd et al. (2009) clearly demonstrate, *women everywhere want care in their communities*! Community-based care systems are more flexible and adaptable to the upheaval caused by disasters, more likely to be able to provide high-quality care, more economically sustainable, and also more adaptable to women's actual needs–which most often do not include technological surveillance and intervention but do include skilled, low-tech care and hands-on physical and emotional support. We conclude by also reiterating that in all birthing models, the Principles and 12 Steps of the *International Childbirth Initiative* should be used as the template for best practice, as their woman-centered, low-tech approach can be fully implemented in any birth setting, even in the aftermath of devastating disasters. Pregnant women should be fully educated about birth and, when possible, offered the full range of birthing options–which midwives, working collaboratively with obstetricians in cases where they are truly needed, can provide, both under normal circumstances and in the face of multiple types of disasters.

Acknowledgments Robbie Davis-Floyd sincerely thanks her co-editor Kim Gutschow for her careful and helpful edits and improvements to this chapter. She also thanks Springer editor Janet Kim and Series Editor David Schwartz for the encouragement and TLC they have consistently provided during the process of creating this volume.

References

Alliman J, Stapleton SR, Wright J, Bauer K, Slider K, Jolles D (2019) Strong start in birth centers: socio-demographic characteristics, care processes, and outcomes for mothers and newborns. Birth 46(2):234–243

Anderson DA, Daviss BA, Johnson KC (2021) What if another 10% of deliveries in the United States occurred at home or in a birth center? Safety, economics and politics. In: Daviss BA, Davis-Floyd R (eds) Birthing models on the human rights frontier: speaking truth to power. Routledge, London

Cheyney M, Bovbjerg M, Everson C et al (2014) Outcomes of care for 16,984 planned homebirths in the United States: The Midwives Alliance of North America Statistics Project, 2004-2009. J Midwifery Womens Health 59(1):17–27

Davis-Floyd R (2001) The technocratic, humanistic, and holistic paradigms of childbirth. Int J Gynecol Obstet 75(S1):5–23

Davis-Floyd R (2003) Birth as an American rite of passage, 2nd edn. University of California Press, Berkeley

Davis-Floyd R, Barclay L, Daviss BA et al (eds) (2009) Birth models that work. University of California Press, Berkeley

Davis-Floyd R, Gutschow K, Schwartz D (2020) Pregnancy, birth, and the COVID-19 pandemic in the United States. Med Anthropol. https://doi.org/10.1080/01459740.2020.1761804

Davis-Floyd R, Gutschow K eds. (2021) The Global Impacts of COVID-19 on Maternity Care Practices and Childbearing Experiences, a Special Issue of Frontiers in Sociology, in press.

Fortun K, Frickel S (2012) Making a case for disaster science and technology studies. An STS Forum on the East Japan Disaster. https://fukushimaforum.wordpress.com/onlineforum-2/online-forum/making-a-case-for-disaster-science-and-technology-studies/

Hoffman SM (2005) Katrina and Rita: a disaster anthropologists' thoughts. Anthropol News 46:19

Ivry T, Takaki-Einy R, Murotsuki J (2019) What disasters can reveal about techno-medical birth: Japanese women's stories of childbirth during the 11 March, 2011 earthquake. Health Risk Soc 21(3–4):164–184. https://www.tandfonline.com/doi/full/10.1080/13698575.2019.1643827

Japanese Nursing Association (JNA) (2013) Bunben shisetsu ni okeru saigai hasseiji no taiou manyuaru sakusei gaido [A guide for the creation of a response manual in maternity facilities at times of disaster]. Medica Shuppan, Osaka

Johnson KC, Daviss BA (2005) Outcomes of planned homebirths with certified professional midwives: large prospective study in North America. Br Med J 330:1416

Lalonde A, Herschderfer K, Pascali-Bonaro D et al (2019) The international childbirth initiative: 12 steps to safe and respectful motherbaby-family maternity care. Int J Gynecol Obstet 146:65–73

Lawrence A, Lewis L, Hofmeyr GJ, Styles C (2013) Maternal positions and mobility during first stage labour. Cochrane Database Syst Rev 8

Lim IR, Davis-Floyd R (2021) Implementing the international childbirth initiative (ICI) in disaster zones: Bumi Sehat's experiences in Indonesia, Haiti, the Philippines, and Nepal. In: Daviss BA, Davis-Floyd R (eds) Birthing models on the human rights frontier: speaking truth to power. Routledge, London

Lim IR, Leggett S (2021) Bumi Sehat Bali: birth on the checkered cloth. In: Daviss BA, Davis-Floyd R (eds) Birthing models on the human rights frontier: speaking truth to power. Routledge, New York/London. in press

Matsuoka E (2019) Japanese independent midwives and the 3/11/11/ Great East Japan Earthquake: an update on chapter 8 of Birth models that work, Maternity homes in Japan: reservoirs of normal childbirth. Available at www.understandingbirthbetter.com

Menezes DC, Leite IC, al SJM (2006) Evaluation of antenatal peregrination in a sample of postpartum women in Rio de Janeiro, Brazil, 1999-2001. Cad Saude Publica 22(3):553–559

Monteblanco AD, Leyser-Whalen O (2019) Thinking outside of the hospital and nurse-midwife paradigm: a qualitative examination of midwifery in times of natural disasters. Int J Mass Emerg Disasters 37(2):138–173

Namikawa S, Kobayashi K (2012) Happy birthday 3.11: Ano hi shinsaichi de umareta kodomotachi to kazoku no monogatari [happy birthday 3.11: the stories of the children who were born on that day and their families]. Asukashinsa, Tokyo

Penwell V (2020) A birth model for disaster care in the Philippines. An update on chapter 12 of Birth models that work, Mercy In Action: bringing mother- and baby-friendly birth centers to the Philippines. www.understandingbirthbetter.com

Pinkert M, Dar S, Goldberg D et al (2013) Lessons learned from an obstetrics and gynecology field hospital response to natural disasters. J Obstetr Gynecol 122(3):532–536

Turkewitz J, Herrera I (2020) Childbirth in Venezuela, where women's deaths are a state secret New York Times, April 10. https://www.nytimes.com/2020/04/10/world/americas/venezuela-pregnancy-birth-death.html

UNICEF (2017) Levels and trends in child mortality, report 2017. Estimates developed by the United Nations inter-agency group for child mortality estimates. UNICEF, New York

White Ribbon Alliance National Working Group for Women and Infant Needs in Emergencies (2006) Women and Infants Service Package, December

Williamson KE, Matsuoka E (2018) Comparing childbirth in Brazil and Japan: social hierarchies, cultural values, and the meaning of place. In: Davis-Floyd R, Cheyney M (eds) Birth in eight cultures. Waveland Press, Long Grove, pp 89–128

Chapter 19
Sustainable Newborn Care: Helping Babies Breathe and Essential Newborn Care

Chiamaka Aneji and George Little

19.1 Introduction

Adverse birth outcomes are some of the biggest drains on global human capital, especially in low resource settings (Lawn et al. 2014). The neonate (the first 28 days of life) faces unique challenges. In 2018, the 2.5 million neonatal deaths across the globe represented 47% of global under-5 year-deaths. One-third of all neonates who died did so on their day of birth (UNICEF 2019). Importantly, a majority of neonatal deaths have preventable causes (Liu et al. 2016; Akseer et al. 2015). This chapter will review the origin of Helping Babies Breathe (HBB)[a] a revolutionary, successful newborn resuscitation program that has expanded into the Helping Babies Survive (HBS)[a] suite of programs. There is strong evidence that low cost, low-technology interventions like neonatal resuscitation (NR), kangaroo mother care (KMC) for thermal stability, and proper hand washing, can produce significant reductions in neonatal mortality (Bhutta et al. 2014). For sustainable progress in the global fight against neonatal morbidity and mortality, the focus has to be on systematic scaling up of such interventions in the hardest hit areas of the world. We draw your attention to the following observations.

C. Aneji (✉)
Department of Pediatrics, McGovern Medical School at the University of Texas Health Science Center at Houston, Houston, TX, USA
e-mail: Chiamaka.aneji@uth.tmc.edu

G. Little
Pediatrics and Obstetrics and Gynecology, Geisel School of Medicine at Dartmouth, Hanover, NH, USA
e-mail: George.A.Little@dartmouth.edu

© Springer Nature Switzerland AG 2021
K. Gutschow et al. (eds.), *Sustainable Birth in Disruptive Times*, Global Maternal and Child Health, https://doi.org/10.1007/978-3-030-54775-2_19

19.2   Neonatal Resuscitation at Birth and Subsequent Stabilization

The day of birth is the most dangerous for mothers and their babies, resulting in nearly half of maternal and neonatal deaths and stillbirths (Lawn et al. 2009; Mason et al. 2014). Transition from fetal to extrauterine neonatal life is the most complex human adaptation that occurs, involving a series of well-orchestrated changes. All human body systems are involved at some level in this process. Maternal conditions can affect the success of transition (Swanson and Sinkin 2015). The most essential neonatal birth adaptation is breathing (Hillman et al. 2012).

Birth complications can result in adverse neonatal outcomes. Most neonates transition without help and initiate spontaneous breathing at birth, but up to 10% require varying degrees of assistance to initiate breathing. Three to 6% positive pressure ventilation (PPV) is required for apnea (absence of breathing) or poor respiration after stimulation and suctioning have been done. Less than 1% of newborns require highly complex resuscitation including endotracheal intubation, chest compressions, and medications (Kattwinkel et al. 2010).

In 2018, there were 2.5 million neonatal deaths and 2.6 million stillbirths (Healthy Neonatal Network 2020). Intrapartum-related events are the second leading cause of neonatal morbidity and mortality, accounting for almost one-quarter of newborn deaths (Berkelhamer et al. 2016). They can lead to long-term consequences such as cerebral palsy, epilepsy, and learning disabilities (Kattwinkel et al. 2010; Ahearne et al. 2016; Lee et al. 2013). Stillbirth data are limited in low resource settings. We know that many stillbirths that occur in late labor and delivery are related to hypoxia. These babies may be in the process of dying and might respond if timely resuscitative efforts were implemented by skilled providers who correctly recognize the situation (Nelson et al. 2011).

19.2.1   Neonatal Resuscitation Program (NRP)®

Neonatal resuscitation and stabilization are evidence-based interventions that have seen significant advancement and implementation. First developed in 1987 by the American Academy of Pediatrics (AAP), NRP recommendations originally were based predominantly on expert opinions. Now in its 7th edition, NRP is a global standard of care for NR (Guiding the Way Forward 2017), with millions of health workers trained and courses taught in more than 130 countries and over 24 languages (NRP 2017). It is important to note that comprehensive NRP is intended for advanced, appropriately equipped facilities staffed with skilled providers and an array of technologies including monitoring and endotracheal intubation.

Every five years, the International Liaison Committee on Resuscitation (ILCOR), first organized in the 1980s, develops and publishes a consensus on resuscitation science based on the best available evidence. This commitment is necessary for systematic and ongoing development of knowledge and quality improvement that are the core of sustainable care (AAP 2017a, b). Despite the professional acceptance of NRP, it became clear that a gap existed between the available resuscitation programs and needs in regions with the highest neonatal mortality. Experts expressed a strong opinion that NRP, while effective in resourced environments, was perceived widely to be too complex, expensive, and not realistic for large, low-resource populations (Little et al. 2014). Programs like the NRP, though effective for addressing intrapartum-related events, were not feasible or sustainable in resource-limited environments due to lack of adequately trained staff and limited availability of the technology and supplies needed at each resuscitation. Yet evidence shows that lack of access to trained, skilled health care providers correlates strongly with high global maternal, neonatal, and child mortality rates. The AAP first gave permission to develop and teach simplified versions of NRP in 2004. In 2006, the AAP NRP committee convened a subcommittee to specifically address the challenge of NR in low resource settings. The result was a new NR program known as Helping Babies Breathe (HBB).

19.2.2   Helping Babies Breathe (HBB) [a]

HBB is an innovative, hands-on, and cost-effective educational curriculum specifically developed for birth attendants working in low-resource settings. It is built on evidence and recommendations clarified by ILCOR. HBB recommends interventions that are effective for most NR challenges while not being able to address resource-demanding circumstances like the birth of an extremely low birthweight neonate. Its main principle is that every infant deserves initial evaluation and resuscitation if needed (Little et al. 2011).

The hallmark of HBB training is a focus on the "Golden Minute"[b] as the most important time of a newborn's life. This concept states that the first minute after birth must be focused on ensuring that a baby either breathes spontaneously, or a skilled birth attendant initiates NR steps to help the baby initiate breathing, including providing PPV within 60 s after birth using bag-mask ventilation (Little et al. 2014). Research has shown that many neonates with failure to initiate spontaneous breathing at birth (primary apnea) respond with prompt interventions like drying, stimulation, and clearing the airway when indicated. Some 2% of all neonates require PPV within the first minute.

A unique aspect of HBB is curriculum design. HBB was designed to be part of comprehensive neonatal care and developed to be implemented across systems and organizations of any size. The program has three basic components: an evidence-based resuscitation clinical curriculum that emphasizes the initial steps of resuscitation; a well-designed educational curriculum that is understandable regardless of level of formal education; and purpose-built educational and clinical equipment that includes a low-cost, high-fidelity neonatal simulator to enhance skill development (Little et al. 2011).

The design of the curriculum repeats evaluation-decision-action cycles and for ease is presented in symbols and words (see Fig. 19.1 HBB action plan). Cultural and linguistic influences are also taken into account. The program utilizes carefully developed universally recognizable pictorial representations. The provider manual, flip chart, and action plan are all coordinated and divided by colored zones that signify level of help needed: green–routine care; yellow–caution—initiate initial steps to help the newborn breath; and red zone—danger–continue ventilation and seek advanced care.

The equipment included in the HBB course is focused on the initial steps of neonatal resuscitation. The curriculum stresses the importance of clean hands to reduce the risk of infection; a clean, warm environment to enhance thermoregulation; and dedicated space for resuscitating the newborn. A timer ensures that the birth attendant is cognizant of time elapsed. Where available, attendants should wear gloves to protect themselves, the mother, and the baby by decreasing the risk of infection. Clean, dry cloths for drying and swaddling with a head covering to help keep the baby warm are included, along with ties or cord clamp and a clean pair of scissors to tie off and cut the cord in a clean manner. A re-useable penguin suction device to clear oral and nasal secretions is available. The suction device is made of clear silicone and opens up for cleaning and disinfecting. Also included are a reusable positive pressure ventilation (PPV) bag with a mask to initiate PPV if the newborn is not breathing or has irregular, poor respiratory pattern. This is also designed to be taken apart for cleaning and disinfecting between patients. The program emphasizes cleaning and disinfecting all equipment immediately after use to ensure they are ready for the next birth. The learning materials included in the HBB equipment list also double as clinical tools (Little et al. 2011). Other course materials include a facilitator flipchart, provider guide, and action plan.

HBB uses the "Train-the-Trainer" model. Learners or trainees participate in pairs with each taking turns as the trainer (teacher) and trainee/provider (learner). The learner is taken through clinical case scenarios throughout the course of training. At the end of the curriculum, there is an objective structured clinical examination (OSCE). Each learner is required to attain a minimum score and show proficiency in acquired skills including bag-mask ventilation skills. Field testing of the educational curriculum and program implementation was done prior to rollout in 2010 (Little et al. 2011).

Physicians, midwives, and nurses with skills to care for neonates are often in short supply in areas with high neonatal mortality. Neonatal nursing is a key discipline in maternal, neonatal, and child health (MNCH) but is severely under-staffed and also undervalued in many settings (Little et al. 2011). Collaboration of nursing and medicine has been dynamic and continues to be instrumental in the development, teaching, and management of the long-standing NRP program. This important collaboration has served as a model for HBB implementation and needs emphasis in the field (Little et al. 2011). There is a need to train more staff including nurses and to improve the availability of equipment/supplies used in basic resuscitation, especially in low-resource environments.

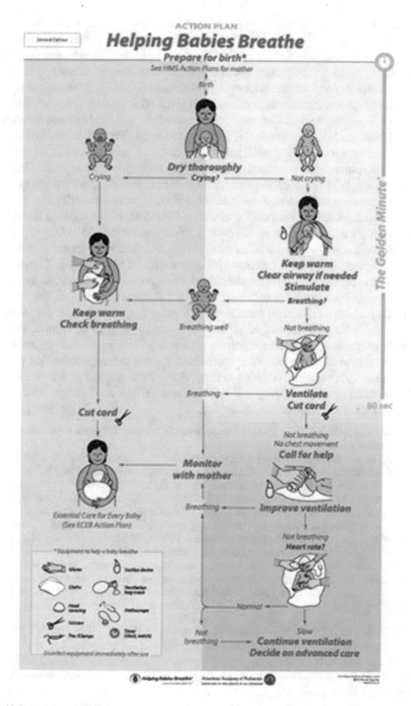

Fig. 19.1 Helping Babies Breathe action plan. (Source: Reprinted with permission from the American Academy of Pediatrics (AAP). Retrieved from https://www.aap.org/en-us/advocacy-and-policy/aap-health-initiatives/helping-babies-survive/Pages/Helping-Babies-Breathe-2nd-Edition-Summmary-of-Changes.aspx)

The HBB Global Development Alliance (GDA) was formed in 2010 to address the challenges of newborn resuscitation program development and implementation. It is an excellent, effective model of public-private partnership between the private and public sectors. Participants include governmental organizations such as the United States Agency for International Development (USAID), professional organizations and non-governmental organizations (NGOs) including the AAP, Save the Children, Laerdal Medical Company and Foundation, and the National Institute of Child Health and Development (NICHD). Between 2010 and 2015, the HBB GDA strove to disseminate HBB globally through policy, increase of uptake of newborn resuscitation in national programs, creation of resuscitation indicators, and increase in global supply of resuscitation equipment (Guiding the way forward 2017).

The implementation and dissemination of HBB was very effective as HBB became the gold standard of care for newborn resuscitation and training birth attendants globally (Chaudhury et al. 2016). In 10 years, more than 850,000 providers in over 80 countries have been educated to help provide life-saving care to newborns and the curriculum has been translated into more than 20 languages. In 2016 following field testing, the HBB Program launched a second edition (Kamath-Rayne et al. 2018), updated to harmonize with the 2015 ILCOR recommendations and the 2012 WHO Guidelines on Basic Newborn Resuscitation. Changes include de-emphasizing routine suctioning, which can be potentially harmful, as well as emphasizing the hazards of prolonged or over-vigorous suctioning. The first edition conditional action step of routine aspiration, if meconium stained amniotic fluid was present, was deleted. A statement was added to support that PPV may occur with the umbilical cord intact or after clamping and cutting the umbilical cord, in line with recommendations around delayed cord clamping.

Personal experience at a secondary level hospital in Southeast Nigeria as described by Chiamaka Aneji

As an HBB Master Trainer, I witnessed firsthand the lifesaving impact of HBB on a rural community in Nigeria. In 2016, I trained trainers and providers in a village in Anambra State. At a secondary level hospital, less than 20% of the healthcare providers were capable of providing effective PPV using bag and mask. Following the training, all the staff demonstrated 100% efficacy in this life-saving skill. This came in use a few nights later when a baby was delivered and did not cry despite being warmed, dried, and stimulated. The medical officer and nurse, working together, initiated PPV by 45 seconds (see Fig. 19.1) and within a minute the baby's strong cry filled the delivery room air! Later, they would recount this experience with a mixture of elation and a sense of accomplishment. In the 3 years that the facility has been providing delivery services following HBB training, there have been no reported cases of delivery room neonatal deaths, a stellar record for a facility in a region with very high neonatal mortality especially in the first day of life.

HBB has maintained a commitment to dynamic quality improvement and has strengthened educational advice and put in guidance on program implementation. There is an emphasis on low-dose, high-frequency skills practice with self-reflection, debriefing, and case reviews. The curriculum includes more detailed, clear resources for facilitators for workshop planning and facilitation. Sustainability of the program is important, and the curriculum addresses this by providing a road map for quality improvement and mentoring. To enhance cleaning and disinfecting equipment after each birth, the curriculum has included equipment reprocessing guidelines. Additionally, HBB put together resources to aid facilitators and in-country health authorities in disseminating the updated edition (HBB second Edition FAQs).

The curriculum is freely available for global use, intended for implementation within micro- and macro-systems of care, and integrated and harmonized with the WHO Essential Newborn Care (ENC) program. After its rollout in Tanzania in 2009, HBB has resulted in a 47% reduction in neonatal deaths within 24 h and a 24% decrease in fresh stillbirths (Msemo et al. 2013). The program has also helped health facilities by providing much-needed resuscitation equipment (Arlington et al. 2017). In Nepal, Ashish et al. (2012) sought to improve adherence to HBB protocols and to reduce perinatal mortality through quality improvement cycles. They reported a reduction in the odds of intrapartum stillbirth and first day mortality. Other studies have reported reduction in fresh stillbirth and neonatal deaths in the first 24 h after birth, but mortality after the first day or week has been less affected by HBB, which is primarily directed at neonatal resuscitation. Resuscitation training has reduced pre-discharge death from intrapartum-related events and has improved recognition that not all infants who initially fail to breathe are stillborn (Goudar et al. 2013).

HBB and NRP are similar because both are based on ILCOR guidelines, stress importance of expeditious newborn assessment and initiation of appropriate action for newborns at birth, and emphasize the importance of initial steps in and referral of patients for higher level of care. Table 19.1 emphasizes the intent of NRP and HBB. NRP is designed for the entire population of newborns while HBB is focused

Table 19.1 Differences between NRP and HBB programs

	Neonatal Resuscitation Program (NRP)	Helping Babies Breathe (HBB)
Program focus	Comprehensive neonatal resuscitation including advanced cardiopulmonary resuscitation	Basic neonatal resuscitation
Timeline	Provides respiratory and cardiovascular support as needed	Focuses on respiratory resuscitation especially in the first minute after birth—The Golden Minute®
Educational curriculum	Designed for well-resourced environments	Designed specifically for low-resource environments
		Includes a quality improvement module
Training style	Team training	Train-the-Trainer cascade
		Paired/dyad learning
Learner	Skilled, educated	Learner with any level of training or education
Personnel	Resuscitation team	Often a sole birth attendant caring for both mother and newborn
Scope	Detailed teaching on advanced resuscitative measures for all babies	Basic resuscitative measures for most babies

on select populations to make the most efficient and effective use of limited human and material resources.

HBB and NRP both face several challenges related to attrition of both knowledge and skills over time. Ongoing skills practice and monitoring, more frequent retesting, and refresher trainings help to maintain proficiency (Bang et al. 2014). A Tanzanian program reported using short (5–10 min), mandatory HBB simulation-based training sessions over 6 years. Approximately 40% more newborns survived when changes in perinatal risk factors were adjusted. The report concluded that short refresher HBB sessions are an important factor for improved perinatal survival (Mduma et al. 2019).

HBB providers face challenges in its real-life utilization when they must recognize need and implement ventilation within the golden minute. Moshiro et al. (2018) explored both barriers and facilitators to effective bag mask ventilation—a critical skill taught in the HBB program during actual newborn resuscitation in rural Tanzania. They found that midwives thought that their anxiety and fear due to the stress of ventilating a non-breathing child often led to poor resuscitation performance. In addition, the midwives experienced difficulty in assessment of babies at birth and providing appropriate initial care. The authors concluded that training efforts should be focused on accurate assessment immediately after birth and that frequent simulation training with emphasis on teamwork training is essential (AAP 2017a, b).

19.3 The Neonatal Period

The majority of neonatal deaths – 77.7%—occur in the first week of life, 11.1% in the 2nd week, and 11.2% in weeks 3 and 4 (Sankar et al. 2016). For gains to be sustained beyond initial stabilization and resuscitation, neonatal care programs must focus on days 2–28, and simplify existing care programs like Essential Newborn Care. The majority of maternal, newborn, and child deaths are preventable and can be treated with already existing cost-effective interventions. The HBB GDA recognized that maternal and child wellbeing are inextricably connected. To tackle this continuing challenge, the HBB GDA expanded its scope and partner base, leading to the launch of the Survive and Thrive (S&T) GDA in 2012 to address this continued challenge.

Building on the successes of HBB, the GDA leveraged $120 million and in-kind contributions from 2010 to 2017. The partners agreed on two key objectives: (1) To support, sustain, and strengthen high-quality, facility-based interventions and clinical competence through training, quality improvement (QI) approaches and application of effective innovations and technology; (2) to mobilize and equip professional association members to champion and improve the quality of high-impact MNCH interventions in their national health facilities. The GDA used the principle of country-led and owned initiatives, working closely and in coordination with ministries of health and the host-country stakeholder. All activities are implemented within the national maternal and newborn plans developed and owned by each country (Guiding the way forward 2017). HBB served as the model module for Helping Mothers Survive (HMS), launched in 2013, Essential Care for Every Baby (ECEB) and Essential Care for Small Babies (ECSB), both launched in 2014. HMS includes educational modules that strengthen critical skills for care in pregnancy, labor, delivery, and postpartum.

By adding ECEB and ECSB to the groundbreaking HBB program, the Helping Babies Survive (HBS) initiative included evidence-based hands-on training curricula to address the three leading causes of neonatal mortality: prematurity/low birth weight (LBW), intrapartum-related events, and sepsis. *Improving Care of Mothers and Babies: a guide for improvement teams* is the 4th program in the HBS suite. Low birthweight (LBW), defined as birthweight less than 2500 g, has adverse effects on neonatal survival and development, including increased risk of hypothermia, early growth retardation, infections, developmental delays, and death (Barker 1995). LBW is a result of preterm birth or intra-uterine growth restriction, or both. Conventional neonatal care of LBW infants in intensive care units is expensive and requires skilled staff and resources not available in many low-resource areas of the world. Every year over 20 million LBW babies are born across the globe, 96% of them in developing countries (WHO 2019).

19.3.1 Essential Care for Every Baby (ECEB) ®

ECEB teaches healthcare providers essential newborn care practices to keep all babies healthy from the time of birth to discharge (AAP 2020). ECEB trains providers to assess all newborns soon after birth to determine if they require routine or special care. ECEB ensures thermal regulation for all babies, adequate and appropriate nutrition, disease prevention, ongoing assessment for danger signs and proper referral procedures in low-resource settings. It includes a timeline for care.

Neonatal hypothermia is under-recognized and has been shown to increase neonatal mortality in a dose-dependent manner. It can occur in both cold and hot climates, in facilities and in the community (Bhutta et al. 2014; Niermeyer 2017). ECEB teaches health care providers to maintain normal body temperature by regularly assessing a baby's temperature by touch and with a thermometer, providing environmental support and skin-to-skin care—a component of kangaroo mother care (KMC) (see also page 12)—to keep the baby warm, and interventions to prevent both heat loss and overheating. The program emphasizes early and exclusive breastfeeding with practical advice on problem detection and ways to provide support.

To prevent infection, ECEB stresses the importance of hand hygiene for all who come in contact with the baby, application of eye ointment to prevent serious eye infections, and umbilical cord care to prevent bleeding and infection. Sterile or clean umbilical cord cutting, securing the umbilical ties/clamp to prevent bleeding, and keeping the cord clean by following acceptable cord practices—including the application of antiseptics like chlorhexidine—and discussing and discouraging harmful cord care practices are known to be effective. A Cochrane review by Sinha et al. (2015) concluded that chlorhexidine—a broad-spectrum topical antiseptic agent for skin or cord care in the community setting results in a 50% reduction in the incidence of omphalitis (inflammation of the cord stump, usually due to a bacterial infection) and a 12% reduction in neonatal mortality. Initiation of immunizations to prevent serious childhood illnesses is strongly emphasized. Ongoing assessments and classification into normal, problem, or danger zones are continued throughout the facility stay and appropriate actions implemented. Finally, guidance is provided to the family for home care (see Fig. 19.2 ECEB action plan).

19.3.2 Essential Care for Small Babies (ECSB) ®

ECSB builds on the essential newborn care of ECEB. The program focuses on thermal regulation, alternative feeding methods and recognition, initiation of treatment, and timely referral for danger signs. Mothers are important to temperature management of their babies and are taught skin-to-skin care. This concept of maternal care-providing is an integral part of Kangaroo Mother Care (KMC). LBW and preterm babies may have feeding problems including poor latch to the breast or bottle nipple. To ensure adequate nutrition, other feeding methods including spoon, cup, and nasogastric tube feeding are used till these babies are ready for nipple feeding. Referral of very low birth weight (VLBW or less than 1500 g) babies and sick babies with guidance on safe and effective referral is emphasized. The course curriculum resources for ECEB and ECSB include a facilitator flipchart, a provider guide, and an action plan like HBB and in addition, a parent guide.

19.3.3 Quality Improvement (QI)

This HBS curriculum provides a step-by-step guide for those new to QI and also supports those who are experienced in implementation and management of improvement projects. The QI curriculum is versatile and can be utilized by facilitators to help learners in both clinical and workshop settings, or as a self-study manual for teams or individuals. Sarin et al. (2017) evaluated a QI initiative to provide better care to women and babies before, during, and immediately after delivery. The study reported that QI had a positive impact on 8 of 9 care elements of maternal and newborn care.

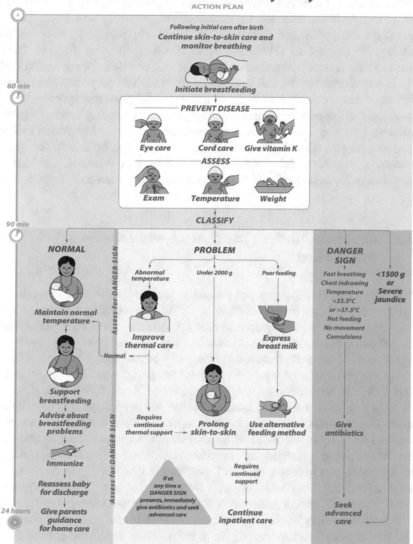

Fig. 19.2 Essential care for every baby action plan. (Source: Reprinted with permission from the American Academy of Pediatrics (AAP). Helping Babies Breathe, 2nd Edition. Retrieved from https://www.aap.org/en-us/advocacy-and-policy/aap-health-initiatives/helping-babies-survive/Pages/Helping-Babies-Breathe-Edition.aspx)

19.3.4   The Survive and Thrive Alliance (S&T) ®

The S&T Alliance played an important role in improving newborn and maternal health globally via an emphasis on collaboration, health system strengthening, improvement of quality and availability of health services and resources, and increasing the number of skilled providers (Guiding the way forward 2017). Through lessons learned, the Alliance articulated best practices for successful HMS and HBS implementation for partners into national MNCH programs. For sustainability, the alliance continues to build on its successful programs by providing an array of tools to support implementation and maintains a strong focus on quality improvement science. This includes mentoring and continuous monitoring to identify and address gaps (Guiding the way forward 2017). The program added a quality improvement workbook that guides both newborn and maternal providers to improve the quality of care in facilities and systems to support program implementers.

19.3.5   Kangaroo Mother Care (KMC)—An Important Intervention

In 1978, Edgar Rey (1983) developed Kangaroo Mother Care (KMC) as an alternative to conventional care for LBW infants to replace the warming function of incubators, which were in short supply in Colombia at the time. KMC constitutes prolonged and continuous skin-to-skin contact started early between a mother (or caregiver) and her newborn, frequent and exclusive breastfeeding, parental support, and early hospital discharge regardless of weight or gestational age, with strict follow-up. KMC can be continuous, defined as skin-to-skin care (SSC) throughout the day without any break in contact between a mother and her baby except for maternal activities like restroom breaks and bathing, or intermittent when SSC between a mother and her baby is alternated with either a radiant warmer or an incubator. It can be done in a sitting, reclining, or lying down position. KMC is recommended by WHO as routine care in babies with birthweights less than 2000 g, as continuously as possible (WHO 2019). KMC is different from kangaroo care (sometimes referred to as SSC) which is recommended by WHO immediately after delivery for every baby to ensure they stay warm in the first 2 h of life; it is also practiced in newborn special care units to facilitate bonding for ill infants (Kangaroo Mother Care 2012).

Caregivers, defined as mothers, fathers, and families are key to KMC. In most cases, the mother is intimately involved in KMC, being the primary caregiver in KMC. However, there are situations like maternal illness, distance between the mother and the referral center where her LBW baby is, or maternal death, that make it impossible for mothers to carry out this important intervention. In those cases, the family is called upon to identify a caregiver to take on this role.

For KMC to be effectively implemented, several resources have to be in place. This includes appropriate space that ensures privacy, where the mother or caregiver and baby will stay, furniture like a bed, table, and chair, and supplies like cloths that are adequate for wrapping the infant to the caregiver's chest. Staff training materials with job aids, family education, and training aids including pictures with details on how to initiate and sustain KMC are necessary. Policies and guidelines on KMC with community education are also important. Comprehensive support for the facility staff, caregiver, and the community as a whole is crucial for program buy-in and sustainability.

A Cochrane review of 21 studies included 3042 LBW infants, 16 evaluated intermittent KMC, and 5 evaluated continuous KMC (Conde-Agudelo and Diaz-Rossello 2016). The study found that continuous KMC initiated within 10 days after birth in LMIC resulted in a statistically significant decrease in mortality at discharge, at 40–41 weeks postmenstrual age and also at latest subject follow-up. KMC was also associated with significant reduction in severe infections/sepsis, nosocomial infections/sepsis at discharge, and decrease in hypothermia at discharge. It also resulted in increased exclusive or any breastfeeding at discharge and at 1–3 months follow up. In addition, studies found increased infant growth, maternal satisfaction with the infant care method, and mother-infant interaction and attachment. However, there was no difference between KMC and conventional care infants in psychomotor development at 12 months. One study reported that mother's sense of competence, mother's feelings of worry and stress, her sensitivity and her infant's responsiveness were significantly increased in KMC compared to mothers in the conventional care group. KMC also resulted in increased father involvement. The authors concluded that KMC is an effective and safe alternative to conventional neonatal care in stabilized LBW infants in resource-limited countries. Boundy et al. (2016) reported similar findings in their study comparing KMC to conventional care. In addition, the authors found that KMC led to other benefits to the infant including decreased hypoglycemia and hospital readmission, lower mean respiratory rates and pain measures, higher oxygen saturation and temperature, and increased head circumference growth. KMC can reduce postpartum depression in mothers and enhance mother-baby bonding (Conde-Agudelo and Diaz-Rossello 2016). An economic analysis in Bogota found that KMC was more effective and cost saving than conventional care.

KMC has proven to be a cost-effective intervention and aspects of it have been integrated into ECEB and ECSB of the HBS suite. The practice is recommended by WHO for LBW <2000 g; however, less than 5% of these infants receive it. KMC is currently underutilized worldwide for various reasons, one of them being the timing of its initiation. Many studies of KMC were initiated 3–24 days after birth, when the infant was assessed as clinically stable. However, 70.1% of neonatal deaths in developing countries due to prematurity occur by day of life 3, with 83.2% mortality in this group by the first week of life. This means that a large proportion of preterm babies will not have opportunity for KMC. An immediate KMC group study to explore the impact of continuous KMC initiated immediately after birth on survival of 1000–1800 g infants is in progress. This will provide valuable information on timing to optimize the clear benefits of KMC. Other barriers to caregiver adoption of KMC are lack of buy-in by caregivers, poor social support, lack of time at home or at the hospital, maternal or infant medical conditions, finances, traditional newborn practices, and social stigma around preterm infants (Smith et al. 2017).

Personal experience at a secondary level hospital in Southeast Nigeria as described by Chiamaka Aneji

The hospital routinely cares for small babies in incubators. My suggestions of KMC had not gained traction due to the barriers cited above. This changed in early 2018 when twins born at 30 weeks were referred to the hospital by a midwife from a birth center for "incubator care." They were delivered vaginally 2 hours earlier, both cried at birth, were dried, dressed and swaddled in clean blankets and transported by taxi to the hospital in the arms of their worried parents, accompanied by an anxious-looking grandmother. Initial evaluation revealed a boy 900 grams and a girl 950 grams in weight, both were breathing spontaneously but barely moving, had weak cries on stimulation, were cold and had low blood glucose levels. Essential newborn care including temperature stabilization was initiated. Due to financial constraints however, their father was vehemently against hospital admission. I suggested SSC would be perfect and both staff and family agreed. Working with the hospital staff, the mother and grandmother were supervised in providing SSC. Their mother had a small amount of colostrum, so the twins were started on prenatal formula through nasogastric tubes. They were treated for 2 days for suspected bacterial infection which blood cultures did not confirm. They were able to start on expressed breastmilk by day of life 3 and transition off formula as mother's milk supply got established. The mother was quick at learning and by the end of the first week, she became very comfortable and competent in providing continuous SSC for her twins and coaching her relatives to effectively assist her with minimal supervision from the medical staff. The twins were discharged after 5 weeks. At the most recent follow-up appointment, the children were 2 years old and thriving, and mom was back in business as a retailer. This experience galvanized the clinical leadership to develop a protocol for KMC and champion this.

KMC or SSC are complex and their successful scale up hinges on high caregiver engagement and the health system and society enabling caregivers to successfully adopt this program. Bergh et al. (2016) illustrated the complexities of implementing KMC in different countries, with differences in adoption, training, and implementation. The authors concluded that concerted country-led scale-up strategies with associated operational plans and budgets will be essential to program success.

19.4 Conclusion

For countries in the very low perinatal mortality stratum, there is plenty of room for improvement in outcomes of problems such as stillbirths, preterm births and congenital abnormalities, as well as narrowing the gaps in health care accessibility and quality to the poor. With available evidence-based interventions and international commitment and collaboration in tackling the problems of neonatal morbidity, mortality and stillbirth, the future success of sustainable neonatal care is feasible.

To attain truly sustainable improvements in stillbirth and neonatal mortality rates, a multi-faceted approach must be embraced. Key elements must include clear goal setting, upscaling of evidence-based effective "low cost with high impact" interventions, upscaling of available human power, provision of necessary tools and equipment to deliver care, publicizing available care and ensuring its accessibility to those who need it most. Just as important as implementing change is the ability to track the progress accomplished. Work needs to be focused on data collection and tracking to ensure that no matter which tracking system a country uses, it will not hinder that country's ability to attain the Sustainable Development Goals. With the collaboration of governments, researchers/scientists, and international donor agencies, combined efforts will result in truly sustainable birth.

References

Ahearne C, Geraldine B, Deirdre M (2016) Short and long term prognosis in perinatal asphyxia: an update. World J Clin Pediatr 5(1):67–74. https://doi.org/10.5409/wjcp.v5.i1.67

Akseer N, Lawn J, Keenan W et al (2015) Ending preventable newborn deaths in a generation. Int J Gynecol Obstet 13:S43. https://doi.org/10.1016/j.ijgo.2015.03.017

American Academy of Pediatrics (2017a) Global neonatal resuscitation program. https://www.aap.org/en-us/continuing-medical-education/life-support/NRP/Pages/International-Overview.aspx

American Academy of Pediatrics (2017b) Neonatal resuscitation program. http://www2.aap.org/nrp/global.html. Accessed 30 Jan 2017

American Academy of Pediatrics (2020) About helping babies survive. https://www.aap.org/en-us/advocacy-and-policy/aap-health-initiatives/helping-babies-survive/Pages/About.aspx. Accessed 01 Apr 2020

Arlington L, Kairuki K, Isangula K et al (2017) Implementation of "Helping babies breathe": a 3-year experience in Tanzania. Pediatrics 139(5):e20162132. https://doi.org/10.1542/peds.2016-2132

Ashish KC, Malqvist M, Wrammert J et al (2012) Implementing a simplified neonatal resuscitation protocol-helping babies breathe at birth (HBB) – at a tertiary level hospital in Nepal for an increased perinatal survival. BMC Pediatr 12:159. https://doi.org/10.1186/1471-2431-12-159

Bang A, Bellad R, Gisore P (2014) Implementation and evaluation of the helping babies breathe curriculum in three resource limited settings: does helping babies breathe save lives? A study protocol. BMC Pregnancy Childbirth 14(1):1. https://doi.org/10.1186/1471-2393-14-116

Bergh A, Joseph D, Neena K et al (2016) The three waves in implementation of facility-based KMC: a multi-country case study from Asia. BMC Int Health Hum Rights 16:4. https://doi.org/10.1186/s12914-016-0080-4

Berkelhamer S, Kamath-Rayne B, Niermeyer S (2016) Neonatal resuscitation in low-resource settings. Clin Perinatol 43(3):573–591. https://doi.org/10.1016/j.clp.2016.04.013

Bhutta Z, Das J, Bahl R et al (2014) Can available interventions end preventable deaths in mothers, newborn babies, and stillbirths, and at what cost? Lancet 384(9940):347–370. https://doi.org/10.1016/s0140-6736(14)60792-3

Bloom R, Cropley C (1987) Textbook of neonatal resuscitation. American Heart Association, American Academy of Pediatrics, Dallas

Boundy E, Dastjerdi R, Spiegelman D et al (2016) Kangaroo mother care and neonatal outcomes: a meta-analysis. Pediatrics 137(1):1–16. https://doi.org/10.1542/peds.2015-2238

Conde-Agudelo A, Diaz-Rossello JL (2016) Kangaroo mother care to reduce morbidity and mortality in low birthweight infants. Cochrane Database Syst Rev 2016(8):CD002771. https://doi.org/10.1002/14651858.CD002771.pub4

Goudar S, Somannavar M, Clark R et al (2013) Stillbirth and newborn mortality in India after 'helping babies breathe' training. Pediatrics 131:e344–e352

Guiding the way forward. 5 Year Report 2012–2017. https://www.surviveandthrive.org/about/Documents/Survive%20%20Trive%205%20year%20report%20FINAL.pdf

HBB 2nd Edition FAQs. The golden minute. https://internationalresources.aap.org/Resource/ShowFile?documentName=HBB%202nd%20Edition%20FAQs.pdf

Healthy Neonatal Network (2020) Database: global and national newborn health data and indicators. https://www.healthynewbornnetwork.org/resource/database-global-and-national-newborn-health-data-and-indicators/. Accessed 5 May 2020

Hillman N, Kallapur S, Jobe A (2012) Physiology of transition from intrauterine to extrauterine life. Clin Perinatol 39(4):769–783. https://doi.org/10.1016/j.clp.2012.09.009

Kamath-Rayne B, Thukral A, Visick M et al (2018) Helping babies breathe, second edition. A model for strengthening educational programs to increase global newborn survival. Glob Health Sci Pract 6(3):538–551. https://doi.org/10.9745/GHSP-D-18-00147

Kangaroo Mother Care Implementation Guide (2012) http://resources.jhpiego.org/system/files/resources/MCHIP%20KMC%20Guide_English.pdf. Accessed 5 May 2020

Kattwinkel J, Perlman J, Aziz K et al (2010) Neonatal resuscitation: 2010 American heart association guidelines for cardiopulmonary resuscitation and emergency cardiovascular care. Pediatrics 126(5):e1400. https://doi.org/10.1542/peds.2010-2972e

Lawn J, Lee A, Kinney M et al (2009) Two million intrapartum-related stillbirths and neonatal deaths: where, why, and what can be done? Int J Gynecol Obstet 107:S5–S19. https://doi.org/10.1016/j.ijgo.2009.07.016

Lawn J, Blencowe H, Oza S et al (2014) Every newborn: progress, priorities, and potential beyond survival. Lancet 384(9938):189–205. https://doi.org/10.1016/s0140-6736(14)60496-7

Lee A, Kozuki N, Blencowe H et al (2013) Intrapartum-related neonatal encephalopathy incidence and impairment at regional and global levels for 2010 with trends from 1990. Pediatr Res 74(S1):50–72. https://doi.org/10.1038/pr.2013.206

Little G, Keenan W, Niermeyer S et al (2011) Neonatal nursing and helping babies breathe: an effective intervention to decrease global neonatal mortality. Newborn Infant Nurs Rev 11(2):82–87. https://doi.org/10.1053/j.nainr.2011.04.007

Little G, Keenan W, Singhal N et al (2014) International perspectives: helping babies breathe: evolution of a global neonatal resuscitation program for resource-limited areas. NeoReviews 15(9):369–380

Liu L, Oza S, Hogan D et al (2016) Global, regional, and national causes of under-5 mortality in 2000–15: an updated systematic analysis with implications for the sustainable development goals. Lancet 388(10063):3027–3035. https://doi.org/10.1016/s0140-6736(16)31593-8

Mason E, Mcdougall L, Lawn J et al (2014) From evidence to action to deliver a healthy start for the next generation. Lancet 384(9941):455–467. https://doi.org/10.1016/s0140-6736(14)60750-9

Mduma E, Kvaloy J, Soreide E et al (2019) Frequent refresher training on newborn resuscitation and potential impact on perinatal outcome over time in a rural Tanzanian hospital: an observation study. BMJ Open 9(9):e0305072. https://doi.org/10.1136/bmjopen-2019-030572

Moshiro R, Ersdal H, Mdoe P et al (2018) Factors affecting effective ventilation during newborn resuscitation: a qualitative study among midwives in rural Tanzania. Glob Health Action 11(1):1423862. https://doi.org/10.1080/16549716.2018.1423862

Msemo G, Massawe A, Mmbando D et al (2013) Newborn mortality and fresh stillbirth rates in Tanzania after helping babies breathe training. Pediatrics 131(2):E353–E360. https://doi.org/10.1542/peds.2012-1795d

Nelson K, Simonsen S, Henry E et al (2011) The apparently stillborn infant: risk factors, incidence and neonatal outcomes. Am J Perinatol 28(1):75–82. https://doi.org/10.1055/s-0030-1262906

Niermeyer S (2017) Global gains after 'Helping babies breathe'. Acta Paediatr 106:1550. https://doi.org/10.1111/apa.13999

Perlman J, Risser R (1995) Cardiopulmonary resuscitation in the delivery room: associated clinical events. Arch Pediat Adolesc Med 149(1):20–25. https://doi.org/10.1001/archpedi.1995.02170130022005

Sankar M, Natarajan C, Das R et al (2016) When do newborns die? A systematic review of timing of overall and cause-specific neonatal deaths in developing countries. J Perinatol 36:S1–S11. https://doi.org/10.1038/jp.2016.27

Sarin E, Kole S, Patel R et al (2017) Evaluation of a quality improvement intervention for obstetric and neonatal care in selected public health facilities across six states in India. BMC Pregnancy Childbirth 17:134. https://doi.org/10.1186/s12884-017-1318-4

Sinha A, Sazawal S, Pradhan A et al (2015) Chlorhexidine skin or cord care for prevention of mortality and infections in neonates. Cochrane Database Syst Rev. https://doi.org/10.1002/14651858.cd007835.pub2

Smith ER, Bergelson I, Constantian S et al (2017) Barriers and enablers of health system adoption of kangaroo mother care: a systematic review of caregiver perspectives. MBC Pediatrics 17:35. https://doi.org/10.1186/s12887-016-0769-5

Swanson J, Sinkin R (2015) Transition from fetus to newborn. Pediatr Clin N Am 62(2):329–343. https://doi.org/10.1016/j.pcl.2014.11.002

UNICEF (2019) Levels & trends in child mortality report 2019: estimates developed by the UN Inter-agency Group for Child Mortality Estimation. UNICEF Publications, New York

World Health Organization (2014) Every newborn: an action plan to end preventable deaths. http://apps.who.int/iris/bitstream/10665/127938/1/9789241507448_eng.pdf. Accessed 24 Mar 2017

World Health Organization (2019) Kangaroo mother care to reduce morbidity and mortality in low birth weight infants. https://www.who.int/elena/titles/kangaroo_care_infants/en/. Accessed 09 Apr 2020

Chapter 20
Conclusion: Sustainable Maternity Care in Disruptive Times

Kim Gutschow, Robbie Davis-Floyd, and Betty-Anne Daviss

20.1 Disruptive Times

> The anthropologist in me wants to argue that caregiving is one of the crucial means by which humans have adapted over tens of thousands of years to a cold and impersonal natural world replete with both dangers and opportunities. And it is also how *we have sustained and developed societies in response to the very real threats of social suffering and historical change.* (Kleinman 2019: 245, emphasis ours)

Written in response to a decade of caregiving during his wife Joan's decline from Alzheimer's, and 50 years of service in medicine and academics caring for patients, students, and their families, Arthur Kleinman (2019) describes caregiving as a means of sustaining and adapting human societies in response to social suffering and chaotic human and historical changes. His observations—that caregiving is a sustainable response and evolutionary adaptation to the unpredictable and emergent threats of social suffering-echo themes from our introduction to which we now return. His meditation and lament on the diminished role of caring in medicine today points to the role of caregiving as a way of managing human suffering in response to birth, death, disease, and other disruptions.

Midwifery discourse considers birth as nature's opportunity for resilience, renewal, and regeneration. Yet modern obstetric discourse often depicts birth as a moment of risk and danger that needs to be controlled rather than a physiological

K. Gutschow (✉)
Department of Anthropology and Religion, Williams College, Williamstown, MA, USA
e-mail: Kim.Gutschow@williams.edu

R. Davis-Floyd
Department of Anthropology, University of Texas Austin, Austin, TX, USA
e-mail: davis-floyd@outlook.com

B.-A. Daviss
The Pauline Jewett Institute of Women's and Gender Studies, Carleton University, Ottawa, ON, Canada

© Springer Nature Switzerland AG 2021
K. Gutschow et al. (eds.), *Sustainable Birth in Disruptive Times*, Global Maternal and Child Health, https://doi.org/10.1007/978-3-030-54775-2_20

process that can be disrupted by biomedical interventions. Our volume has shown how humanistic and midwifery models of care can offer a sustainable response to birth in ways that allow mothers, newborns, and providers to thrive. We now return to our themes of sustainability and disruption, as we describe what makes a model of birth sustainable in both stable and unstable times. We believe the time is ripe for widespread implementation of new/old models of maternity care that are low-tech, high-touch, and flexibly adaptable to a variety of settings. We acknowledge the overwhelming consensus that we are living in an era of profound disruptions that already have threatened the very stability of human lives and livelihoods as we know them (Wallace-Wells 2019). Our focus on humanistic care amidst disruptive times directly relates to the global disruptions and social suffering we are seeing during the COVID-19 pandemic (Davis-Floyd, Gutschow, and Schwartz, 2020).

A consortium of over 11,000 climate scientists recently declared that the climate emergency we face will require "an immense increase in scale of endeavors to conserve our biosphere…to avoid untold suffering" (Ripple et al. 2020:8). The annual economic losses due to climate events rose from less than $20 billion/year in 1980 to over $200 billion/year in 2020, an 83% increase in 40 years (Ripple et al. 2020). Globally, a rise of two degrees Celsius by 2100 (nearly inevitable) will translate into 400 million people suffering from extreme water scarcity, many cities near oceans being rendered uninhabitable, and thousands dying in heat waves (Wallace-Wells 2019). A rise of three degrees (highly likely if we don't change our patterns) would mean much of Southern Europe would reside in permanent drought, while the average drought period in Central America and Africa would last 21 months and five years longer five than current droughts in these respective regions (Wallace-Wells 2019). It is not unreasonable to expect that there will be 200 million climate refugees by 2050 as the UN projects (Wallace-Wells 2019), although the World Bank has a lower estimate of 140 million climate refugees by 2050 (UNICEF 2020). Regardless of which projection is right, climate migration will disrupt existing systems that provide healthcare access, food security, and work for millions of people.

By the end of 2019, of the 80 million refugees across the globe, 47 million people were internally displaced within their own countries (UNICEF 2020). Roughly 25 million or half of the internally displaced population were newly displaced in 2019 alone by natural disasters, and 8.5 million were newly displaced by conflict and violence (UNICEF 2020). The climate refugees in 2019 included 12 million people displaced by storms, nearly ten million by floods, and nearly a million by earthquakes (UNICEF 2020). Most of the newly displaced people in 2019 lived in Asia: five million people in India, 4.1 million people in Bangladesh, 4.1 million people in the Philippines, and four million in China. Much of this internal migration affects children and women disproportionately, with about 19 million children displaced in 2019 (UNICEF 2020). The growth in climate refugees has been tremendous. Every year, between 2015 and 2020, nearly 20 million people were newly displaced by disasters, or double the 8.5 million displaced by conflict in 2019. Between 2006 and 2013, 75 natural disasters affected the Philippines alone, including the horrific destruction wrought by Hurricane Haiyan/Yolanda. In high-income countries (HIC) such as the United States and Australia, wildfires are a pressing and immediate reminder of our climate crisis (Sanderson and Fisher 2020). Rising population pressure, internal and external migration, disasters, and raising livestock close to forests have all contributed to an increased threat of emerging infectious diseases. An essay in *Nature* that analyzed 335 emerging infectious disease (EID) events between 1960 and 2004 determined that the vast majority of EID events are caused by viruses or bacteria that spread from animals to people (Jones et al. 2008).

The climate crisis will exacerbate social suffering, food security, and maternal and child health on a planet where too many people already suffer from food deficits. Roughly 800 million people are undernourished, and roughly 127 million children under 5 years of age will have stunted growth by 2025 because of nutrient deficiencies (WHO 2014). Around one billion people already have micronutrient deficiencies that contribute to congenital defects and other poor pregnancy outcomes. Long before COVID-19, it was estimated that by 2050, one billion people––1/8th of the planet's population—will be so vulnerable from climate-related disasters or conflict that they will have little choice but to flee or fight for survival (Wallace-Wells 2019).

While there have been some descriptions of the direct costs to human life and infrastructure from the rising tide of disasters including global pandemics, local epidemics, shifting disease patterns, hurricanes, floods, tsunamis, earthquakes, and other extreme weather events, we have not fully calculated the short-term and long-term shocks to health outcomes and healthcare systems. Integrated and adaptable healthcare systems will be all the more necessary given rising migration, increasing conflict, and predicted global declines in agrarian yields.

The profound disruptions across the globe due to the COVID-19 pandemic have revealed the systemic weaknesses of healthcare systems in a wide range of countries, regardless of income level or human development index. In nearly every country, regardless of COVID-19 related mortality rates, the COVID-19 crisis exacerbated existing social dysfunctions and led to systemic calls for reform. In the US, these demands for social reform included demands for racial and social justice, as nearly 25 million people marched to protest police brutality and systemic racism. Many countries across the globe enacted sweeping public assistance programs to stem rising social and economic disruption. Broader demands for healthcare reform included efforts to improve testing and treatment of COVID-19 in the early months of the crisis, as well as broader efforts to improve healthcare access increase healthcare equipment like personal protective equipment (PPE) and ventilators, provide essential medicines, and offer improved healthcare screening and technologies including testing, contact tracing, and methods of protecting both providers and patients from contagion. As with the Ebola crisis of 2013–2015), the disruptions of the COVID-19 pandemic revealed profound inequities in our health systems and their ability to adapt in times of disruption or stress (Mukherjee 2020, Strong and Schwartz 2019).

Across the globe, between 88 and 115 million people—representing baseline versus downside scenarios—will be pushed into extreme poverty by Covid-19 by the end of 2020 (World Bank 2020). with another 35 million forced into extreme poverty by the end of 2021 (World Bank 2020). The global rate of extreme poverty rose in 2020 for the first time since 1998 due to Covid-19 (World Bank 2020). Climate change and conflict had already slowed the progress on poverty decline, (World Bank 2020). South Asia is hardest hit, with between 49-57 million falling into extreme poverty in 2020, while 26-40 million will fall into extreme poverty in Sub-Saharan Africa. In the baseline scenario, some 70 million people (82%) pushed into extreme poverty by Covid-19 live in middle income countries. In the United States, COVID-19 has resulted in economic shocks not seen since the Great Depression—unemployment reaching 20%, 20 million jobs lost in the month of April alone, and only 51% of the adult population employed (Schwartz et al. 2020). Further, women accounted for 55% of the job losses in April, although they only make up 49% of the workforce (Ewing-Nelson 2020). COVID-19 further revealed the longstanding gender and racial inequities in the U.S. workforce that leave women of color doubly vulnerable. For Black women, the official unemployment rate increased to 16.4% while for Latina women it was 20.2%, compared to 12.4% for White men. Disturbingly, *the employment gains for women in the decade* since the Great Recession ended in July 2010 were wiped out *in a single month* (Ewing-Nelson 2020). In each work sector, women lost a disproportionate share of jobs—a higher proportion of job losses than the share of women holding jobs in that sector. In short, men held on to their jobs while women lost theirs during the COVID-19 pandemic. In Education and Health Services, where women hold 77% of the jobs, women made up 83% of the jobs lost (Ewing-Nelson 2020). Although some job losses were recovered by September, there were still 30 million people on unemployment when federal stimulus program for unemployment relief expired at the end of July 2020.

This worrying trend illustrates the vulnerability of women in the workforce and offers an opportunity to reform existing institutional inequities. The marginalization of midwifery and nursing is evidence of deep seated and structural sexism within the U.S. healthcare system that disregards those who shoulder a large burden of caring for patients (Kleinman 2019). Caring has long since ceased to be the soul of medicine and only when health systems recognize and privilege the value of caring, will we begin fix myriad problems in U.S. health care (Kleinman 2019).

It is difficult to predict how we will manage the known and unknown difficulties that COVID-19 and future pandemics or disasters will produce. Yet it is clear that maternity care will need to become more mobile, flexible, and adaptable. Within the United States, attitudes about hospitals—already perceived as sites of contagion—quickly shifted as women sought alternative sites for births. As Davis-Floyd et al. (2020) describe in a rapid-response article, the rising appeal of out-of-hospital (OOH) or community births resulted in home birth midwives and birth clinics being inundated in the United States with requests from pregnant women who wanted to shift their site of birth. Yet only a fraction of pregnant women could be accommodated by home birth midwives and its birth centers—since many birth centers had closed across the country in recent decades. These closures were due to many factors, and systemic dysfunctions in the U.S. maternity care system have made small-scale, decentralized birthing options less affordable than centralized birthing options. Even as some hospitals were turning some women away in places like New York City, some in the medical establishment continued to resist the evidence of the safety of community births (Davis-Floyd et al. 2020). Given the numerous studies that out-of-hospital births involve fewer interventions, fewer maternal morbidities, similar neonatal outcomes, and far lower costs (Cheyney et al. 2014; Anderson et al. 2021), the continued resistance toward OOH births has little basis in clinical evidence.

During COVID-19, high-pitched rhetoric from some hospitals about the contagion dangers that doulas or birth partners might present magnified already existing distrust between technocratic providers and doulas (Davis-Floyd et al. 2020), whose presence has been shown to improve outcomes (Motti-Santiago et al. 2008), lower cesarean rates (Kozhimannil et al. 2013), increase women's agency over the birthing process, and mitigate the racism and sexism found within American obstetrics (Bakal and McLemore, this volume). Providers' denials of the evidence for positive outcomes from OOH births and their continued obstruction to midwifery models of care that we illustrate in this book have potentially factored into why the United States has the worst maternal and neonatal outcomes in the Organisation for Economic Co-operation and Development (OECD) (Wagner 2006, WHO 2019).

Yet disruptions and crises can provide a turning point or a moment of reflection where new solutions are sought, out of desperation or frustration. We argue that the COVID-19 pandemic offers such a moment, when new solutions must be sought as the failures of fragmented medical systems across the globe are laid bare. Although there is much despair over the loss of life in these disruptive times, there is also hope that more sustainable models of maternity care can emerge.

20.2 Sustainable and Lean Maternity Care

While it can appear that fragmented systems of maternity care are sustainable simply because they persist, in fact they consume more resources and cause more harm than benefit. As such, poor maternity care is not sustainable in our definition, where "sustainable" implies an ecological balance that avoids depleting resources, health, and lives. Birth by definition is the opposite of depletion as a life has been added, with all of its potential. We build on the World Commission on Environment and Development (1987), which claims that sustainable development "meets the needs of the present generation without compromising the ability of future generations to meet their needs" (Sadler, this volume). A concept that tries to harmonize human development with the protection of nature is encapsulated in the term "Sustainable Development Economy," suggesting that environmental problems must be tackled by considering their relationship with both the economy and societal well-being (Wealth 2018). Schroeder et al. (2012) define the concept of "sustainable health care" as lean systems of clinical care that use the minimum of resources to maximize their efficiency in promoting health and humanity.

Lean maternity care will be needed in this era of rising scarcity due to the disruptions of disease, socio-economic stressors, declining crop yields and food security, and rising socio-economic inequality. In the United States, pregnancy, childbirth, and newborn care were the second and third highest diagnostic categories for hospital discharges in 2016, after circulatory disorders (AHRQ 2017). The median facility charge for a vaginal delivery without complications was $10,580, while the median charge for a cesarean was double that at $21,704 in the United States (AHRQ 2017). Indeed, the total charges for hospital births in 2014 in the United States were roughly $62 billion, nearly four times the cost two decades earlier in 1994 (AHRQ 2017). There is no overwhelming clinical reason for such dramatic price increases for birth, which is a normal physiological process it must be stressed. These price increases in the United States were driven by structural and economic factors including overhead costs due to fragmentation, high charges from the insurance and pharmaceutical industries, and hospitals seeking to recoup shortages via increased costs of birth.

In this context, shifting toward the lower-cost and more evidence-based midwifery care in high-, middle-, and low-income countries is the only sustainable and logical solution. We will need to train 300,000 midwives just to have enough providers for skilled birth attendance at the next generation of births across sub-Saharan Africa (Renfrew et al. 2014; Homer et al. 2014). There is a consensus that high-income countries will also need to shift away from obstetric models of care toward midwifery models of care in the next century if we are to improve birth outcomes and keep costs low most efficiently (Shaw et al. 2016; Koblinsky et al. 2014).

20.3   Perspectives on Sustainable Models of Maternity Care

All of our chapters offer sustainable solutions or lessons that can be translated to other settings. Our authors' analyses call into question the sustainability of a strategy of universal institutional delivery and obstetric models of care as the best means to reduce maternal mortality and morbidity. Many of our chapters describe hospital resource constraints and bureaucratic processes that will only worsen with increased patient volume should more low-risk births be moved into hospitals. We demonstrate that midwifery care is more sustainable and feasible given its low-tech and low-cost approaches. Unfortunately, many low- and middle-income countries (LMIC) still promote an unsustainable push toward over-medicalized obstetric models of care in hospitals that may be under-equipped to provide high-quality care. Further, too many hospital administrators and obstetricians remain resistant to midwifery models of care.

Our book provides evidence that women are highly motivated to pursue care in facilities when those facilities offer respectful, skilled, and timely care. Examples abound from Ladakh, Guatemala, Mexico, India, the Netherlands, the United States, or Indonesia, where we show midwifery models of care used in or outside of hospitals in remote or marginalized settings outperforming nation-wide maternal and newborn outcomes. Our chapters illustrate that when women and midwives collaborate, they can shift maternity care *toward* normal birth physiology or upright vaginal breech delivery, *toward* sustainable transfers of care, *toward* doula and *dai* care that counters the racism within mainstream maternity care, and *toward* holistic or femifocal models of care that empower women and reduce obstetric violence.

These models of maternity care work for both women and providers. Their successes speak for themselves, but their lessons need to be applied more widely. As we show throughout, models are sustainable when the *entire team is on board*, including all staff and policy makers. To be sustainable, successful models need to plan for dissemination and continuity after their original protagonists retire.

In Chap. 2, Davis defines sustainable midwifery as characterizing "midwifery practice for millennia, plus new skills and approaches that have proven useful since midwifery's resurgence in the last century." She explains that midwifery autonomy and empowerment are critical to effective practice and teaching, and that midwives must apply humanistic and holistic approaches to themselves as well as to their clients in order to avoid exhaustion and burnout. Her description of how midwives should deal holistically with trauma and vulnerability in birth shows that sustainable care is built on the emotional skills of honesty, compassion, empathy, and interpersonal awareness.

In Chap. 3, midwives and clinical researchers researchers Daviss, Hedditch, Krishnan, and Dresner Barnes describe the key elements of a sustainable model for vaginal breech delivery, arguing that the language of risk should give way to the language of choice, and that breech should not be considered a pathology but rather a variant of normal. Daviss and co-authors present the data for the advantages of upright or all-fours positions for vaginal breech delivery, which widen the pelvic outlet and facilitate normal birth physiology. They discuss how obstetricians adhering to older supine positions ultimately deskilled themselves in vaginal breech in favor of performing cesareans despite the downstream maternal consequences. They show how obstetricians and administrators are brought on board, bolstered by the new recognition that what women and traditional midwives have been doing for millennia—birthing in upright positions—is now scientifically proven to be far more beneficial that the supine positions so routinely used in hospitals around the world (Gupta et al. 2012).

In Chap. 4, Dunham and Hall describe a coordinated and sustainable model for peripartum transfers that was developed by the Home Birth Summit in the form of "Best Practice Guidelines" for transfers of planned home births to hospital settings. They show how this approach smooths the formerly inevitable inefficiencies that arise in transfers and thereby promotes better newborn and maternal outcomes, while supporting needs of the mother, newborn, and providers. Dunham and Hall have defined transfers as sustainable when they conserve resources and avoid redundancies of care or interventions that can produce further iatrogenic harm. Their model depicts transfers of care as sustainable when they are humanistic and holistic, and place the laboring person's physical, emotional, and social needs at the center of evidence-based care, while preserving the needs of newborns and providers.

In Chap. 5, Bommarito shows how collaborative dynamics in the form of monthly regional meetings and shared allegiance to national guidelines both produce and maintain a sustainable maternity care system in the Netherlands, despite the challenges and disagreements faced by midwives and obstetricians today. She notes that such exchanges, in which midwives and obstetricians speak directly to one another on equal footing, do not occur in most countries. Bommarito argues that they should, because mutual trust, collaboration, and communication among obstetricians and autonomous community midwives are essential to sustainable models of maternity care.

In Chap. 6, Bakal and McLemore explore how doula work can link women of color seeking meaningful employment to improved outcomes for vulnerable populations. They argue that doula work is sustainable because it provides doulas, women of color, and previously incarcerated women with employment, while lowering costs for Medicaid or other programs due to reduced interventions. They show that widespread access to doula care in the United States could lead to a savings of $58.4 million each year for Medicaid in the Midwest alone—partly because doula care reduces the high risks and costs of preterm birth. They propose nationwide Medicaid coverage for doula care, the integration of doula services into other social programs, and vocational trainings to equip formerly incarcerated individuals to serve their own communities as doulas. Together such measures would systemically address the lack of social support in maternity care for women of color and low-income women.

In Chap. 7, Pine and Morton delineate how quality improvement helps produce sustainable models of maternity care in the United States by providing a practical guide to the landscape of quality measurement. They show that high-quality maternity care can be made more sustainable by improved metrics, as well as by improved methods for creating and analyzing those metrics. They describe the pitfall of the inordinate time needed to enter metric data and note that the subsequent provider burnout and frequent inaccuracies work against sustainability. To make quality measurement and metrics sustainable requires attention to the needs of end users such as providers, while the "wicked problems" that are too complex to be dealt with by metrics must be broken down into "tame problems" that can actually be solved. Sustainability in metrics collection and dissemination requires functional and efficient data infrastructure that supports patient care by fading into the background, rather than obstructing patient care with inefficiencies of use. Their arguments mirror broader critiques about the inefficiencies of electronic patient records that suck time and energy from providers while doing little to assist providers seeking rapid answers to complex scientific questions (Mukherjee 2020).

In Chap. 8, Teman and Berend compare the sustainable surrogacy program in Israel to the unsustainable surrogacy practices of the United States. They argue that unified regulation that protects the rights of both surrogate mothers and the intended parents is needed for surrogacy practices to become sustainable in any nation. Essential mechanisms for surrogacy sustainability include standardization and regulation of contracts and clinical practices; mandatory screening of intended parents to ensure their viability as parents; and encouraging open communication between the surrogates and the intended parents.

In Chap. 9, Sadler, Leiva, and Gomez describe a public hospital in Chile that made rapid and remarkable changes in lowering cesarean rates from 40% to 5% by promoting humanistic and sustainable models of maternity care. They also describe a 20-year sustainable movement for the humanization of birth and against obstetric violence that has been spread across Latin America by activists using legal, medical, and social movement methods. They highlight the results in improved outcomes for mothers and providers and the passing of favorable legislation that makes humanistic and woman-centered birth care sustainable in five Latin American countries.

In Chap. 10, Jerez shows how sustainable shifts in maternity care require collaborative and participatory models of change at the Maternidad Estela de Carlotto, a public hospital in Argentina. She illustrates a hospital landscape where providers learned to shift their practices in ways that avoid excess interventions and obstetric violence while promoting humanization of care. Jerez shows that when staff were allowed to collaborate in shifting the hospital protocols rather than forcing change through top-down orders, hospital staff became empowered to make truly transformative changes in care. This process was sustainable and successful because the self-affirming process allowed behavioral change to percolate through all levels of the staff.

In Chap. 11 on the Luna Maya birth centers in Mexico, Alonso, Murray de López, Lucas-Danch, and Tryon present a humanized, "femifocal,"and community-based model of maternity care that provides full continuity of care—including infant and child health, well-woman care, and post-menopausal care. These authors argue that their model is the most sustainable way to care for Indigenous and non-Indigenous women in two widely differing settings—Mexico City and San Cristóbal de Las Casas, Chiapas. The femifocal model of care they describe is adaptable because it integrates evidence-based care into the local context. Furthermore, this model emphasizes human rights, collaborative care, and participatory processes, as it is continuously shaped by the women from the communities it serves. The authors identify eight characteristics that make the Luna Maya model sustainable: (1) femifocal care that supports women's agency; (2) integrated and alternative care practices; (3) a humanistic midwifery model of care with a rights-based approach; (4) informed consent; (5) client-directed care; (6) the strength and commitment of staff; (7) continuity of care and provider; and (8) self-care for both mothers and staff.

In Chap. 12 on Maya women in Guatemala, Austad, Chary, Hawkins, Martinez, and Rohloff understand sustainability as the "the strategic use of resources to meet human needs while promoting ecological harmony and balance". They argue that a sustainable model of birth will deploy local expertise while creatively innovating within local resource constraints. The authors identify the current obstetric model of care in Guatemala as unsustainable, in particular for those Maya women with high-risk pregnancies, who were being turned away at the very facilities that local policies and the state were pushing them toward. To push Maya women toward facility-based delivery while denying them entrance to those same facilities because of class and racial bias is the very definition of unsustainable. To help high-risk

Maya women navigate this institutional bureaucracy that denied them the care they were told to seek, these authors helped create a system of "obstetric care naviga- tors." These patient navigators would translate for and help Maya women receive much-needed facility-based care and essential medicines that they were required to purchase before being admitted into the hospital. The navigators also served as dou- las, modeling respectful care for hospital staff, including techniques to support women during labor that staff otherwise would not learn. This pilot program is designed to be scalable across Guatemala as it requires little funding, given that obstetric patient navigators could be funded from within the community or work as volunteers.

In Chap. 13, McCauley and van den Broek argue that sustainable efforts to improve the quality of maternity care will require addressing prevailing gaps in accountability in ways that would ensure the existence of basic and emergency obstetric care in facilities. They argue that sustainable improvements in maternity care require identifying bottlenecks that better assess postnatal and prenatal care, which have been somewhat neglected during the focus on intrapartum care. They also argue that sustainable maternity care requires focus not just on maternal deaths, but also on near-misses and maternal morbidities, which present a far larger burden of disease for women globally. They explain that sustainable maternity care improvements will require working with local and national stakeholders to ensure that maternity care is safe, effective, woman-centered, and equitable.

In Chap. 14, Gutschow, Dolma, and Gonbo describe a team that has nurtured 40 years of woman-centered maternity and newborn care in a public hospital in the remote Himalayan region of Ladakh, India. The district hospital in Leh, Ladakh priv- ileges vaginal delivery while providing skilled emergency obstetric care to produce outcomes that are equal to those found in Latin America. The hospital's average MMR of 37 between 2000 and 2020 is less than one-sixth India's average MMR and better than both Mexico's and Argentina's average MMRs of 45 and 51 respec- tively between 2000 and 2017 (WHO 2019).[1] This team of obstetricians, nurse- midwives, and other staff developed a sustainable model for nurturing women's reproductive rights in the face of increasing pro-natalism in the region, while flexi- bly adapting to shifting circumstances, new technologies, and policies within India's rural health system. The model is sustainable because it has remained responsive to its community's needs, while providing outcomes that were recognized as optimal across the region and the nation.

In Chap. 15, Roy, Qadeer, Sadgopal, Chawla, and Gautam illustrate how the *dais* of India provide a local, low-tech, high touch, humanistic birth model that is acces- sible to the most marginalized Indian women. They note that the dais' monitoring of labor is sustainable because it is more woman-centered, pelvic-friendly, and evi- dence-based than the obstetric care found in many primary care clinics in the four

---

[1] Gutschow calculated SNM hospital's MMR using data from SNMH, namely 27,318 live births and 10 deaths between 2000 and 2020. India's, Argentina's, and Mexico's average MMRs between 2000 and 2020 were calculated using WHO data and MMR estimates for 2000, 2005, 2010, 2015, and 2017 (WHO 2019).

Indian districts they studied. They affirm that it is unsustainable to push low-risk births to poorly managed first referral units because that increases the burden both on institutions and on families who cannot afford costly transport or risks of poor, often abusive maternity care. They argue for national acceptance of home births attended by dais, and suggest that dais' knowledges be considered essential resources within India's maternity care system. With health budgets dropping in India and inequality rising in the face of climate change, drought, and other disasters, these authors argue that dais are essential to sustainable improvements in maternal and newborn care across rural India.

In Chap. 16, Adams, Craig, Samen, and Bhatta insist that a sustainable model of community-based maternal and newborn care involves local stakeholders, initiatives, and social networks. They describe their development of a model called the Network of Safety (NOS) in Nepal that emphasizes cultural respect, local ownership, ongoing education, and the creation of both physical and social infrastructures. Their aim is to *scale across* rather than simply scale up. "Scaling across" means prioritizing bonds of knowledge, trust, and infrastructure that move from households to referral hospitals and the halls of government—and back again—as opposed to exporting and imposing standardized status quo tactics across diverse regions and communities without local buy-in. Their innovative approach is flexible and sustainable because it responds to the particular needs of each community, Hindu or Buddhist, while also attending to individual experience. For them, an "n of one" is still a crucial index of success, rather than simply looking at numbers of facility-based births or other quantitative indices that fail to measure quality of care or degree of empowerment. They describe an NGO, One Heart Worldwide, that works with the Nepal government to support the cost of training local skilled birth attendants (SBAs), using municipal budgets. For them, *community ownership is vital to sustainability*, and public-private partnerships can foreground viable, ethical, and sustainable exit plans for their progress.

In Chap. 17, McDougall argues that inefficient interventions and medicines waste time and money in scarce economies of care within South Africa, while also producing further need for interventions to treat the iatrogenic harm they have created. This model of costly but ineffective obstetric care that generates requirements for further care is both unsustainable and ineffective, yet still widely practiced across the globe, as other chapters in our book have shown. Safely localizing birthing at home or in non-medical freestanding birth centers helps increase access to midwifery care. The "tranquil birth" model that McDougall outlines offers compassionate, rights-based care in post-apartheid settings where interventions and excess medicalization constitute generational trauma. Her chapter illustrates that home births and birth center births offer woman-centered care that makes better use of existing human and financial resources.

As Davis-Floyd, Lim, Penwell, and Ivry show in Chap. 18, when providing maternity care in a disaster zone, it can be wise not to have an exit strategy, but rather to enter with the intention to build long-term and sustainable maternity care. Even years after the multiple disasters that Bumi Sehat and Mercy in Action staff addressed, the clinics staffed by the midwives they trained are still providing community-based care—in collaboration with local TBAs where possible. As their statistics demonstrate, a model of care based on the 12 Steps of the *International Childbirth Initiative* (ICI) can be cost-effective, life-saving, and sustainable, even in the context of utter devastation. As with our chapter on the dais of India, Robin Lim of Bumi Sehat issues a clarion call for including and collaborating with local TBAs who have earned the trust of the families they serve, to foster long-term growth and sustainability within communities.

In Chap. 19, Aneji and Little argue that for sustainable progress in the global fight against neonatal morbidity and mortality, focus would be best applied to systematic scaling up of low cost, low technology interventions like neonatal resuscitation (NR), kangaroo mother care (KMC), and proper hand washing. These measures all result in significant reductions in neonatal mortality in the hardest hit areas of the world. The authors state that systemic development of knowledge, skills, and quality improvement is critical to sustainable newborn care.

The accounts of sustainable maternity and newborn care in our volume help us recognize the value of skilled community midwives who are flexible, mobile, and thus less tied to bureaucratic hospital settings and their technologies than obstetricians or facility-based midwives. Our authors show that *de-centralizing birth care in favor of localized systems of support for normal physiologic birth will better prepare LMIC and high-resource nations alike for effective disaster care and pandemic responses.*

We single out sustainability as embodied in models where providers deserve to experience sanctuary and safety in their sites of care, thereby avoiding staff dissatisfaction and burnout. Our authors describe how caring for women and meeting their needs, listening to their voices, and applying informed consent at every step provides a sustainable environment where both staff and women can learn and feel listened to and honored for who they are.

20.4   Characteristics of Sustainable Maternity Care

Each chapter in our volume describes an individual model of birth that is sustainable and resilient in its local context or setting, while addressing the ways in which the model offers wider lessons for scaling up or across different settings or world regions. We now summarize what characteristics are most essential in sustainable maternity care:

- Humanized, evidence-based midwifery model care that honors women's rights and agency
- Recognition of the rights and needs of mothers and providers
- Midwifery autonomy and collaboration with other providers
- Low-tech, high-touch, and lean models of midwifery care
- Scalability, replicability, and flexibility across varied and similar settings
- Maternal and neonatal outcomes that demonstrate success

- Cost-effectiveness that promotes access for the most marginalized persons
- Collaboration among providers and families within and beyond the health-care system
- Provision of culturally appropriate and evidence-based care
- Fully integrated and collaborative maternity care systems that include all levels of providers
- Decentralized care based in and responsive to community needs and local context
- Care that embraces emergent realities of birth while downplaying risk and illusion of control

In conclusion, we highlight our previous statement that disruptions can provide a turning point or a moment of reflection where new solutions are sought. We argue *that this is such a time*. The failures of many medical systems across the globe to deal with COVID-19 pandemic effectively, especially in relationship to pregnant and laboring women whose support systems were disrupted, offer proof that the sustainable models of maternity care we illustrate are needed, now more than ever.

We have identified multiple aspects of sustainability and have shown that low-cost, low-tech, high-quality models match these criteria. We re-emphasize that the effects of the rapidly escalating climate crisis will soon *demand* such models and *demand* the decentralization of maternity care. Centralized health care and the bureaucratic inertia of large facilities are vulnerable to the disruptions of pandemics and other disasters that can destroy infrastructure. Smaller, localized facilities and models of care may be able to function during disasters and should be supported and expanded across the globe. Our mothers, our babies, and our providers deserve the chance to experience high-quality and sustainable maternity care in the face of future disruptions.

References

AHRQ (2017) HCUPnet, Healthcare cost & utilization project. AHRQ, Rockville. http://hcupnet. ahrq.gov. Accessed 18 Feb 2017

Anderson DA, Daviss BA, Johnson KC (2021) What if another 10% of deliveries in the United States occurred at home or in a birth center? Safety, economics and politics. In: Daviss BA, Davis-Floyd R (eds) Birthing models on the human rights frontier: speaking truth to power. Routledge, New York/London. in press

Cheyney M, Bovbjerg M, Everson C et al (2014) Outcomes of care for 16,984 planned homebirths in the United States: The Midwives Alliance of North America Statistics Project, 2004–2009. J Midwifery Womens Health 59(1):17–27

Davis-Floyd R, Gutschow K, Schwartz D (2020) Rapid changes in US birthing practices: the effects of COVID-19. Med Anthropol. https://doi.org/10.1080/01459740.2020.1761804

Ewing-Nelson C (2020) After a full month of business closures women were hit hardest by April's job losses. National Women's Law Center Fact Sheet, May 2020. Available via https://nwlc. org/resources/women-were-hit-hardest-by-aprils-job-losses/

Gupta JK, Hofmeyr GJ, Shehmar M (2012) Position in the second stage of labour for women without epidural anaesthesia. Cochrane Database Syst Rev 5:CD002006

Homer CSE et al (2014) The projected effect of scaling up midwifery. The Lancet 384: 1146-57. https://doi.org/10.1016/S0140-6736(14)60790-X

Johnson KC, Daviss BA (2005) Outcomes of planned homebirths with certified professional midwives: large prospective study in North America. Br Med J 330:1416

Jones E, Patel NG, Levy M et al (2008) Global trends in emerging infectious diseases. Nature 451:990–993

Kleinman A (2019) The soul of care: the moral education of a husband and a doctor. Penguin, New York

Koblinsky et al (2014) Quality maternity care for every woman, everywhere: a call to action. Lancet 388:2307–2320. https://doi.org/10.1016/S0140-6736(16)31333-2

Kozhimannil KB, Hardeman RR, Attanasio LB et al (2013) Doula care, birth outcomes, and costs among medicaid beneficiaries. Am J Public Health 103(4):e113–e121

Lalonde A, Herschderfer K, Pascali Bonaro D et al (2019) The international childbirth initiative: 12 steps to safe and respectful motherbaby-family maternity care. Int J Gynecol Obstet 146:65–73

Motti-Santiago J, Walker C, Ewan J et al (2008) A hospital-based doula program and childbirth outcomes in an urban, multicultural setting. Matern Child Health J 12:372–377

Mukherjee S (2020) What the coronavirus reveals about American medicine. The New Yorker, May 4

Renfrew MJ, McFadden A, Bastos MH et al (2014) Midwifery and quality care: findings from a new evidence-informed framework for maternal and newborn care. The Lancet 384:1129-45. https://doi.org/10.1016/S0140-6736(14)60789-3

Ripple WJ, Wolf C, Newsome TM et al (2020) World scientists' warning of a climate emergency. Bioscience 70(1):9–12

Sanderson BM, Fisher RA (2020) A fiery wake-up call for climate science. Nat Clim Chang 10:175–177

Schroeder K, Thompson T, Frith K et al (2012) Sustainable healthcare. Wiley, London

Schwartz ND, Casselman B, Koeze E (2020) How bad is unemployment? 'literally off the charts'. New York Times, May 8

Shaw et al (2016) Drivers of maternity care in high-income countries: can health systems support women-centered care? Lancet 388:2285–2295

Strong A, Schwartz D (2019) Effects of the Ebola epidemic on health care of pregnant women: stigmatization with and without infection. In Schwartz DA (ed) Pregnant in the time of Ebola. Springer Nature, New York

UNICEF (2020) Lost at home: the risks and challenges for internally displaced children and the urgent actions needed to protect them. UNICEF Publications, New York

Wagner M (2006) Born in the USA: how a broken maternity system must be fixed to put women and children first. University of California Press, Berkeley

Wallace-Wells D (2019) The uninhabitable earth: life after warming. Random House, London

Wealth L (2018) Principles of sustainable environment. https://www.sustainable-environment.org.uk/Principles/Definitions.php

WHO et al (2019) Trends In Maternal Mortality 2000–2017: estimates Developed by WHO, UNICEF, UNFPA, The World Bank, and the United Nations Population Division. WHO Publications, Geneva. Available via: https://apps.who.int/iris/handle/10665/327596

World Health Organization (2014) WHO global nutrition targets 2025: stunting policy brief. https://www.who.int/nutrition/publications/globaltargets2025_policybrief_stunting/en/

World Bank (2020) Poverty and Shared Prosperity 2020: Reversals of Fortune. World Bank, Washington, DC. https://openknowledge.worldbank.org/bitstream/handle/10986/34496/9781464816024.pdf

Correction to: Introduction: Sustainable Birth in Disruptive Times

Kim Gutschow and Robbie Davis-Floyd

Correction to:
Chapter 1 in: K. Gutschow et al. (eds.), *Sustainable Birth*
in Disruptive Times, **Global Maternal and Child Health,**
https://doi.org/10.1007/978-3-030-54775-2_1

The chapter was published inadvertently with half of the country names missing on the Y-axis of Fig 1.1. This has now been corrected.

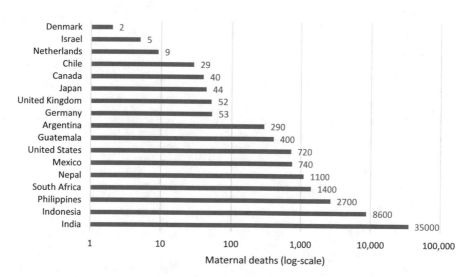

Fig. 1.1 Total maternal deaths in 2017 in our case countries. (Data from WHO 2019)

The updated online version of this chapter can be found at
https://doi.org/10.1007/978-3-030-54775-2_1

Index

A

Acehnese midwives, 265
Adams, V., 233–247
Alonso, C., 157–168
American Academy of Pediatrics (AAP), 102,
    207, 278, 279, 281, 284, 285
American College of Obstetrics and
    Gynecology (ACOG), 11, 67,
    106, 111
Aneji, C., 277–291
Antenatal care, 8
Argentina, 3, 8–10, 13, 16–19, 134, 145–147,
    149, 151–154, 303, 304
Austad, K., 171–182
Autonomous midwifery practice, 39
Auxiliary nurse midwife (ANM), 199, 219,
    229, 240

B

Bakal, R.L., 85–97
Barnes, H.D., 43–59
Basic Emergency Obstetric Care (BEmOC),
    220, 229, 304
Berend, Z., 115–126
Best Practice Guidelines, 61, 63–67
Bhatta, S., 233–247
Birth
    decentralized approach, 2
    on hands and knees, 57
    hospital-based, 2
    innovative birth practices, 4
    intervention and obstetric models, 11
    models, 4, 5
    OOH births, 11
    patterns and complications, 224
    physiologic, 19
    quality of care, 12
    safety, 5
    SGA, 14
    stillbirths, 13
    sustainable models, 6
Bommarito, R.K., 73–83
Brain wave patterns, 36, 37
Breech birth
    breech clinic, 50–51
    CS, 44
    "future alternatives", 45
    hospital in Ottawa, 52
    labor and birth, 51
    management, breech delivery, 52
    by midwife with obstetrician in the
        room, 56–57
    multidisciplinary planning, 50
    multi-professional service, 54
    by obstetricians, with midwives/doulas as
        support, 57–58
    patient and provider preferences, 46
    practice as midwives, 44
    research and conferences, 47
    risk perception, 46
    Sanctum Birth Center, 53
    societal norms, 46
    SOGC protocols, 46
    TBT, 44, 45 (*see also* Vaginal breech birth)
    vaginal *vs.* cesarean breech birth, 47
Bumi Sehat's disaster relief efforts
    disaster relief, 264
    post-disaster birth, 264
    solar lanterns, 264
    traditional midwives, 266
    tsunami and earthquake, 265

© Springer Nature Switzerland AG 2021
K. Gutschow et al. (eds.), *Sustainable Birth in Disruptive Times*, Global
Maternal and Child Health, https://doi.org/10.1007/978-3-030-54775-2

C

Canada, 4, 8, 12, 16, 18, 44–46, 51–52
Caseload midwifery, 34
Center for Disaster Philanthropy, 269
Center for Disease Control and Prevention
        (CDC), 15, 103
Certified professional midwives
        (CPMs), 56, 64
Cesarean section (CS), 44, 249
Chary, A., 171–182
Chawla, J., 217–230
Childbirth activism, 133–135
Childbirth, Chile
    home birth, 137–139
    landscape, 139
    maternity care, 132
    professional midwives, 132
    RELACAHUPAN, 133
    technocratic model, 131
    territories of birth, 135–137
Childbirth risk, 255
Chile, 3, 8, 10, 13, 16–19, 131–141, 303
Client-directed care, 165
Climate change, 3, 8, 261, 298
Climate crisis, 7, 20, 264, 273, 297, 307
Climate refugees, 296
Clinical detachment, 31, 38
Communication, 63, 64, 66, 69, 82, 109,
        136, 242
Community-based participatory programs, 212
Community Health Centers (CHCs), 211,
        219, 220
Competency-based curriculum, 241
Comprehensive Emergency Obstetric Care
        (CEmOC), 220, 230
Conditional Cash Transfer, 161
Continuous positive airway pressure (CPAP),
        208, 211
Contraceptive prevalence rates (CPRs), 198
Conventional obstetrics, 5
COVID-19, 271
    crisis, 2
    disruptions, 2
    maternal deaths, 15
    maternal mortality, 15
    on maternity care, 271
    pandemic, 1, 4, 15
    public health responses, 1
    transfer of care, 67
Craig, S.R., 233–247
Cross-cultural communication, 68
Cultural capital, 179, 180
Culture of quality, 192, 193

D

Dais, 10, 217–230, 304–306
    physical assessments, 223
Davis, E., 29–41
Davis-Floyd, R., 1–24, 261–274, 295–307
Daviss, B.-A., 43–59, 295–307
"Deep physiology" of birth, 31
Denmark, 8, 16, 18, 47, 56–57
Direct Relief International, 267
Disaster care, 262
    Aceh tsunami, 20, 265–266
    Bumi Sehat, 262–267, 305, 306
    climate-related shocks, 262
    government health centers, 267
    Great Japanese Earthquake of
        3/11/11, 270–271
    Lombok, 267
    Mercy in Action, 268
    Nepal, 3, 8, 10, 12–14, 16–18, 20, 126,
        213, 233–247, 264, 283, 305
    nonprofit board members, 269
    statistical outcomes, 268
    Sulawesi, 267
    typhoon Haiyan, 268
    violent flooding, 267
Disruption, 8, 18, 20, 38, 61, 64, 67, 210,
        295–297, 299, 300, 307
    COVID-19, 2
    models of birth, 4
    political, 8
Disruptive times, 295–299
Dolma, P., 197–214
Donor-NGO-community dynamics, 245
Doula training
    birth doulas, 87
    birthing spaces, 88–89
    challenges to sustainability, 90–95
    changes in network, 89–90
    EBCBSP (*see* East Bay Community Birth
        Support Project (EBCBSP))
    experience and impact, 87–88
    policy implications (*see* Roots of labor
        collective)
    racial disparities, 86–87
    reentry training programs, 97
Dunham, B., 61–70

E

East Bay Community Birth Support Project
        (EBCBSP), 85, 87–89, 91, 92, 95
Electronic fetal monitoring (EFM), 9, 104,
        136, 189, 202, 204, 207

Electronic health record (EHR) systems, 99
Emergency obstetric care (EmOC), 10, 19,
        160, 177, 178, 180, 189, 194, 202,
        220, 230, 262, 304
"Emergency talk", 251
Emerging infectious disease (EID) events, 297
Environmental transitions, 8
Essential Care for Every Baby (ECEB), 19,
        285–287, 289
Essential Care for Small Babies (ECSB), 19,
        285, 286, 289
Essential newborn care (ENC), 12–15, 23,
        204, 206, 208, 211, 213, 277–291
Evidence-based activism, 134, 135
Evidence-based care, 8, 21, 22, 64, 133, 136,
        189, 191
Evidence-based interventions, 8, 21, 194,
        278, 290
Evidence-based practices, 3, 4, 23, 104,
        134, 191
External cephalic version (ECV), 50, 55
Eye Movement Desensitization and
        Reprocessing (EMDR), 37

F
Female Community Health Volunteers
        (FCHVs), 235, 238, 242
Femifocal care, 164
Femifocal model
    female experiences, 162
    storytelling and space-sharing, 163
    sustainable, 163, 164
First-line maternity care, 80
First-line midwife, 76, 78–80
Formative Tibet experience, 246
Freebirth, 39

G
Gautam, S., 217–230
Germany, 8, 16, 18, 30, 35, 57–58
Gestational diabetes mellitus (GDM), 202
Global COVID-19 pandemic, 264
Global Development Alliance (GDA),
        282, 284
Gómez, R., 131–141
Gonbo, S., 197–214
Great Depression, 298
Great Japanese Earthquake, 270
Guatemala, birth, 171–182
Guatemala's Indigenous Maya traditions
    analysis, 172

biomedical institutions, 172
biomedical settings, 172
care navigation, 178–181
health care providers, 171
home birth, 171
"institutional bureaucracy", 172
Latin American countries, 171
maternal health, 181
maternal mortality, 171, 173, 174
methodology, 174
midwifery, 171
obstetric violence, 172
patient accompaniment, 178–181
policymakers, 171
public biomedical institutions, 172
scholars, 171
sustainability, 172
systems of care, 176–178
Telma, 175, 176
Gutschow, K., vii, ix, xxii, 1–24,
        197–214, 295–307

H
Hall, S., 61–70
Happiness, 36
Hawkins, J., 171–182
Hedditch, A., 43–59
Helping Babies Breathe (HBB), 13, 19, 207,
        209, 277–291
Helping Babies Survive (HBS), 285
Helping Mothers Survive (HMS), 285
High-income countries (HICs), 2, 3, 9, 11, 14,
        16, 18, 21, 189, 191, 213, 271,
        296, 300
Holistic care, 30, 166
    autonomous midwifery practice, 39
    clinical detachment, 38
    holistic model, 30, 31
    misdiagnosis, 38
    nutritional counseling, 33
    oxytocin, 36
    partly holistic, 32
    perinatal care, 30
    practicing midwifery, 34–36
    practitioners, 33
    provider/client relationship, 31
    routine postdates screening, 40
    teaching/practicing, 32
    technocratic model, 41
    theta, 37, 38
    trauma, 37
Holistic classroom, 33

Holistic education, 32
Homebirth midwives, 62, 63, 67
Homebirths, 30, 35, 61, 62, 66, 67
    cultural safety, 218
    dais continue, 218
    facility-based care, 218
    healthcare systems, 219
    institutional births, 217
    referral centers, 220
    retrospective survey, 219
    women's everyday hardships, 219
Home Birth Summit (HBS), 61, 63–67, 69, 70,
        277, 285, 286, 288, 289, 301
Hospital births, 65
Hospital transfers, 62
Humanism, 31–33
Humanistic education, 32
Humanistic model, 30, 32
Humanized care, 165
    Argentina, 145–147, 151, 152, 154
    feminist anthropology, 146, 154
    sustainable birth principles (see
            Sustainable birth principles)
    sustainable changes, 146, 154
Human rights framework, 1

I
Immigrant women, 68
India
    childbirth, 197
    MMR, 9, 11, 16–18, 197, 198, 304
    neonatal care, 203, 205, 209, 211–214,
            218, 229, 279
Indian government cash transfer scheme, 217
Indonesia, 3, 4, 8, 16–18, 20, 262,
        264–267, 300
Infant mortality ratio (IMR), 131
Information and communication technologies
        (ICTs), 99
Informed consent-based care, 165
Integral Preparation for Motherhood
        (IPM), 145
Integrated care, 164
Intended parents (IPs), 115–126
International Childbirth Initiative (ICI), 3, 6,
        20–22, 136, 193, 262–264, 268,
        273, 274, 306
International Federation of Gynecology and
        Obstetrics (FIGO), 20, 69, 136
International Liaison Committee on
        Resuscitation (ILCOR), 278, 279,
        282, 283

Interprofessional collaboration, 63, 64, 66, 67
Interprofessional education, 64
Intrahepatic cholestasis of pregnancy
        (IHCP), 202
Intrapartum care, 9
Intraventricular hemorrhage (IVH), 213
In vitro fertilization (IVF), 74
Israel, 8, 16–19, 48, 116–126, 263, 302
Israeli Defense Forces, 263
Ivry, T., 261–274

J
Janani Suraksha Yojana (JSY), 217
Japan, 8, 16–18, 20, 29, 125, 262,
        263, 270–271
Japanese Nursing Association (JNA), 271
Jerez, C., 145–154

K
Kangaroo Mother Care (KMC), 14, 204, 205,
        209, 211, 213, 277, 285, 286,
        288–290, 306
Krishnan, V., 43–59

L
Ladakh, vii, xxi, xxii, 11, 13, 14, 197–215
Language of risk, 43
Leh, Ladakh, vii, 9, 197–200, 203–214, 304
Leiva, G., 131–141
Lim, R., 261–274
Little, G., 277–291
López, J.M., 157–168
Low- and middle-income countries (LMICs),
        2, 11, 12, 14, 19, 21, 180, 188–191,
        193, 253, 273, 274, 289, 298,
        300, 306
Low birthweight (LBW), 14, 118, 211, 213,
        233, 279, 285, 286, 288, 289
Lucas-Danch, A., 157–168
Luna Maya Birth Centers, Mexico
    biomedicine and traditional medical
            knowledge systems, 160
    community-informed maternal, 157
    community model of care, 160
    environment, 158
    family health care, 157
    flexibility, 157
    government-sponsored model, 160
    health systems, 167
    institutional values, 158

integration, 167
lack of communication, 167
landscape, 158–160
Latin America, 166
MANA Stats research database, 167
midwifery apprentices, 162
midwifery care, 167
midwifery model of care, 161
policy, 161
practices, 164–166
principles, 164–166
rights-based approach, 160
safe space, 158
scope of practice, 157
self-care, 161, 162
socio-economic survey, 160
sustainable environment, 158
women, 158, 161

M
Manual techniques dais, 226
Martinez, B., 171–182
Maternal and neonatal outcomes, 234
methods, 200
SNMH, 197
Maternal care quality measurement
advances, 104
national organizations, 100–103
state level, 103
Maternal death, 7–9, 11, 13, 15–18, 131, 159, 167, 174, 176
Maternal health, 6, 7, 12, 15, 22
antenatal and postnatal care, 188
complications, 188
culture of quality, 192, 193
definitions, 189
evidence-based care, 191
healthcare services, 188
indicators, 189
maternal deaths, 188
morbidity, 188–190
mortality, 188
pregnancy-related complications, 188
quality of care, 187, 190, 191
SAMM, 189
sustainable improvements, 193, 194
Maternal morbidity, 187–190
Maternal mortality
causes, 8
grand divergence, 8
MMR, 9, 16, 17
and morbidity, 7

private facilities, 11
ratios, 16
Maternal mortality ratio (MMR) (maternal deaths/100,000 live births), 9, 16–18, 29, 131, 149, 158, 159, 171–173, 189, 197, 198, 235, 236, 304
Maternal, neonatal and child health (MNCH), 280
Maternity care, 218, 230, 272
birth models, 5
community-driven, 1
conventional policies, 2
COVID-19 crisis, 2, 12
ICI, 20–22
innovative approaches, 8
interventions, 6
models, 3
MotherBaby-Family Maternity Care Model, 21, 22
sustainability, 3
systemic racism, 19
transfers, 62
Maternity care system, 228
McCauley, M., 187–194
McDougall, K.L., 249–259
McLemore, M.R., 85–97
Measurement based quality measurement
data-driven accountability, 99, 100
designing
actionable problem, 105–106
clinician burden, 107–108
data issues, 107
ICT-embedded accountability, 99
infrastructure pitfalls, 108–110
maternal care
QI, 100
quality measurement (*see* Maternal care quality measurement)
methodological pitfalls, 110–112
public-facing accountability, 104
Mexico, 3, 8, 10, 12, 13, 16–19, 46, 115, 126, 134, 146, 157–168, 300, 303, 304
Mexico's national maternal mortality ratio (MMR), 158
Midwife classes, 33
Midwifery
caseload, 34
holistic education, 32
holistic midwifery, 39–41
human evolution, 29
humanism, 33
humanistic education, 32

Midwifery (*cont.*)
  humanistic practitioner, 33
  one-on-one, 34
  practice midwifery holistically, 34
  risks and challenges, 36
  shift, 34
  teaching/practicing holistically, 32
  technocratic medical education, 32
Midwifery care, 2
  on "birth models that work", 6
  birth safety, 5
  community-based, 11
  for low-risk women, 2
  high-quality models of care, 11
  innovative hospitals, 3
  maternity care, 20
  midwifery model of care, 11
  in OECD, 11
Midwifery Education Accreditation Council
  (MEAC), 73
Midwife skills, 30, 38, 41
Midwives
  generous use, 29
  in Germany, 30
  home birth, 35
  independent, 34
  and nurses, 270
  and obstetrician interactions, 73
  PCP, 82
  professional autonomy, 30
  resilience, 30
  senior midwife, 74
  survival, 30
  working on caseload basis, 34
Midwives Alliance of Washington State
  (MAWS), 63, 64
Mobile health, 174
Morton, C.H., 99–112
MotherBaby-Family maternity care, 21, 22
Mother's attitudes
  dais, 220, 221
  supportive environment, 220
Mountain environments, 234, 236

N
National Rural Health Mission (NRHM), 211
Natural disasters, 235, 267, 272, 296
Navjaat Shishu Suraksha Karyakram
  (NSSK), 204
Necrotizing enterocolitis (NEC), 203, 213
Neonatal health, 6, 15, 95
Neonatal Intensive Care Units (NICUs), 47,
  53, 106, 118, 138, 151, 204, 211

Neonatal mortality ratio (NMR) (neonatal
  deaths/1000 live births), 16, 18, 202
Neonatal resuscitation (NR), 14, 207, 209,
  213, 220, 277–284, 306
Neonatal Resuscitation Program (NRP),
  278–280, 283, 284
Nepal, 3, 8, 10, 12–14, 16–18, 20, 126, 213,
  233–247, 264, 283, 305
Nepali programs, 235, 236
Netherlands, 3, 4, 8, 13, 16–19, 30, 35, 63,
  73–83, 300, 302
  community midwives, 73
  IVF, 74
  organization, maternity care, 75
Network of Safety (NOS), 20, 233–247, 305
Newborn care, 145, 192, 214, 227, 277–291
Newborn Care Corners (NCCs), 211
Newborns, 2, 4–7, 12–15, 18, 91, 102, 103,
  151, 197–214, 226, 227, 277–291
Newborn Stabilization Units (NBSUs), 211
NGO's Network of Safety, 234
Nongovernmental organizations (NGOs),
  263, 282
Nourishment, 36

O
Objective structured clinical examination
  (OSCE), 280
Obstetric and Midwifery Manual (OMM),
  74–76, 81
Obstetric care
  EmOC, 10
  LMICs, 19
  midwifery care, 2
Obstetric care navigator program, 174, 178,
  180, 181
Obstetric disaster responses, 263
Obstetric Indications List, 76, 77
Obstetric models, 2, 8, 11, 31, 61, 161,
  300, 303
"Obstetric paradox", 31
Obstetric violence (OV), 132–134, 138, 140,
  141, 146, 152, 154
One Heart Worldwide (OHW), 235
  approach, 238, 242
  in Baglung, 244
  continuum of care, 236
  cultural diversity, 239
  governmental partners, 236
  healthcare accessibility, 242
  knowledge and resources, 244
  larger-scale program building, 238
  and local government leaders, 241

Nepal programs, 238
organizations, 246
partners, 243
pollution, 239
rural locations, 237
SBA course, 241
SBA trainings, 240
staff, 239
sustainability, 245
villages, 240, 244
work in Nepal, 238
One-on-one midwifery, 34
Out-of-hospital (OOH), 2, 11, 12, 21, 34, 62, 64, 65, 67, 68, 138, 140, 158, 160, 161, 166–168, 271, 298–300
Organisation for Economic Co-operation and Development (OECD), 299
Oxytocin, 36, 38–40, 77, 109

P
Penwell, V., 261–274
Perinatal Care Partnerships (PCPs)
board meeting, 78, 79, 81
face-to-face communication and negotiation, 82
first- and second-line care providers, 82
health professionals, 78
maternity care, 81
midwives and obstetricians, 74
norms, organizational structure, 78
obstetrics department, 77
postpartum care facility, 80
Perinatal quality collaboratives (PQCs), 103
Peripartum transfers, 61, 62, 64, 65, 68, 69, 301
Personal communication, 64
Personal fulfillment, 36, 97
Personal protective equipment (PPE), 297
Philippines, 3, 8, 16–18, 20, 262, 264, 268, 269, 296
Pine, K.H., 99–112
Positive pressure ventilation (PPV), 208, 278–280, 282
Postpartum care, 9, 79, 80, 96, 160, 187, 205, 229, 230
Prematurity, 14, 41, 176, 182
Preregistration, 67
Primary Health Centres (PHC), 220
Professional organizations, 81, 83

Q
Qadeer, I., 217–230

Quality improvement (QI), 63, 66, 70, 99–112, 192, 193, 279, 282–284, 286–288, 302, 306
Quality of care, 187, 188, 191–194

R
Remote mountain communities, 233
Respiratory distress syndrome (RDS), 203
Right amount at the right time (RART), 8, 31
Risk, 253–255
aversion, 45
with breech birth, 44
concepts, 58
CS, 44
"high risk", 44
language, 43
medical/clinical, 46
neonatal, 45
perceptions, 43
TBT, 44
vaginal *vs.* cesarean breech birth, 47
in VBB, 50
Risk management, 52, 63, 255
Rituals comfort, 228
Rohloff, P., 171–182
Roots of labor collective, 95–97
Roy, B., 217–230

S
Sadgopal, M., 217–230
Sadler, M., 131–141
Samen, A., 233–247
Scheduled Caste (SC), 11, 212
Scheduled Tribe (ST), 11, 198, 212
Secondary care, 63
Security, 36
Severe acute maternal morbidity (SAMM), 189
Sexual satisfaction, 36
Sexual trauma, 68
Shift midwifery, 34
Skilled birth attendants (SBAs), 236, 305
Skin-to-skin care (SSC), 285, 286, 288, 290
Small for gestational age (SGA), 13, 14, 203, 233
Smooth articulation, 63
Socioeconomic transitions, 8
Sonam Norboo Memorial Hospital (SNMH), 197
Dr. Padma's story, 203–206
Dr. Spalchen's story, 206–209
Ladakh, India, 211, 212

Sonam Norboo Memorial Hospital
  (SNMH) (cont.)
  maternal and newborn outcomes, 197, 198
  maternity care, 200–203, 214
  methods, 199
  neonatal care, 211, 212
  neonatal survival, 212–214
  SNCU, 209, 211
  sustainable newborn, 214
South Africa, 3, 4, 8, 10, 16–18, 20, 249–255,
  258, 259, 305
Special Newborn Care Unit (SNCU), 204,
  209, 211
Superficial humanism, 30
Surrogacy
  altruistic practices, 115
  commercial/compensated, 115
  legal and regulatory contexts, 117–119
  methods, 116–117
  open surrogacy relationship, 123–125
  outsourcing pregnancy and childbirth, 115
  screening of IPs, 122–123
  sociocultural and political contexts, 116
  standardized and regulated
    contracts, 119–122
Surrogacy contracts, 118, 119, 121, 126
Surveillance of the normal, 59
Survey population, 220
Survive and Thrive (S&T) Alliance, 284, 288
Sustainability, 234
  adopting practices, 3
  birth models, 5
  definition, 2
  Dutch maternity care, 75
  femifocal model of care, 3
  holistic and humanistic care, 3
  maternity care, 3
  models of childbirth, 6
  paradigm/model of care, 3
  SDGs, 2
  transfers of care, 68
Sustainable birth principles
  importance of name, 146–148
  protagonists of paradigm shift, 150–152
  reorganizing complex childbirth
    care, 148–150
  sexual and reproductive healthcare
    setting, 152–154
Sustainable breech delivery models, 48, 49
Sustainable Development Economy, 299
Sustainable development goals (SDGs), 2,
  187, 190, 236, 255, 291
Sustainable healthcare
  COVID-19 pandemic, 3

  maternity care models, 3
  OOH births, 2
  sustainability, 2
Sustainable maternity care
  characteristics, 306, 307
  climate crisis, 297
  climate emergency, 296
  collaborative dynamics, 302
  community births, 298, 299
  COVID-19, 297, 299
  crop yields, 300
  disruption, 296
  economy and societal wellbeing, 299
  food security, 300
  holistic/femifocal models, 301
  human development, 299
  human lives and livelihoods, 296, 297
  infrastructure, 297
  innovative approach, 305
  integrated and adaptable healthcare
    systems, 297
  internal migration, 296
  Medicaid, 302
  medicine and academics caring, 295
  micronutrient deficiencies, 297
  morbidity, 300
  mortality, 300
  natural disasters, 296
  navigators, 304
  newborn care, 306
  out-of-hospital (OOH), 298
  pandemics/disasters, 298
  peripartum transfers, 301
  physiological process, 300
  pregnant women, 298
  quality, 304
  sustainable midwifery, 301
  sustainable surrogacy program, 302
  tranquil birth, 305
  U.S. maternity care system, 298
  vulnerability of women, 298
  woman-centered care, 304
  women and providers, 301
Sustainable midwifery, 29–41
Sustainable newborn care
  adverse birth outcomes, 277
  birth complications, 278
  ECEB, 285, 286
  ECSB, 286
  HBB, 279, 280, 282, 283
  intrapartum-related events, 278
  KMC, 288–290
  maternal conditions, 278
  neonatal deaths, 277

neonatal period, 284, 285
NRP, 278, 279
QI, 286
S&T Alliance, 288

T
Technocratic medical education, 32
Technocratic model, 30, 31, 261
Technocratic training, 31
Teman, E., 115–126
Term Breech Trial (TBT), 44, 45, 49, 58
Theta, 36–38
Three-line maternity care system, 75
Too little too late (TLTL) care, 8, 22, 31, 132,
        159, 188, 250
Too much too soon (TMTS) care, 8, 10, 22,
        31, 132, 159, 167, 188, 250, 253
Total parenteral nutrition (TNP), 208
Traditional and professional midwives, 272
Traditional midwives, 171, 173, 174,
        178–181, 229
Tranquil birth
    attitude and ideology, 250
    Cape Town, 250
    COVID-19, 250
    CS, 249
    decision-making authority, 250
    ethnographic fieldwork, 250
    fearfulness and institutional
            apartheid, 251–253
    fieldwork, 250
    financial resources, 251
    maternity care system, 250
    non-medical workers, 250
    psychological well-being, 249
    risk, 253–255
    sustainable birth, 255–257
Transfer of care
    accurate diagnostic information, 65
    Best Practice Guidelines, 63, 64
    communication, 64
    community- and hospital-based
            providers, 66
    COVID-19 pandemic, 67
    disarticulation, 62
    elective obstetric interventions, 66
    fractured articulations, 62, 66
    fragmentation of care, 66
    home to hospital, 61
    interprofessional collaboration, 63, 64
    maternity care, 62
    pregnant client's support personnel, 65
    seamless articulation, 62
    smooth articulation, 62

sustainable and humanized
        approach, 62, 63
Trauma, 36, 37, 39
Trauma therapy, 37
Tryon, J., 157–168
Typhoon Haiyan, 268

U
United Kingdom (UK), 4, 8, 18, 43, 45, 50,
        51, 54, 55, 58, 66, 115, 116,
        139, 204
United States, 3–5, 8–12, 16–20, 29, 35,
        61–70, 85–97, 100, 103, 115–117,
        119, 122–126, 140, 235, 271, 274,
        282, 296, 298–300, 302
United States Agency for International
        Development (USAID), 235, 282
Unnecessary cesareans, 10, 38, 47, 249
Upright birthing position, 46, 47

V
Vaginal births after cesareans
        (VBACs), 249
Vaginal breech birth
    conservative elements, 47
    deliveries, 44, 45
    delivery in facilities, 49, 50
    national guidelines, 44
    obstetric community, 56
    premature babies, 56–57
    program, 48
    and teaching, 47
    24/7 on call service, 55
    safety, 46
    skilled provider, 45
    SOGC protocols, 46
    as VBACs, 54
van den Broek, N., 187–194
Vitality, 36
Volcanic eruptions, 20, 261, 267

W
Wadah Foundation, 264, 265
Women-centric approach, 217–230
World Commission on Environment and
        Development, 299
World Health Organization (WHO), 3, 8, 11,
        12, 14–17, 29, 102, 131, 158, 161,
        166, 173, 188–190, 192–194, 198,
        205, 211, 213, 217, 220, 222, 223,
        229, 235, 236, 241, 249, 282, 283,
        285, 288, 289, 297, 299, 304